ECHOCARDIOGRAPHY REVIEW GUIDE

D1379471

ECHOCARDIOGRAPHY REVIEW GUIDE

COMPANION TO THE TEXTBOOK OF CLINICAL ECHOCARDIOGRAPHY

CATHERINE M. OTTO, MD

J. Ward Kennedy-Hamilton Endowed Professor in Cardiology

Director, Training Program in Cardiovascular Disease
University of Washington School of Medicine

Associate Director, Echocardiography Laboratory
Co-Director, Adult Congenital Heart Disease Clinic
University of Washington Medical Center
Seattle, Washington

REBECCA GIBBONS SCHWAEGLER, BS, RDCS

Cardiac Sonographer
University of Washington Medical Center
Seattle, WA

SAUNDERS

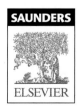

ELSEVIER

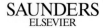

1600 John F. Kennedy Blvd.
Ste 1800
Philadelphia, PA 19103-2899

ECHOCARDIOGRAPHY REVIEW GUIDE: COMPANION TO THE TEXTBOOK OF CLINICAL ECHOCARDIOGRAPHY
First Edition   ISBN: 978-1-4160-2970-0

Copyright © 2008 by Saunders, an imprint of Elsevier, Inc.

All rights reserved. No part of this publication may be reproduced or transmitted in any form
or by any means, electronic or mechanical, including photocopying, recording, or any information
storage and retrieval system, without permission in writing from the publisher.

Permissions may be sought directly from Elsevier's Health Sciences Rights Department in Philadelphia, PA, USA: phone:
(+1) 215 239 3804, fax: (+1) 215 239 3805, e-mail: healthpermissions@elsevier.com. You may also complete your
request on-line via the Elsevier homepage (http://www.elsevier.com), by selecting 'Customer Support' and then 'Obtaining
Permissions'.

Notice

Neither the Publisher nor the Authors assume any responsibility for any loss or injury and/or damage to persons or
property arising out of or related to any use of the material contained in this book. It is the responsibility of the treating
practitioner, relying on independent expertise and knowledge of the patient, to determine the best treatment and
method of application for the patient.

The Publisher

Library of Congress Cataloging-in-Publication Data
Otto, Catherine M.
  Echocardiography review guide: companion to the Textbook of clinical
echocardiography / Catherine M. Otto, Rebecca G. Schwaegler. — 1st ed.
    p. cm.
  ISBN 978-1-4160-2970-0
  1. Echocardiography—Outlines, syllabi, etc. 2.
Echocardiography—Examinations, questions, etc. I. Schwaegler, Rebecca
G. II. Otto, Catherine M. Textbook of clinical echocardiography. III.
Title.

RC683.5.U5O87 2004 Suppl.
616.1'207543—dc22
                                    2007029181

Acquisitions Editor: Natasha Andjelkovic
Developmental Editor: Pamela Hetherington
Design Direction: Karen O'Keefe Owens

Cover image created by Starr Kaplan

Printed in China

Last digit is the print number: 9 8 7 6 5 4 3 2 1

Working together to grow
libraries in developing countries

www.elsevier.com | www.bookaid.org | www.sabre.org

ELSEVIER   BOOK AID
             International   Sabre Foundation

INTRODUCTION

This *Echocardiography Review Guide* complements the *Textbook of Clinical Echocardiography,* providing a review of basic principles, additional details of data acquisition and interpretation, a step-by-step approach to patient examination for each diagnosis, and self-assessment questions to involve the reader actively in the learning process.

This book will be of interest to practicing cardiologists and sonographers as a quick update on echocardiography and will be of value for cardiology fellows and cardiac sonography students who are mastering the material for the first time. Cardiac anesthesiologists will find helpful information about details of the examination. In addition, primary care physicians using handheld echo can use this book to get started and to improve their echocardiography skills. Multiple-choice questions provide a review and self-assessment for those preparing for echocardiography examinations and may be useful in echocardiography laboratory continuous quality improvement processes.

The chapters are arranged in the same order as in the *Textbook of Clinical Echocardiography,* and we recommend that these two books be used in parallel. As in the textbook, there are introductory chapters on basic principles of image acquisition, transthoracic and transesophageal echocardiography, other echocardiographic modalities, and clinical indications. Each of the subsequent chapters focuses on a specific clinical diagnosis, including ventricular systolic and diastolic function, ischemic cardiac disease, cardiomyopathies, valve stenosis and regurgitation, prosthetic valves, endocarditis, cardiac masses, aortic disease, and adult congenital heart disease.

At the beginning of each chapter, the "Echo Exam" summary from the *Textbook of Clinical Echocardiography* is included for quick reference. Then, a step-by-step approach to patient examination is detailed. Information is conveyed in bulleted points, with each set of major principles followed by a list of key points. Potential pitfalls are identified, and approaches to avoiding errors are provided. Data measurements and calculations are explained with specific examples. Numerous illustrations with detailed figure legends demonstrate each major point and guide the reader through the teaching points. Self-assessment questions are included with each chapter to help the reader consolidate the information and identify areas where further study is needed. Along with the correct answer to each question, there is a brief discussion of how that answer was determined and why the other potential answers are not correct.

This *Review Guide* is intended as a supplement to formal training programs in echocardiography; a book does not replace hands-on training or practical experience. Both authors fully endorse current standards for education and training of physicians and sonographers in clinical cardiac ultrasound as provided by the American Society of Echocardiography, American Heart Association, American College of Cardiology, and the Society of Cardiovascular Anesthesiologists. We support training in accredited programs with formal certification of sonographers and physician competency. The material in this book reflects the clinical practice of echocardiography at one point in time. Cardiac imaging is a rapidly changing field, and we encourage our readers to stay up to date by reading journals and other online sources and by attending national meetings and continuing medical education courses.

ACKNOWLEDGMENTS

It is never possible to fully acknowledge all those who help make a book possible; however, we would like to thank some of those who helped along the way. First, the cardiac sonographers at the University of Washington deserve our special appreciation for the excellence of their imaging skills and the time they dedicated to acquiring additional images for us and discussing the finer points of data acquisition: Dan Bergman, RDMS; David Diedrick, RDCS; Caryn D'Jang, RDCS; Michelle Fujioka, RDCS; Yelana Kovalenko, RDCS; Amy Loscher, RDCS; Ren Singh, RDCS; Erin Trent, RDCS; and Todd Zwink, RDCS.

We also thank our Cardiology Fellows for their diligence in providing feedback on beta-versions of the self-assessment questions. Anna Leach provided outstanding computer graphics design support and preparation of images for publication. Thoughtful reviews of the chapters were provided by Rosario V. Freeman, MD; Peter Cawley, MD; Karen K. Stout, MD; and Michelle Z. Gurvitz, MD. Special thanks to Edward A. Gill, MD, for providing the three-dimensional echocardiography images. Sharon A. Kemp and Angie Frederickson provided essential administrative support. Our appreciation extends to Natasha Andjelkovic and Pamela Hetherington at Elsevier, who supported this project and helped us make it a reality.

Finally, we both want to sincerely thank our families, not only our husbands for their unwavering and continual encouragement, but even the youngest members—Sarah, Claire, and Jack—for their support and patience in the book writing process. This book would not have been possible without their help in finding the time to complete the book.

Catherine M. Otto, MD
Rebecca Gibbons Schwaegler, BS, RDCS

CONTENTS

ABBREVIATIONS USED IN FIGURES, TABLES, AND EQUATIONS

2D–two-dimensional

3D–three-dimensional

A–late (atrial) diastolic velocity peak

A-long–apical long-axis

A-mode–amplitude mode (amplitude versus depth)

A2C–apical two-chamber

A4C–apical four-chamber

AcT–acceleration time

a_{dur}–duration of pulmonary venous atrial reversal velocity

A_{dur}–duration of atrial filling velocity

AF–atrial fibrillation

A_m–myocardial tissue late diastolic velocity

AMVL–anterior mitral valve leaflet

ant–anterior

Ao–aortic or aorta

AR–aortic regurgitation

AS–aortic stenosis

ASD–atrial septal defect

ASH–asymmetrical septal hypertrophy

ATVL–anterior tricuspid valve leaflet

AV–atrioventricular

AVA–aortic valve area

AVR–aortic valve replacement

BAV–balloon aortic valvuloplasty

BP–blood pressure

BSA–body surface area

c–propagation velocity of sound in tissue

C-TGA–congenitally corrected transposition of the great arteries

CAD–coronary artery disease

cath–cardiac catheterization

cm–centimeters

C_m–specific heat of tissue

cm/s–centimeters per second

CO–cardiac output

Cont eq–continuity equation valve area

cos–cosine

CS–coronary sinus

CSA–cross-sectional area

CT–computed tomography

CW–continuous wave

Cx–circumflex coronary artery

D–diameter

DA–descending aorta

dB–decibels

dP/dt–rate of change in pressure over time

DT–deceleration time

dT/dt–rate of increase in temperature

dyne·s·cm^5–units of resistance

E–early diastolic peak velocity

ECG–electrocardiogram

echo–echocardiography

ED–end-diastole

EDD–end-diastolic dimension

EDV–end-diastolic volume

EF–ejection fraction

E_m–myocardial tissue early diastolic velocity

endo–endocardium

epi–epicardium

EPSS–E-point septal separation

ES–end-systole

ESD–end-systolic dimension

ESPVR–end-systolic pressure-volume relationship

ESV–end-systolic volume

ETT–exercise treadmill test

Δf–frequency shift

f–frequency

FL–false lumen

F_n–near field

FN–false negative

F_o–resonance frequency

FP–false positive

F_s–scattered frequency

FSV–forward stroke volume

F_t–transmitted frequency

fx–function

HCM–hypertrophic cardiomyopathy

HPRF–high pulse repetition frequency

HR–heart rate

HV–hepatic vein

I–intensity of ultrasound exposure

IAS–interatrial septum

inf–inferior

IV–intravenous

IVC–inferior vena cava

IVCT–isovolumic contraction time

IVRT–isovolumic relaxation time

kHz–kilohertz

L–length

LA–left atrium

LAA–left atrial appendage

LAD–left anterior descending coronary artery

LAE–left atrial enlargement

lat–lateral

LCC–left coronary cusp

LLAT–left lateral

LMCA–left main coronary artery

LPA–left pulmonary artery

LSPV–left superior pulmonary vein

LV–left ventricle

LVE–left ventricular enlargement

LV-EDP–left ventricular end-diastolic pressure

LVH–left ventricular hypertrophy

LVI–left ventricular inflow

LVID–left ventricular internal dimension

LVO–left ventricular outflow

LVOT–left ventricular outflow tract

M–myxoma

M-mode–motion display (depth versus time)

MAC–mitral annular calcification

MB–moderator band

MI–myocardial infarction

MR–mitral regurgitation

MRI–magnetic resonance imaging

MS–mitral stenosis

MV–mitral valve

MVA–mitral valve area

MVL–mitral valve leaflet

MVR–mitral valve replacement

n–number of subjects

NBTE–nonbacterial thrombotic endocarditis

NCC–noncoronary cusp

ΔP–pressure gradient

P–pressure

PA–pulmonary artery

pAn–pseudoaneurysm

PAP–pulmonary artery pressure

PD–pulsed Doppler

PDA–patent ductus arteriosus or posterior descending artery (depends on context)

PE–pericardial effusion

PEP–preejection period

PET–positron-emission tomography

PISA–proximal isovelocity surface area

PLAX–parasternal long-axis

PM–papillary muscle

PMVL–posterior mitral valve leaflet

PR–pulmonic regurgitation

PRF–pulse repetition frequency

PRFR–peak rapid filling rate

PS–pulmonic stenosis

PSAX–parasternal short axis

PTCA–percutaneous transluminal coronary angioplasty

PV–pulmonary vein

PV_a–pulmonary venous atrial reversal velocity

PV_D–pulmonary venous peak diastolic velocity

PV_S–pulmonary venous peak systolic velocity

PVC–premature ventricular contraction

PWT–posterior wall thickness

Q–volume flow rate

Q_p–pulmonic volume flow rate

Q_s–systemic volume flow rate

RA–right atrium

RAE–right atrial enlargement

RAO–right anterior oblique

RAP–right atrial pressure

RCA–right coronary artery

RCC–right coronary cusp

Re–Reynolds number

RF–regurgitant fraction

RJ–regurgitant jet

R_o–radius of microbubble

ROA–regurgitant orifice area

RPA–right pulmonary artery

RSPV–right superior pulmonary vein

RSV–regurgitant stroke volume

RV–right ventricle

RVE–right ventricular enlargement

RVH–right ventricular hypertrophy

RVI–right ventricular inflow

RVO–right ventricular outflow
RVOT–right ventricular outflow tract
SAM–systolic anterior motion
SC–subcostal
SPPA–spatial peak pulse average
SPTA–spatial peak temporal average
SSN–suprasternal notch
ST–septal thickness
STJ–sinotubular junction
STVL–septal tricuspid valve leaflet
SV–stroke volume or sample volume (depends on context)
SVC–superior vena cava
SWMA–segmental wall motion abnormality
$T_{1/2}$–pressure half-time
T–thrombus
TEE–transesophageal echocardiography
TGA–transposition of the great arteries
TGC–time gain compensation

TL–true lumen
TN–true negatives
TOF–tetralogy of Fallot
TP–true positives
TPV–time to peak velocity
TR–tricuspid regurgitation
TS–tricuspid stenosis
TSV–total stroke volume
TTE–transthoracic echocardiography
TV–tricuspid valve
v–velocity
V–volume or velocity (depends on context)
VAS–ventriculo-atrial septum
Veg–vegetation
V_{max}–maximum velocity
VSD–ventricular septal defect
VTI–velocity-time integral
WPW–Wolff-Parkinson-White syndrome
Z–acoustic impedance

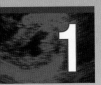

1 Principles of Echocardiographic Image Acquisition and Doppler Analysis

THE ECHO EXAM

BASIC PRINCIPLES
Ultrasound Waves
Transducers
Ultrasound Imaging
Principles
Imaging Artifacts

Doppler
Pulsed Doppler
Color Doppler
Continuous Wave Doppler
Doppler Artifacts
Bioeffects and Safety

SELF-ASSESSMENT QUESTIONS

THE ECHO EXAM: BASIC PRINCIPLES

SOUND WAVES

f = frequency
λ = wavelength
c = velocity of propagation
$c = \lambda \times f$

ULTRASOUND–TISSUE INTERACTION

Reflection	Imaging
Scattering	Doppler
Refraction	Beam focusing
	Artifacts
Attenuation	Penetration

RESOLUTION

Axial	Transducer frequency
	Bandwidth
	Pulse length
Lateral	Depth
Elevational	Depth

FRAME RATE

Depth
Sector width

IMAGING INSTRUMENT SETTINGS

Transducer frequency
Power output
Gain
Time gain compensation (TCG)
Depth
Dynamic range
Sector width

DOPPLER MODALITIES

Pulsed	Spectral display
	Anatomic location
	Signal aliasing
Continuous wave (CW)	Spectral display
	High velocity flow
	Range ambiguity
Color	Visual 2D display
	Quantitation problematic

DOPPLER EQUATION

$$v = \frac{c(\Delta F)}{[2 F_T (\cos\theta)]}$$

c = speed of sound in blood (1540 m/s)
θ = the intercept angle with flow
F_T = transducer frequency
ΔF = Doppler frequency shift

SPECTRAL DOPPLER INSTRUMENT SETTINGS

Power output
Receiver gain
Wall (high-pass) filters
Baseline shift
Velocity range
Post-processing
Sample volume depth (pulsed)
Sample volume length (pulsed)
Number of sample volumes (HPRF)

ULTRASOUND SAFETY

Bioeffects	Thermal
	Cavitation
	Other

Perform echoes appropriately
Know power output and exposure intensities
Limit power output and exposure, as possible

OPTIMIZATION OF DOPPLER RECORDINGS

MODALITY	DATA OPTIMIZATION	COMMON ARTIFACTS
Pulsed	2D guided with "frozen" image Parallel to flow Small sample volume Velocity scale at Nyquist limit Adjust baseline for aliasing Use low wall filters Adjust gain and dynamic range	Nonparallel angle with underestimation of velocity Signal aliasing; Nyquist limit = $\frac{1}{2}$ pulse repetition frequency (PRF) Signal strength/noise
Continuous wave	Dedicated nonimaging transducer Parallel to flow Adjust velocity scale so flow fits and fills the displayed range Use high wall filters Adjust gain and dynamic range	Nonparallel angle with underestimation of velocity Range ambiguity Beam width Transit time effect
Color flow	Use minimal depth and sector width for flow of interest (best frame rate) Adjust gain just below random noise Color scale at Nyquist limit	Shadowing Ghosting Electronic interference

2D, *Two-dimensional.*

PRINCIPLES OF DOPPLER QUANTITATION

METHOD	ASSUMPTIONS/CHARACTERISTICS	EXAMPLES OF CLINICAL APPLICATIONS
Volume flow $SV = CSA \times VTI$	Laminar flow Flat flow profile Cross-sectional area (CSA) and velocity time integral (VTI) measured at same site	Cardiac output Continuity equation for valve area Regurgitant volume calculations Intracardiac shunts, pulmonary-to-systemic flow ratio
Velocity-pressure relationship $\Delta P = 4v^2$	Flow-limiting orifice CW Doppler signal recorded parallel to flow	Stenotic valve gradients Calculation of pulmonary pressures Left ventricular *dP/dt*
Spatial flow patterns	Proximal flow convergence region Narrow flow stream in orifice (vena contracta) Downstream flow disturbance	Detection of valve regurgitation and intracardiac shunts Level of obstruction Quantitation of regurgitant severity

BASIC PRINCIPLES

- Knowledge of basic ultrasound principles is needed for interpretation of images and Doppler data.
- Appropriate adjustment of instrument parameters is needed to obtain diagnostic information.

Key points:

- ❏ The appropriate ultrasound modality (two-dimensional [2D] imaging, pulsed Doppler, color Doppler, etc.) is chosen for each type of desired clinical information.
- ❏ Current instrumentation allows modification of many parameters during data acquisition, such as depth, gain, harmonic imaging, wall filters, etc.

- ❏ Artifacts must be distinguished from anatomic findings on ultrasound images.
- ❏ Accurate Doppler measurements depend on details of both blood flow interrogation and instrument acquisition parameters.

Ultrasound Waves

- Ultrasound waves are mechanical vibrations, with basic descriptors including:
  - ❏ Frequency (cycles per second = Hz; 1000 cycles per second = MHz)
  - ❏ Propagation velocity (about 1540 m/s in blood)
  - ❏ Wavelength (equal to the propagation velocity divided by frequency)
  - ❏ Amplitude (decibels or dB)

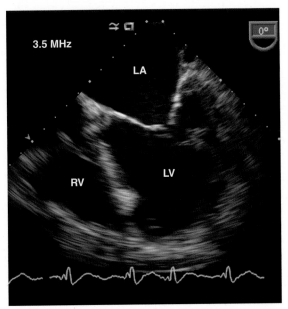
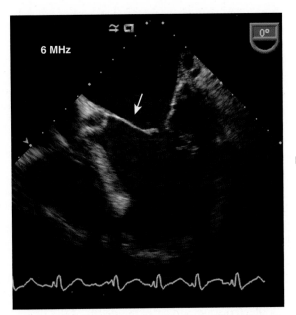

A   B

Figure 1–1 The effect of transducer frequency on penetration and resolution is shown by this transesophageal 4-chamber view recorded at a transmitted frequency of (A) 3.5 MHz and (B) 6 MHz. The higher frequency transducer provides better resolution—for example, the mitral leaflets (*arrow*) look thin, but the depth of penetration of the signal is very poor, so the apical ¹/₂ of the left ventricle is not seen. With the lower frequency transducer, improved tissue penetration provides a better image of the left ventricular apex, but image resolution is poorer, with the mitral leaflets looking thicker and less well defined.

■ Ultrasound waves interact with tissues in four different ways:
1. Reflection (used to create ultrasound images)
2. Scattering (the basis of Doppler ultrasound)
3. Refraction (used to focus the ultrasound beam)
4. Attenuation (loss of signal strength in the tissue)

Key points:

❑ Tissue penetration is greatest with a lower frequency transducer (e.g., 2 to 3 MHz).

❑ Image resolution is greatest (about 1 mm) with a higher frequency transducer (e.g., 5 to 7.5 MHz) (Fig. 1–1).

❑ Amplitude ("loudness") is described using the logarithmic decibel scale; a 6 dB change represents a doubling or halving of signal amplitude.

❑ Acoustic impedance depends on tissue density and the propagation velocity of ultrasound in that tissue.

❑ Ultrasound reflection occurs at smooth tissue boundaries with different acoustic impedances (such as between blood and myocardium); reflection is greatest when the ultrasound beam is *perpendicular* to the tissue interface.

❑ Ultrasound scattering that occurs with small structures (such as red blood cells) is used to generate Doppler signals; Doppler velocity recordings are most accurate when the ultrasound beam is *parallel* to the blood flow direction.

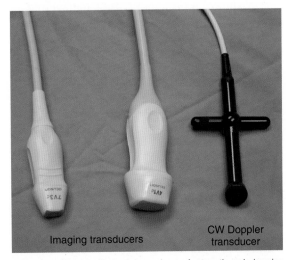

Imaging transducers   CW Doppler transducer

Figure 1–2 The specific transducer chosen for transthoracic imaging depends on the transmitted frequency, transducer size, and the specific application. A small phased array imaging transducer used in children and to view the apex in adults; a larger lower frequency phased array imaging transducer for better ultrasound penetration; and a nonimaging dedicated dual-crystal continuous wave Doppler transducer are shown here. Typically, multiple transducers are used during the examination.

❑ Refraction of ultrasound can result in imaging artifacts caused by deflection of the ultrasound beam from a straight path.

Transducers

■ Ultrasound transducers use a piezoelectric crystal to alternately transmit and receive ultrasound signals (Fig. 1–2).

- Transducers are configured for specific imaging approaches: transthoracic, transesophageal, intracardiac, and intravascular.
- The basic characteristics of a transducer are:
  - Transmission frequency (from 2.5 MHz for transthoracic to 20 MHz for intravascular ultrasound)
  - Bandwidth (range of frequencies in the transmitted ultrasound pulse)
  - Pulse repetition frequency (number of transmission-received cycles per second)
  - Focal depth (depends on beam shape and focusing)
  - Aperture (size of the transducer face or "footprint")
  - Power output

Key points:

- The time delay between transmission of an ultrasound burst and detection of the reflected wave indicates the depth of the tissue reflector.
- The pulse repetition frequency is an important factor in image resolution and frame rate.
- A shorter transmitted pulse length results in improved depth (or axial) resolution.
- A wider bandwidth provides better resolution of structures distant from the transducer.
- The shape of the ultrasound beam depends on several complex factors. Each type of transducer focuses the beam at a depth appropriate for the clinical application. Some transducers allow adjustment of focal depth.
- A smaller aperture is associated with a wider beam width; however, a smaller "footprint" may allow improved angulation of the beam in the intercostal spaces. This is most evident clinically with a dedicated nonimaging continuous wave (CW) Doppler transducer.

Ultrasound Imaging

Principles

- The basic ultrasound imaging modalities are:
  - M-mode—a graph of depth versus time
  - 2D—a sector scan in a tomographic image plane with real-time motion
  - Three-dimensional (3D)—a selected cut-away real-time image in a 3D display format (see Chapter 4)
- System controls for 2D imaging typically include:
  - Power output (transmitted ultrasound energy)
  - Gain (amplitude of the received signal)
  - Time-gain compensation (differential gain along the ultrasound beam)

- Depth of the image (affects pulse repetition frequency and frame rate)
- Gray scale/dynamic range (degree of contrast in the images)

Key points:

- M-mode recordings allow identification of very rapid intracardiac motion compared with a 2D frame rate, because the sampling rate is about 1800 times per second (Fig. 1–3).
- Ultrasound imaging resolution is more precise along the length of the ultrasound beam (axial resolution) compared with lateral (side to side) or elevational ("thickness" of the image plane) resolution.
- Lateral resolution decreases with increasing distance from the transducer (Fig. 1–4).
- Harmonic imaging improves endocardial definition and reduces near-field and side-lobe artifacts (Fig. 1–5).

Imaging Artifacts

- Common imaging artifacts result from:
  - A low signal-to-noise ratio
  - Acoustic shadowing
  - Reverberations
  - Beam width
  - Refraction
  - Range ambiguity
  - Electronic processing

Key points:

- A shadow occurs distal to a strong ultrasound reflector because the ultrasound wave does not penetrate past the reflector (Fig. 1–6).
- Ultrasound reflected back and forth between two strong reflectors creates a reverberation artifact.

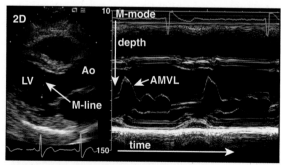

Figure 1–3 M-mode echocardiography. The location of the M-mode beam is guided by the two-dimensional (*2D*) image to ensure the M-mode line is perpendicular to the long axis of the ventricle and centered in the chamber. This M-mode (M for motion) tracing of time (on the horizontal axis) versus depth (on the vertical axis) shows the rapid diastolic motion of the anterior mitral valve leaflet (*AMVL*) in a patient in atrial flutter.

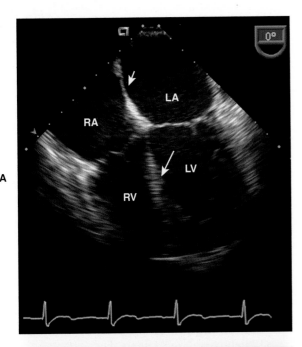

A

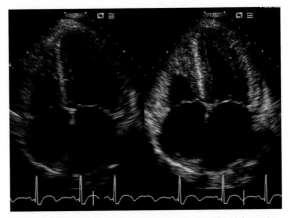

Figure 1–5 Harmonic imaging improves identification of the left ventricular endocardial border, as seen in this apical four-chamber view recorded with a 4-MHz transducer using (*left*) fundamental frequency imaging and (*right*) harmonic imaging.

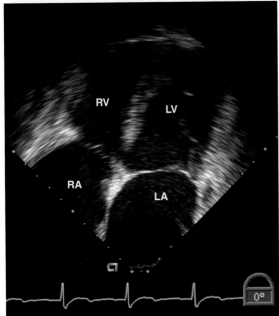

B

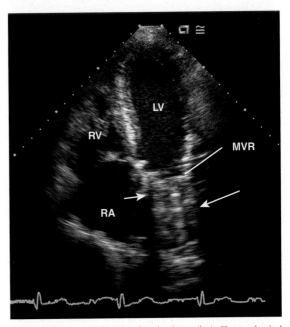

Figure 1–6 This apical four-chamber view in a patient with a mechanical mitral valve replacement (*MVR*) illustrates the shadowing (dark area, *small arrow*) and reverberations (white band of echoes, *large arrow*) that obscure structures (in this case the left atrium) distal to the valve.

Figure 1–4 Lateral resolution with ultrasound decreases with the distance of the reflector from the transducer. In this transesophageal echocardiography image oriented with the origin of the ultrasound signal at the top of the image (*A*), thin structures close to the transducer, such as the atrial septum (*small arrow*) appear as a dot because lateral resolution is optimal at this depth. Reflections from more distant structures, such as the ventricular septum (*large arrow*), appear as a broad line due to poor lateral resolution. When the image is oriented with the transducer at the bottom of the image (*B*), the effects of depth on lateral resolution are more visually apparent. The standard orientation for echocardiography, with the transducer at the top of the image, is based on considerations of ultrasound physics, not on cardiac anatomy.

- Signals originating from the edges of the ultrasound beam or from side lobes can result in imaging or Doppler artifacts.
- Deviation of the ultrasound beam from a straight pathway due to refraction in the tissue results in the structure appearing in the incorrect location across the sector scan.
- Reflected ultrasound signals received at the transducer are assumed to originate from the preceding transmitted pulse. Signals from very deep structures or signals that have been re-reflected will be displayed at one half or twice the actual depth of origin.

Doppler

- Doppler ultrasound is based on the principle that ultrasound backscattered (F_s) from moving red blood cells will appear higher or lower in frequency than the transmitted frequency (F_T) depending on the speed and direction of blood flow (v).
- The Doppler equation is:

$$v = c(F_s - F_T)/[2\,F_T\,(\cos\,\theta)]$$

- Accurate blood flow measurements depend on a parallel intercept angle (θ) between the ultrasound beam and direction of blood flow.

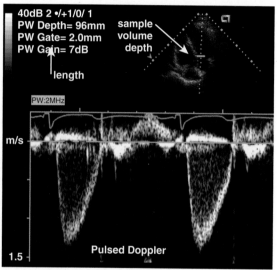

Figure 1–7 Doppler spectral tracing of left ventricular outflow recorded with pulsed Doppler ultrasound from the apex. The sample volume depth (time for transmission and reception of the signal) is shown on a small 2D image with the length (sampling duration) indicated by the pulsed wave (PW) gate size. The spectral tracing shows time (horizontal axis), velocity (vertical axis), and signal strength (gray scale). The baseline has been shifted upward to show the entire velocity curve directed away from the transducer; some diastolic left ventricular inflow is seen above the baseline, directed toward the transducer.

- There are three basic Doppler modalities: pulsed Doppler, color flow imaging, and CW Doppler ultrasound.

Key points:

- ☐ The speed (c) of ultrasound in blood is about 1540 m/s.
- ☐ Blood flow will be underestimated with a nonparallel intercept angle; the error is only 6% with an angle of 20 degrees but increases to 50% at a 60-degree angle.
- ☐ When the ultrasound beam is perpendicular to flow, there is no Doppler shift, and blood flow is not detected, even when present.
- ☐ The standard Doppler velocity display (or spectral recording) shows time on the horizontal axis and velocity on the vertical axis, with signal amplitude displayed using a decibel gray scale (Fig. 1–7).
- ☐ Standard Doppler instrument controls are:
  - ☐ Power output
  - ☐ Receiver gain (Fig. 1–8)
  - ☐ High-pass ("wall") filters (Fig. 1–9)
  - ☐ Velocity range and baseline shift
  - ☐ Post-processing options

Pulsed Doppler

- Pulsed Doppler allows measurement of blood flow velocity at a specific intracardiac site.
- The depth of interrogation (or sample volume) is determined by the time interval between transmission and sampling of the backscattered signal.
- Signal aliasing limits the maximum velocity measurable with pulsed Doppler.

Key points:

- ☐ A pulse of ultrasound is transmitted, then the backscattered signal is analyzed at a time interval corresponding to the transit time from the depth of interest.

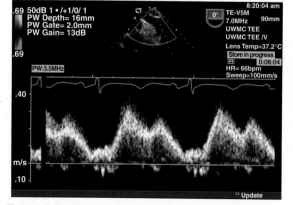

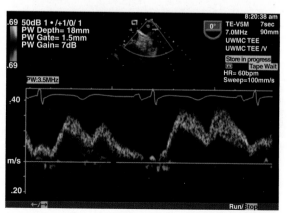

Figure 1–8 The effect of Doppler gain settings are shown for a transesophageal echocardiography recording of pulmonary vein inflow. Excess noise is eliminated when the gain is decreased from 13 dB (*A*) to 7 dB (*B*).

- ❑ The pulsed Doppler interrogation line and sample volume are displayed on the 2D image, with the transducer switched to Doppler only during data recording.
- ❑ Pulse repetition frequency is the number of transmission/receive cycles per second, which is determined by the depth of the sample volume.
- ❑ The maximum frequency detectable with intermittent sampling is one half the pulse repetition frequency (or Nyquist limit).
- ❑ The direction of blood flow for frequencies in excess of the Nyquist limit is ambiguous, a phenomenon called signal aliasing (Fig. 1–10).
- ❑ The effective velocity range for pulsed Doppler can be doubled by moving the baseline to the edge of the spectral display.
- ❑ The sample volume length can be adjusted to localize the signal (short length) or improve signal strength (long length).
- ❑ Pulsed Doppler is used to measure normal intracardiac transvalvular flow velocities.
- ❑ Variations of the pulsed Doppler principle are used to generate color Doppler flow images and tissue Doppler recordings.

Color Doppler

- ■ Color Doppler uses the pulsed Doppler principle to generate a 2D image or "map" of blood flow velocity superimposed on the 2D real-time image.
- ■ Color Doppler signals, like all pulsed Doppler velocity data, are angle dependent and are subject to signal aliasing.

- ■ The frame rate for color Doppler imaging depends on:
  - ❑ Pulse repetition frequency (depth of color sector)
  - ❑ Number of scan lines (width of color sector and scan line density)
  - ❑ Number of pulses per scan line (affects accuracy of mean velocity calculation)

Key points:

- ❑ Color Doppler is recorded in real time simultaneous with 2D imaging.
- ❑ Flow toward the transducer typically is shown in red and flow directed away from the transducer in blue (Fig. 1–11).
- ❑ When velocity exceeds the Nyquist limit, signal aliasing occurs so that faster flows toward the transducer alias from red to blue and from blue to red for flow away from the transducer.
- ❑ The amount of variation in the velocity signal from each site can be coded on the color scale as variance.
- ❑ Variance reflects either signal aliasing (high velocity flow) or the presence of multiple flow velocities or directions (flow disturbance).
- ❑ Color Doppler is most useful for visualization of spatial flow patterns; for this purpose, examiner preference determines the most appropriate color scale.
- ❑ For color Doppler measurements, such as vena contracta width or proximal isovelocity

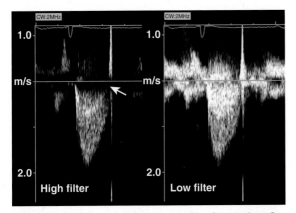

Figure 1–9 Continuous wave Doppler recording of an aortic outflow signal with the high pass ("wall") filter set at a high and low level. With the higher filter, low velocity signals are eliminated, reflected in the blank space adjacent to the baseline. This tracing enhances identification of the maximum velocity and recognition of the valve closing click. At the lower filter setting, the velocity signals extend to the baseline, making measurement of time intervals more accurate, but there also is more low velocity noise in the signal, related to motion of cardiac structures.

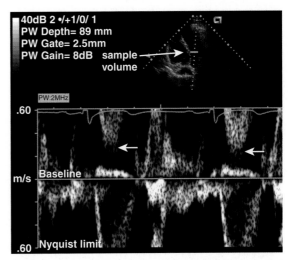

Figure 1–10 Left ventricular outflow velocity recorded from the apical approach with the sample volume on the left ventricular side of the aortic valve. The spectral tracing is shown in the standard format with the baseline in the center of the scale and the Nyquist limit at the top and bottom of the scale. Signal aliasing is present, with the top of the left ventricular outflow signal seen in the reverse channel (*arrows*). This degree of aliasing is easily resolved by shifting the baseline, as seen in Figure 1–7. Aliasing with higher velocity flow is best resolved using continuous wave Doppler ultrasound.

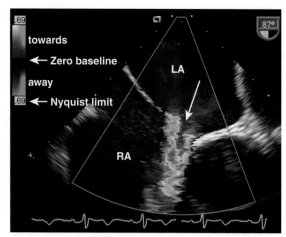

Figure 1–11 Color Doppler flow mapping is illustrated in the transesophageal echocardiography image of an atrial septal defect. The Doppler signal is superimposed on the 2D image using a color scale for flow toward the transducer in red, and flow away from the transducer in blue. The color intensity indicates velocity, as shown by the scale. This scale includes variance as the addition of green to the color scale. The flow (*arrow*) from the left atrium (*LA*) to the right atrium (*RA*) across the septal defect should be blue (away from the transducer) but has aliased to red because the velocity exceeds the Nyquist limit of 60 cm/s.

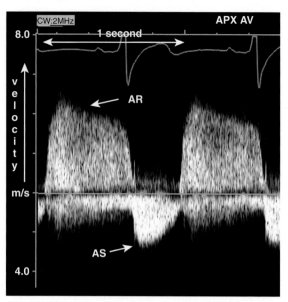

Figure 1–12 Continuous wave Doppler recording of the antegrade (aortic stenosis, *AS*) and retrograde (aortic regurgitation, *AR*) flow across the aortic valve. The spectral recording shows time (horizontal axis in seconds), velocity (vertical axis in m/s), and signal strength (gray scale). High velocity flow can be measured without aliasing using continuous wave Doppler as shown in the aortic regurgitant velocity over 4 m/s in this example.

surface area (PISA) measurements, a color scale without variance is optimal.

❏ The maximum velocity measurable with color Doppler is determined by the Nyquist limit, but the baseline can be shifted or the velocity scale can be reduced.

Continuous Wave Doppler

■ CW Doppler uses two ultrasound crystals to continuously transmit and receive ultrasound signals.
■ CW Doppler allows accurate measurement of high flow velocities, without signal aliasing.
■ Signals from the entire length of the ultrasound beam are included in the spectral CW Doppler recording.

Key points:

❏ CW Doppler is used to measure high velocity flows—for example, across stenotic and regurgitant valves (Fig. 1–12).
❏ The CW Doppler signal is recorded as a spectral tracing, with the scale and baseline adjusted as needed to display the signal of interest.
❏ CW Doppler can be recorded with a standard transducer with the CW interrogation line shown on the 2D image; however, a dedicated nonimaging CW transducer is optimal because of its higher signal-to-noise ratio and better angulation with a smaller transducer.

❏ The lack of range resolution means that the origin of the CW signal must be inferred from:
  ❏ Characteristics of the signal itself (timing, shape, and associated flow signals)
  ❏ Associated 2D imaging and pulsed or color Doppler findings
❏ Underestimation of blood flow velocity occurs when the CW Doppler beam is not parallel to the flow of interest.

Doppler Artifacts

■ Artifacts with pulsed or CW Doppler spectral recordings include:
  ❏ Underestimation of velocity related to a nonparallel intercept angle
  ❏ Range ambiguity
  ❏ Beam width artifacts with superimposition of multiple flow signals
  ❏ Mirror image artifact (Fig. 1–13).
  ❏ Transit time effect
  ❏ Electronic interference
■ Artifacts with color Doppler flow imaging include:
  ❏ Signal aliasing (Fig. 1–14).
  ❏ Shadowing, resulting in inability to detect flow abnormalities
  ❏ Ghosting from strong reflectors leading to flashes of color across the image plane

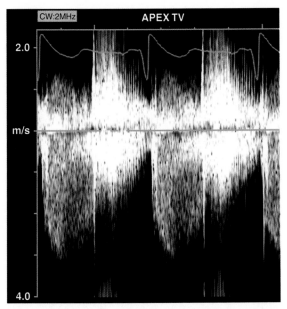

Figure 1–13 Appropriate use of instrumentation allows minimization of many ultrasound artifacts. This recording of tricuspid regurgitant jet velocity shows marked channel cross-talk (signal below the baseline that does not correlate with an actual intracardiac flow) from the diastolic signal across the tricuspid valve. This recording would be improved by a higher wall filter and lower gain setting.

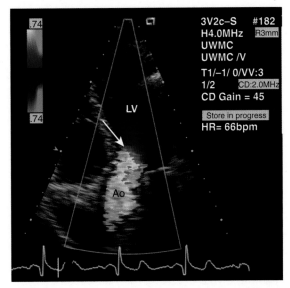

Figure 1–14 In this apical view angulated anteriorly to visualize the aorta, the antegrade flow in the left ventricular outflow tract aliased from blue to orange because the velocity exceeds the Nyquist limit of 74 cm/s. Variance is seen because of signal aliasing.

❏ Lack of signal when the ultrasound beam is perpendicular to flow
❏ Electronic interference

Key points:

❏ The potential for underestimation of velocity is the most important clinical limitation of Doppler ultrasound.
❏ Signal aliasing limits measurement of high velocities with pulsed Doppler and may confuse interpretation of color Doppler images.
❏ Range ambiguity with CW Doppler is obvious. With pulsed Doppler, range ambiguity occurs when signals from 2×, 3×, etc., the depth of the sample volume return to the transducer during a receive cycle.
❏ A mirror image artifact is common on spectral tracings and may be reduced by lowering power output and gain.
❏ As ultrasound propagates through moving blood, there is a slight change in ultrasound frequency, called the transit time effect. The transit time effect results in slight blurring of the edge of the CW Doppler signal, particularly for high velocity flows.
❏ Acoustic shadowing can be avoided by using an alternate transducer position—for example, transesophageal imaging of a mitral prosthetic valve.
❏ Color ghosting is seen in only one or two frames of the cardiac cycle, whereas blood flow signals demonstrate physiologic timing.

Bioeffects and Safety

■ There are two types of ultrasound bioeffects important with diagnostic imaging:
  ❏ Thermal (heating of tissue due to the interaction of ultrasound energy with tissue)
  ❏ Cavitation (the creation or vibration of small gas-filled bodies)
■ Ultrasound exposure is measured by the:
  ❏ Thermal index (TI, the ratio of transmitted acoustic power to the power needed to increase temperature by 1°C)
  ❏ Mechanical index (MI, the ratio of peak rarefactional pressure to the square root of transducer frequency)

Key points:

❏ The degree of tissue heating depends on the ultrasound energy imparted to the tissue and on characteristics of the tissue, including tissue density and blood flow.
❏ The total ultrasound exposure depends on transducer frequency, focus, power output, and depth, as well as the duration of the examination.
❏ Cavitation or vibration of microbubbles occurs with higher intensity ultrasound exposure.
❏ When the TI or MI exceeds 1, the benefit of the ultrasound examination should be balanced against potential biologic effects.
❏ Power output and exposure time should be monitored during the echocardiographic examination.

SELF-ASSESSMENT QUESTIONS

QUESTION 1

The best approach to improve resolution in the near field of a 2D ultrasound image is:

A. Increase gain
B. Decrease power output
C. Increase transducer frequency
D. Decrease dynamic range
E. Narrow the 2D sector

QUESTION 2

The best approach to improve the resolution of a structure at a depth of 9 to 10 cm from the transducer is:

A. Increase gain
B. Decrease depth
C. Increase transducer frequency
D. Decrease dynamic range
E. Narrow the 2D sector

QUESTION 3

Choose the most appropriate Doppler modality (A, B, C) for clinical evaluation of each intracardiac flow signal (I through V).
I.   Left ventricular diastolic inflow
II. Direction of mitral regurgitant jet
III. Aortic stenosis velocity
IV. Pulmonary vein flow velocity
V.   Tricuspid regurgitation velocity

A. Pulsed Doppler
B. Continuous wave Doppler
C. Color Doppler flow imaging

QUESTION 4

Which one of the following would be the best initial approach for increasing the frame rate with color Doppler flow imaging?

A. Decrease depth
B. Widen color sector
C. Shift color baseline
D. Decrease color velocity scale
E. Use a smaller height color box

QUESTION 5

For the Doppler flow shown in Figure 1–15, the most appropriate next step for measuring velocity accurately is:

A. Increase sample volume length
B. Decrease gain
C. Increase the velocity scale
D. Shift the baseline upward
E. Correct for intercept angle

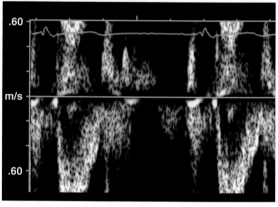

Figure 1–15

QUESTION 6

For the Doppler tracing in Figure 1–16, match the numbered signals with the answers below:

A. Left ventricular diastolic filling
B. Aortic regurgitation
C. Aortic antegrade flow
D. Subaortic left ventricular outflow velocity
E. Doppler artifact

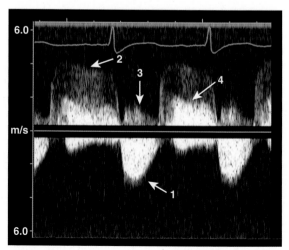

Figure 1–16

ANSWERS

ANSWER 1: C

Resolution is improved with a higher transducer frequency; this effect is most pronounced in the near field because penetration decreases with a higher frequency transducer so distant structures are less well visualized. When the 2D sector is narrowed, scan line density is higher, which improves resolution. However, the wedge shape of the image field limits the value of this approach for near-field structures. Changing the gain, power output, and dynamic range will affect the appearance of the image in terms of brightness and contrast but will not improve image resolution, defined as the ability to separately identify two nearby structures on the ultrasound image.

ANSWER 2: E

At this depth, the first approach to improving resolution is to narrow the 2D sector, which increases the scan line density. The zoom function of many instruments (which eliminates the near and far field as well as narrowing the sector) also may be helpful. The potential benefit of a higher frequency transducer is typically offset by decreased ultrasound tissue penetration at this depth. Decreasing the depth of the image does not substantially affect resolution and is only helpful when the structure of interest is still in the image plane. Gain and dynamic range affect the contrast and brightness of the image but do not affect resolution per se.

ANSWER 3: I, A; II, C; III, B; IV, A; V, B

Normal intracardiac flows (LV inflow and pulmonary vein flow) that have a maximum velocity less than the typical Nyquist limit at that depth are best evaluated with pulsed Doppler ultrasound because this provides localization of the flow signal and a quantitative spectral velocity curve. High velocity flows, either antegrade across a stenotic valve (aortic stenosis) or retrograde across a regurgitant valve (tricuspid regurgitation), are best evaluated with CW Doppler. CW Doppler allows accurate measurement of high velocities without signal aliasing. However, the lack of range resolution means that the origin of the high velocity signal must be inferred from other imaging or Doppler data or from the characteristics of the flow signal itself. Identification of the presence of an intracardiac flow disturbance or characterization of the spatial distribution of flow, for example, the direction and shape of a mitral regurgitant jet, are best evaluated with color Doppler, which provides a "map" of flow superimposed on the 2D image, albeit with only limited velocity data.

ANSWER 4: A

The depth of the color Doppler image determines the pulse repetition frequency, based on the time needed for ultrasound to reach and return from the maximum depth on the image. Thus a decrease in depths means a shorter time interval for generating the color image and a faster frame rate. A wider color sector results in a lower frame rate because of the time needed to generate Doppler data across the image plane. Shifting the color baseline or decreasing the color velocity scale have no effect on frame rate because the total velocity range (and pulse repetition frequency) are unchanged; these parameters simply change the colors assigned to each Doppler velocity value. Pulse repetition frequency and frame rate are determined by the maximum depth displayed on the image; reducing the height of the color box simply removes the color display from the near field—the pulse repetition frequency is unchanged.

ANSWER 5: D

This figure shows signal aliasing with the higher velocities displayed in the opposite channel. Because the top of the velocity curve can be seen "wrapping around" the spectral display, the simplest approach to resolving this velocity is to shift the baseline until the entire velocity curve is intact, directed away from the transducer. Higher velocity flows with severe signal aliasing and no discernible peak velocity would require CW Doppler for accurate velocity measurement. Increasing sample volume length would increase signal strength, and decreasing gain would reduce signal strength, but neither would resolve the aliased signal. The velocity scale cannot be increased past the Nyquist limit with pulsed Doppler and so is not applicable in this case. For cardiac applications, "correction" for intercept angle is not recommended because the exact 3D angle between the ultrasound beam and direction of flow cannot be accurately determined. In any case, a nonparallel intercept angle results in underestimation (not overestimation) of blood flow velocity.

ANSWER 6: 1, C; 2, B; 3, E; 4, A

This is a CW Doppler spectral recording of ante-grade and retrograde flow across the aortic valve recorded with a dedicated CW transducer from the apical window. In systole (after the QRS on the electrocardiogram) the smooth rounded curve of mild aortic stenosis with a maximum velocity of about 3 m/s is seen. In diastole, there is a faint signal of aortic regurgitation with the typical high velocity reflecting the aortic to left ventricular diastolic pressure difference, which declines slightly over the diastolic period. An irregular signal in systole is seen in the channel opposite the aortic jet signal, most consistent with a Doppler recording artifact called channel "cross-talk." The CW Doppler beam is broad at the level of the aortic valve, so the left ventricular inflow signal across the mitral valve, with the typical two-peaked early and late diastolic filling velocity curve, is seen superimposed on the aortic regurgitant signal.

NOTES

2 The Transthoracic Echocardiogram

THE ECHO EXAM

STEP-BY-STEP APPROACH
Clinical Data
Patient Positioning
Basic Instrumentation Principles
Common Aspects of Data Recording
Echocardiographic Examination Sequence
Parasternal Window
Long Axis View
Right Ventricular Inflow View

Right Ventricular Outflow View
Short Axis View
Apical Window
Imaging Four-Chamber, Two-Chamber,
and Long Axis Views
Doppler Data
Subcostal Window
Suprasternal Notch Window
The Echo Report

SELF-ASSESSMENT QUESTIONS

THE ECHO EXAM: CORE ELEMENTS*

MODALITY	WINDOW	VIEW/SIGNAL	MEASUREMENTS
Clinical data		Indication for echo Key history and PE findings Previous cardiac imaging data Blood pressure at time of echo exam	
2D imaging	Parasternal	Long axis Short axis aortic valve Short axis mitral valve Short axis LV (papillary muscle level) Right ventricular inflow Right ventricular outflow	LV dimensions LV wall thickness Aortic root dimension LA dimension
	Apical	Four-chamber Anteriorly angulated four-chamber Two-chamber Long axis	Visual estimate of ejection fraction
	Subcostal	Four-chamber IVC with respiration	
Pulsed Doppler	Apical	Left ventricular inflow at leaflet tips	E velocity A velocity
Color flow	Parasternal	Left ventricular outflow Long axis Short axis of aortic and mitral valves RV inflow and outflow	LV outflow velocity Color flow to identify regurgitation of all four valves. Measure vena contracta if possible.
	Apical	Four-chamber Long axis	Mitral, tricuspid, and aortic valves
Continuous wave Doppler	Parasternal	Tricuspid valve Pulmonic valve	TR-jet velocity
	Apical	Aortic valve Mitral valve Tricuspid valve	Aortic regurgitation Mitral regurgitation TR-jet (PAP)

*A complete echo exam consists of core elements and additional components.

2D, *Two-dimensional;* A, *atrial filling;* E, *early diastolic filling;* IVC, *inferior vena cava;* LA, *left atrium;* LV, *left ventricle;* PAP, *pulmonary artery pressure;* PE, *pericardial effusion;* RV, *right ventricle;* TR, *tricuspid regurgitation.*

THE ECHO EXAM: ADDITIONAL COMPONENTS

ABNORMALITY ON CORE ELEMENTS	ADDITIONAL ECHO EXAM COMPONENTS (CHAPTER)
Reason for Echo	Additional components to address specific clinical question*
Left Ventricle	
Decreased ejection fraction	See Systolic Function and Dilated Cardiomyopathy (6, 9)
Abnormal LV filling velocities	See Diastolic Function (7)
Regional wall motion abnormality	See Ischemic Heart Disease (8)
Increased wall thickness	See Hypertrophic Cardiomyopathy, Restrictive Cardiomyopathy, and Hypertensive Heart Disease (9)
Valves	
Imaging evidence for stenosis or an increased antegrade transvalvular velocity	See Valve Stenosis (11)
Regurgitation greater than mild on color flow imaging or CW Doppler	See Valve Regurgitation (12)
Prosthetic valve	See Prosthetic Valves (13)
Valve mass or suspected endocarditis	See Endocarditis and Masses (14, 15)
Right Heart	
Enlarged right ventricle	See Pulmonary Heart Disease and Congenital Heart Disease (9, 17)
Elevated TR-jet velocity	See Pulmonary Pressures (6)
Pericardium	
Pericardial effusion	See Pericardial Effusion (10)
Pericardial thickening	See Constrictive Pericarditis (10)
Great Vessels	
Enlarged aorta	See Aortic Disease (16)

*The echo exam should always include additional components to address the clinical indication. For example, if the indication is "heart failure," additional components to evaluate systolic and diastolic function are needed even if the core elements do not show obvious abnormalities. If the indication is "cardiac source of embolus," the additional components for that diagnosis are needed.
CW, Continuous wave; LV, left ventricle; TR, tricuspid regurgitation.

STEP-BY-STEP APPROACH

Step 1: Clinical Data

- The indication for the study determines the focus of the examination.
- Key clinical history and physical examination findings and results of any previous cardiac imaging studies are noted.

Key points:

- The goal of the echo study is to answer the specific question asked by the referring provider.
- Blood pressure is recorded at the time of the echo because many measurements vary with loading conditions.
- Knowledge of clinical data ensures that the echo study includes all the pertinent images and Doppler data. For example, when a systolic murmur is present, the echo study includes data addressing all the possible causes for this finding.
- Data from previous imaging studies may identify specific areas of concern—for example, a pericardial effusion noted on computed tomographic (CT) imaging of the chest.
- Detailed information about previous cardiac procedures assists in interpretation of postoperative findings, evaluation of implanted devices (such as prosthetic valves or percutaneous closure devices), and detection of complications.

Step 2: Patient Positioning (Fig. 2–1)

- A steep left lateral position provides acoustic access for parasternal and apical views.
- The subcostal views are obtained when the patient is supine with legs bent (to relax the abdominal wall).
- Suprasternal notch views are obtained when the patient is supine with the head turned toward the left.

Key points:

- Images may be improved with suspended respiration, typically at end-expiration but sometimes at other phases of the respiratory cycle.
- An examination bed with an apical cutout allows a steeper left lateral position, often providing improved acoustic access for apical views.
- Imaging can be performed with either hand holding the transducer and with the exam-

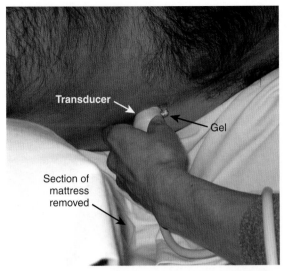

Figure 2–1 The patient is positioned in a steep left lateral decubitus position on an examination bed with a removable section cut out of the mattress to allow placement of the transducer on the apex by the sonographer, as shown. Ultrasound gel is used to enhance coupling between the transducer face and the patient's skin. The sonographer sits on an adjustable chair and uses the left hand for scanning and the right hand to adjust the instrument panel. The room is darkened to improve visualization on the ultrasound instrument display screen.

iner on either side of the patient. However, imaging from the patient's left side avoids reaching over the patient and is essential for apical views when the patient girth is larger than the arm span of the examiner.

❏ Prolonged or repetitive imaging requires the examiner to learn ergonomic approaches to minimize mechanical stress and avoid injury.

Step 3: Basic Instrumentation Principles (Fig. 2–2)

■ A higher transducer frequency provides improved resolution but decreased penetration of the ultrasound signal.
■ Harmonic imaging is commonly used to improve image quality, particularly recognition of endothelial borders.
■ Depth, zoom mode, and sector width are adjusted to optimize the image and frame rate, depending on the structure or flow of interest.
■ Gain settings are adjusted to optimize the data recording while preventing artifacts.

Key points:

❏ Although the control panel varies for each instrument, the basic functions are similar for all ultrasound systems.
❏ The highest frequency that penetrates adequately to the depth of interest is used for optimal imaging.
❏ Flat structures, such as valve leaflets, appear thicker with harmonic imaging than with fundamental imaging.
❏ Frame rate is higher for a shorter depth or a narrower sector; a fast frame rate is especially important with Doppler color flow imaging.

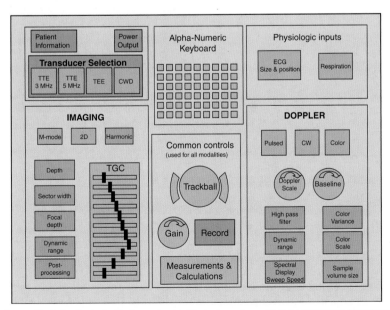

Figure 2–2 Schematic diagram illustrating the typical features of a simplified echocardiographic instrument panel. Many instrument controls affect different parameters depending on the imaging modality. For example, the trackball is used to adjust the position of the M-mode and Doppler beams, sample volume depth, and the size and position of the color Doppler box. The trackball also may be used to adjust two-dimensional image depth and sector width and the position of the zoom box. The gain control adjusts gain for each modality, imaging, pulsed, or CW Doppler. Only a simplified model of an instrument panel is shown. The transducer choices are examples; other transducers are available depending on the system. In addition to the time gain compensation (TGC) controls, a lateral control scale may also be present.

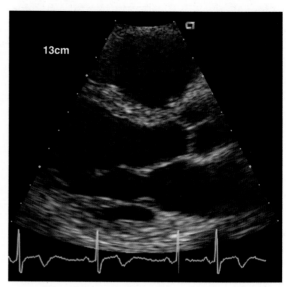

Figure 2–3 Parasternal long axis view recorded at a depth of 18 cm to show the structures posterior to the heart (*A*) and then with the depth decreased to 13 cm (*B*) and the resolution mode used (note that the top of the displayed image now is 2 cm from the skin) to focus on the aortic and mitral valves.

- ❏ Too narrow a sector may miss important anatomic or physiologic findings.
- ❏ Excessive gain results in artifacts with both imaging and Doppler, whereas inadequate gain results in data loss.

Step 4: Common Aspects of Data Recording

- ■ Representative images from the echo study are recorded, usually digitally, to document the findings and for later review and measurement.
- ■ Echo images typically include an electrocardiogram (ECG) tracing for timing purposes.

Key points:

- ❏ Echo images in each view are recorded first with a depth and sector width that encompasses all the structures in the image plane and then at a depth and sector width optimized for the structures of interest (Figs. 2–3*A* and *B*).
- ❏ Additional zoom mode images are recorded, as needed, of normal and abnormal findings.
- ❏ Spectral pulsed and continuous wave (CW) Doppler data are recorded with the baseline and velocity range adjusted so the flow signal fits but fills the vertical axis and the time scale is adjusted to maximize the accuracy of measurements (usually an x-axis of 100 mm/s) (Fig. 2–4).

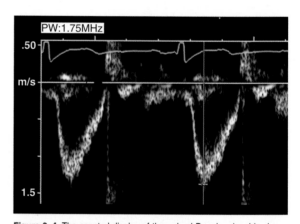

Figure 2–4 The spectral display of the pulsed Doppler signal is shown with the baseline shifted and velocity scale adjusted to avoid aliasing and to use the full vertical axis to improve measurement accuracy (e.g., the signal "fits but fills" the graphical display). The horizontal time scale is 100 mm/s, which is standard for most Doppler recordings.

- ❏ Color Doppler is recorded after sector width and depth are adjusted to optimize frame rate and gain is set just below the level that results in background speckle.
- ❏ The variance mode on the color scale is preferred by many examiners (including the authors) to enhance recognition of abnormal flows.
- ❏ Some normal flows result in a variance display—for example, when left ventricular (LV)

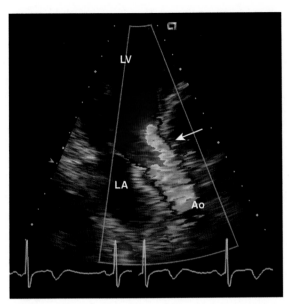

Figure 2–5 This color Doppler image of left ventricular (*LV*) outflow in an apical long axis view shows signal aliasing adjacent to the septum in the subaortic region. Although this appearance may be due to an asymmetric flow profile, the effects of intercept angle also may be important. Even if the velocity is identical across the outflow tract, compared with the region along the anterior mitral valve leaflet, in the region adjacent to the septum the Doppler beam is more parallel to the flow direction. The higher Doppler shift results in signal aliasing. Aliasing at the aortic valve level is expected, as the aortic velocity typically exceeds the Nyquist limit at this depth (0.74 m/s in this example).

outflow velocity exceeds the Nyquist limit and signal aliasing occurs (Fig. 2–5).

❏ Conversely, when variance is not used, it is more difficult to distinguish abnormal flows (such as mitral regurgitation) from normal flows (such as pulmonary vein flow) when both occur in the same anatomic region.

Step 5: Echocardiographic Examination Sequence

■ In subsequent chapters, the elements of the examination for each clinical condition are presented in the order needed for a final diagnosis.

■ Typically, these examination elements are incorporated into a systemic examination sequence.

Key points:

❏ There are several approaches to an examination sequence; any of these are appropriate if a complete systemic examination is performed.

❏ In some clinical situations, a limited examination may be appropriate with the study components selected by the referring or performing physician.

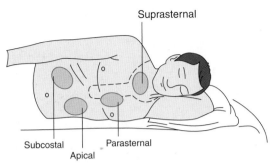

Figure 2–6 The standard acoustic "windows" where ultrasound can reach the cardiac structures without intervening lung or bone include the parasternal, apical, subcostal, and suprasternal notch windows. The parasternal and apical windows typically are optimal with the patient in a steep left lateral position. For the subcostal window, the patient is supine with the knees flexed to relax the abdominal vasculature. For the suprasternal notch window, the patient is supine with the head tilted back and to one side.

❏ The approach suggested here is based on obtaining all data (imaging and Doppler) for each acoustic window (parasternal, apical, subcostal, and suprasternal) before moving to the next acoustic window; this approach minimizes the time needed to reposition the patient between acoustic windows (Fig. 2–6).

❏ Some examiners prefer to obtain all the imaging data and then obtain all the Doppler data; this approach allows the Doppler data recording to be tailored to the imaging findings.

❏ With any approach, the examiner may need to go back to previous acoustic windows at the end of the examination if additional views or measurements are needed based on abnormal findings.

❏ The examination sequence also may need to be modified depending on patient factors (inability to move, bandages, etc.) or the urgency of the examination.

Step 6: Parasternal Window

Step 6A: Long Axis View

■ Many echocardiographers start with the parasternal long axis view with:

❏ Imaging to show the aortic and mitral valves, left atrium and aortic root, the LV base, and the right ventricular (RV) outflow tract

❏ Color Doppler to screen for aortic and mitral regurgitation

■ Standard measurements include:

❏ LV end-diastolic and end-systolic diameters and diastolic thickness of the septum and LV inferior-lateral wall just apical from the mitral leaflet tips (Fig. 2–7)

❏ Aortic diameter at end-diastole (Fig. 2–8)

❏ Left atrial anterior-posterior dimension

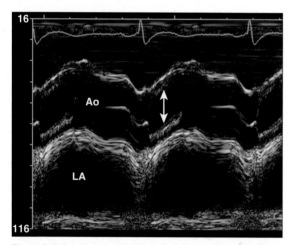

Figure 2–7 Two-dimensional guided M-mode recording of the left ventricle (*LV*) at the mitral chordal level. End-diastolic measurements of wall thickness and cavity dimension are made at the onset of the QRS, as shown. End-systolic measurements are made at the maximum posterior motion of the septum (when septal motion is normal) or at minimal left ventricular size. The rapid sampling rate with M-mode allows more accurate identification of the endocardial border, which is distinguished from chordae or trabeculations as being a continuous line in diastole with the steepest slope during systole.

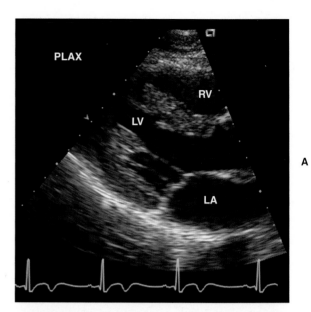

A

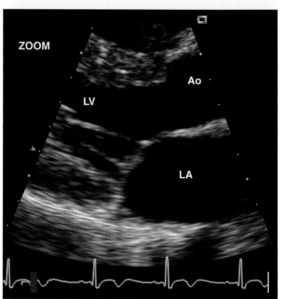

B

Figure 2–8 Two-dimensional guided M-mode recording of the aortic valve (*Ao*) and left atrium (*LA*) allows measurement of aortic root dimension at end-diastole using a leading edge to leading edge approach, the aortic leaflet separation, and the left atrial maximum anterior-posterior dimension in early diastole. The fine fluttering of the aortic valve leaflets is normal.

Figure 2–9 First the mitral valve is examined at a standard depth (*A*), then zoom mode (*B*) is used to optimize visualization of the aortic and mitral valves. The image plane is angled slightly medial and lateral to encompass the medial and lateral aspects of the valve. Some normal thin mitral chords are well seen in this slightly laterally angulated view, extending from the mitral closure plane to the papillary muscle.

❐ Vena contracta width for aortic, mitral, and tricuspid regurgitation

Key points:

❐ Images are initially recorded at a depth that includes the descending thoracic aorta to detect pleural and pericardial effusions.

❐ Then the depth is reduced to the level of the posterior wall for assessment of the size and function of the base of the LV and the RV outflow tract.

❐ The aortic and mitral valves are examined with zoom mode sweeping through the valve planes from medial to lateral to assess valve anatomy and motion (Fig. 2–9).

❐ Left atrial anterior-posterior dimension may underestimate left atrial enlargement; when clinically indicated, additional measurements are made from apical views.

❐ The aortic root (sinuses of Valsalva and sinotubular junction) is visualized first from the standard window and then with the transducer moved up one or more interspaces to visualize the ascending aorta (Fig. 2–10).

❑ Color Doppler of aortic and mitral valves is used to screen for valve regurgitation. If more than physiologic regurgitation is present, further evaluation is needed, as discussed in Chapter 12.

Step 6B: Right Ventricular Inflow View

■ From the long axis view, the image plane is angled medially to show the right ventricular inflow view (Fig. 2–11) with:

❑ Imaging of the right atrium, tricuspid valve, and right ventricle

❑ Color Doppler evaluation of tricuspid regurgitation

❑ CW Doppler recording of tricuspid regurgitant jet velocity

■ Standard measurements include:

❑ Maximum tricuspid regurgitant velocity (Fig. 2–12)

Key points:

❑ Slide apically one interspace if views are not obtained from the standard window.

❑ Adjust depth to include the right atrium (RA), RV, and tricuspid valves.

❑ The entrance of the coronary sinus and the inferior vena cava into the RA are seen in this view.

❑ A small amount of tricuspid regurgitation on color Doppler is seen in most (more than 80%) normal individuals and sometimes is referred to as "physiologic."

❑ The CW Doppler tricuspid regurgitant jet is recorded from multiple views; the highest velocity represents the most parallel intercept angle with flow and is used to estimate pulmonary pressure—the lower velocity recordings are ignored.

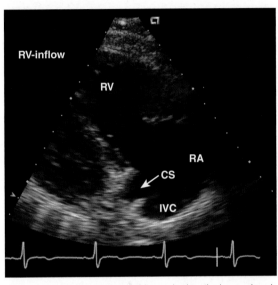

Figure 2–11 From the parasternal long axis view, the image plane is angulated medially to visualize the right ventricular inflow view with the right ventricle (*RV*), right atrium (*RA*), coronary sinus (*CS*), inferior vena cava (*IVC*), and tricuspid valve.

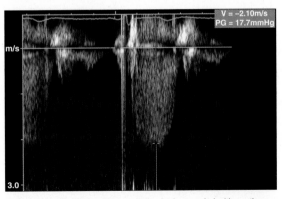

Figure 2–12 The tricuspid regurgitation jet is recorded with continuous wave (CW) Doppler from both the parasternal right ventricular inflow view and from the left ventricular apex. Only the highest velocity is reported, in normal sinus rhythm, because the apparent lower velocity signal is caused by a nonparallel intercept angle between the ultrasound beam and regurgitant jet. This example shows a tricuspid valve closing click and a faint signal of tricuspid regurgitation. Although signal strength is low because regurgitation is only mild, there is a clearly defined velocity curve with a maximum velocity of 2.1 m/s.

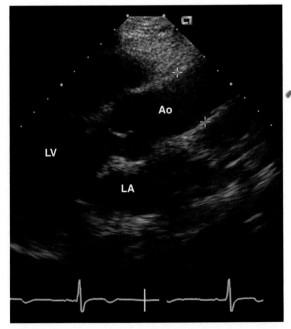

Figure 2–10 The ascending aorta is visualized by moving the transducer up an interspace from the parasternal long axis view.

Step 6C: Right Ventricular Outflow View

- From the long axis view, the image plane is angled laterally to show the right ventricular outflow view (Fig. 2–13) with:
    - Imaging of the RV outflow tract, pulmonic valve, and main pulmonary artery
    - Color Doppler evaluation of pulmonic regurgitation (Fig. 2–14)

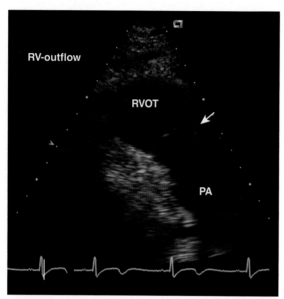

Figure 2–13 Right ventricular outflow tract view, obtained by angulating the transducer laterally from the parasternal long axis view, shows the right ventricular outflow tract (*RVOT*), pulmonic valve (*arrow*), and main pulmonary artery (*PA*).

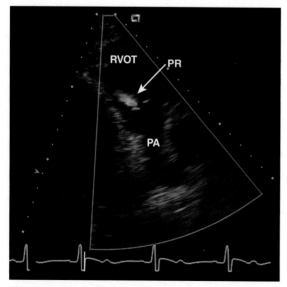

Figure 2–14 Color Doppler in a right ventricular outflow view showing a narrow jet of pulmonic regurgitation (PR) in diastole. Mild pulmonic regurgitation is seen in about 80% of normal adults.

- Pulsed Doppler recording of pulmonary artery flow (Fig. 2–15)
- Standard measurements include:
    - Antegrade velocity in the pulmonary artery

Key points:

- Slide cephalad one interspace if views are not obtained from the standard window.
- Adjust depth to include the RV outflow tract, main pulmonary artery, and pulmonary artery bifurcation.
- The pulmonic valve often is difficult to visualize in adults, but a small amount of pulmonic regurgitation typically is present with a normally functioning valve.
- The pulsed Doppler recording of flow in the main pulmonary artery is helpful for assessment of pulmonary pressures and to exclude pulmonic stenosis or a patent ductus arteriosus.

Step 6D: Short Axis View

- From the long axis view, the image plane is rotated 90 degrees to show the short axis plane with:
    - Imaging and color Doppler at the level of the aortic valve to evaluate the aortic, tricuspid, and pulmonic valves (Fig. 2–16)
    - Imaging at the level of the mitral valve for evaluation of mitral leaflet anatomy and motion and LV size and function (Fig. 2–17)
    - Imaging at the mid-papillary muscle level to evaluate global and regional LV size and function (Fig. 2–18)

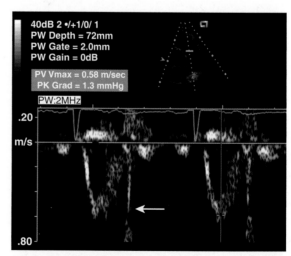

Figure 2–15 Pulsed Doppler recording of normal flow in the right ventricular outflow tract (notice the pulmonic valve closure click indicated the sample volume is on the right ventricular side of the valve) shows a smooth velocity curve that peaks in mid-systole with a velocity less than 1 m/s.

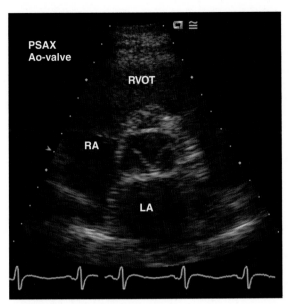

Figure 2–16 Parasternal short axis view of a normal trileaflet aortic valve in systole.

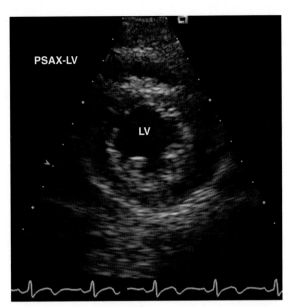

Figure 2–18 Parasternal short axis view of the left ventricle (*LV*) at the papillary muscle level. The LV cavity should appear circular in this view; an elliptical shape suggests an oblique intercept angle. This view sometimes requires the transducer be moved slightly apically from the short axis view of the aortic valve, instead of just tilting the transducer towards the apex from a fixed position on the chest wall.

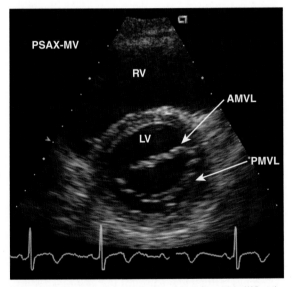

Figure 2–17 Parasternal short axis view of the left ventricle (*LV*) at the level of the mitral valve showing both anterior (*AMVL*) and posterior (*PMVL*) valve leaflets.

- Standard measurements include:
  - ❏ M-mode or two-dimensional (2D) measurements of the aorta, left atrium, and left ventricle using the combination of long and short axis views to ensure the dimensions are measured in the minor axis of each chamber or vessel (Table 2–1)

Key points:

- ❏ The aortic and pulmonic valves normally are perpendicular to each other (when the aortic

valve is seen in short axis view, the pulmonic valve is seen in long axis view).
- ❏ Zoom mode is used to identify the number of aortic valve leaflets, with care taken to visualize the leaflets in systole.
- ❏ A bicuspid aortic valve is a common abnormality, with a prevalence of about 1% of the total population, and often is diagnosed on echocardiography requested for other indications.
- ❏ The atrial septum is seen in the short axis view at the aortic valve level. Color flow imaging may help detect a patent foramen ovale but must be distinguished from normal flow in the right atrium (inflow from the superior and inferior vena cava and regurgitation across the tricuspid valve), all of which are adjacent to the atrial septum.
- ❏ Parasternal views of the left ventricle at the papillary muscle level provide optimal endocardial definition and are used in conjunction with apical views for detection of regional wall motion abnormalities.

Step 7: Apical Window

Step 7A: Imaging Four-Chamber, Two-Chamber, and Long Axis Views

- The apical window usually corresponds to the point of maximal impulse and is optimized with the patient in a steep left lateral position.

TABLE 2–1

BASIC ECHO IMAGING MEASUREMENTS

CARDIAC STRUCTURE	BASIC MEASUREMENTS	ADDITIONAL MEASUREMENTS	TECHNICAL DETAILS
Left ventricle	ED dimension ES dimension Wall thickness	ED volume ES volume 2D stroke volume Ejection fraction LV mass	2D imaging is used to ensure measurements are centered and perpendicular to the long axis of the LV. M-mode provides superior time resolution and more accurate identification of endocardial borders.
Left atrium	AP diameter	LA area LA volume	Left atrial anterior-posterior dimension provides a quick screen but may underestimate LA size. When LA size is important for clinical decision making, measurement of LA volume is helpful.
Right ventricle	Visual estimate of size	Parasternal AP diameter	Quantitation of RV size by echo is challenging due to the complex 3D shape of the chamber.
Right atrium	Visual estimate of size		RA size is usually compared with the LA in the apical four-chamber view.
Aorta	Maximum diameter	Maximum diameter indexed to expected dimension Diameter at multiple sites	With 2D echo, inner edge to inner edge measurements are more reproducible. Measurements are made at end-diastole by convention, but end-systolic measurements also may be helpful.
Pulmonary artery		Diameter	

2D, *Two-dimensional;* 3D, *three-dimensional;* AP, *anterior-posterior;* ED, *end-diastole (onset of the QRS);* ES, *end-systole (minimum LV volume);* LA, *left atrium;* LV, *left ventricle;* RA, *right atrium.*

■ Images are obtained in four-chamber (Fig. 2–19), two-chamber (Fig. 2–20), and long axis (Fig. 2–21) views to evaluate:
  ❑ LV size, wall thickness, and global and regional systolic function
  ❑ RV size, wall thickness, and systolic function
  ❑ Anatomy and motion of the mitral and tricuspid valves
  ❑ Left and right atrial size and coronary sinus anatomy
  ❑ The presence and size of pericardial fluid, if present
■ Standard measurements include:
  ❑ Visual estimate of LV ejection fraction
  ❑ Quantitative apical biplane ejection fraction when clinically indicated (see Chapter 5)
  ❑ Measurement of LA area or volume when clinically indicated (Fig. 2–22)
  ❑ Visual estimate of RV size and systolic function

Key points:

  ❑ The three apical views are at approximately 60 degrees of rotation from each other; however, image planes are based on cardiac anatomy, not external reference points, so slight adjustment of transducer position and angulation often is needed to optimize the image.
  ❑ Initial views are recorded at the maximum depth to see all the cardiac chambers and surrounding pericardium.
  ❑ Evaluation of the left ventricle and right ventricle are based on images with the depth adjusted to just beyond the valve annular plane. The right ventricle is best visualized using zoom mode (Fig. 2–23).
  ❑ From the four-chamber view, the image plane is angled anteriorly to visualize the aortic valve (sometimes called the five-chamber view); this view is useful for Doppler recordings, but image quality is suboptimal at the depth of the aortic valve from the apical window (Fig. 2–24).
  ❑ The image plane is angled posteriorly to visualize the length of the coronary sinus and its entrance into the right atrium (Fig. 2–25).
  ❑ The left atrial appendage is not well visualized on transthoracic imaging, and the sensitivity for detection of left atrial thrombus is low. Transesophageal imaging is needed when atrial thrombus is suspected.
  ❑ The descending thoracic aorta is seen in cross section behind the left atrium in the long axis view and in a longitudinal plane from the two-chamber view with lateral angulation.

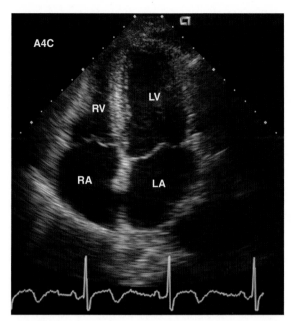

Figure 2–19 Apical four-chamber view with the transducer correctly positioned over the left ventricular apex. Foreshortening of this view results in a more spherical appearance of the left ventricle (*LV*). This older adult has enlargement of both atrium and some benign thickening (lipomatous hypertrophy) of the atrial septum. The loss of signal in the mid-segment of the atrial septum is an artifact because the thin fossa ovalis is parallel to the ultrasound beam at this point, resulting in echo "drop-out."

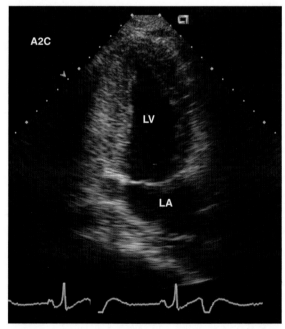

Figure 2–20 Apical two-chamber view obtained by rotating the transducer about 60 degrees counterclockwise from the four-chamber view.

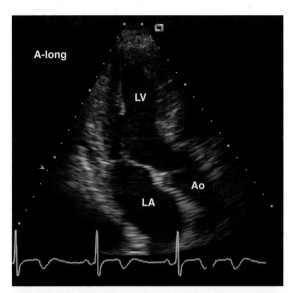

Figure 2–21 Apical long axis view is obtained by rotating an additional 60 degrees counterclockwise to obtain an image similar to the parasternal long axis view.

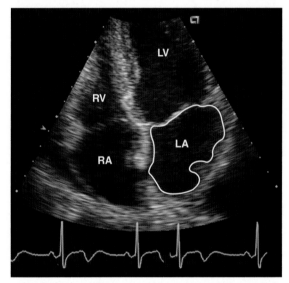

Figure 2–22 Left atrial volume is measured in the apical four-chamber view by tracing the inner edge of the atrial border at end-systole.

Step 7B: Doppler Data

■ The apical window provides an intercept angle that is relatively parallel to flow for the aortic, mitral, and tricuspid valves. Standard data recording includes:

❐ Pulsed Doppler recordings of transmitral flow, pulmonary vein inflow, and LV outflow (Figs. 2–26*A* and *B*)

❐ Color Doppler evaluation of aortic, mitral, and tricuspid regurgitation

❐ CW Doppler recordings of mitral, tricuspid, and aortic antegrade flow and regurgitation (Figs. 2–27*A* and *B*)

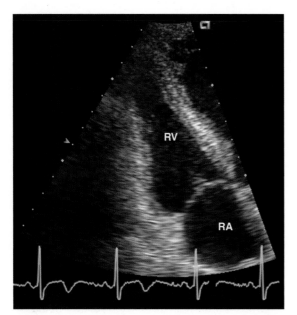

Figure 2–23 Right ventricular size and function are best estimated by centering the right ventricle (*RV*) in the image plane and adjusting depth and zoom appropriately.

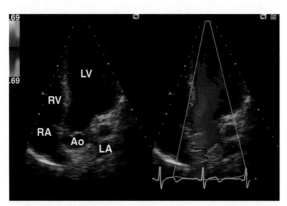

Figure 2–24 Anterior angulation from the four-chamber view allows visualization of the left ventricular (*LV*) outflow tract and an oblique view of the aortic valve. Laminar flow in the LV outflow tract is demonstrated with color Doppler. This view sometimes is colloquially called the "five-chamber view."

■ Standard measurements include:
  ❏ Pulsed Doppler antegrade mitral E and A velocities
  ❏ Pulsed Doppler LV outflow and CW Doppler aortic flow velocities
  ❏ Maximum velocity of the tricuspid regurgitant jet
  ❏ Additional measurements as clinically indicated (see specific chapters for each clinical condition)

Key points:
  ❏ Transmitral and pulmonary venous inflow velocities and tissue Doppler recordings are helpful for evaluation of LV diastolic dysfunction (see Chapter 7).

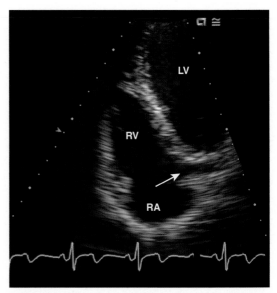

Figure 2–25 The entrance of the coronary sinus (*arrow*) into the right atrium (*RA*) is visualized by posterior angulation from the apical four-chamber view.

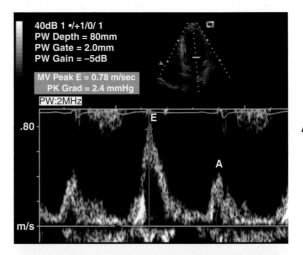

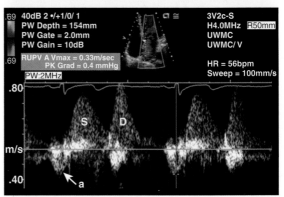

Figure 2–26 *A,* Left ventricular inflow is recorded using pulsed Doppler with the sample volume positioned at the mitral leaflet tips in diastole. The typical early (*E*) diastolic filling velocity and atrial (*A*) velocity are seen. *B,* Left atrial inflow is recorded with the pulsed Doppler sample volume in the right superior pulmonary vein in an apical four-chamber view. The normal pattern of systolic (*S*) and diastolic (*D*) inflow with a small atrial (*a*) flow reversal are seen.

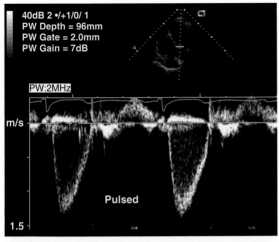
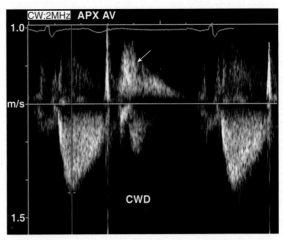

A

B

Figure 2–27 *A,* Left ventricular outflow is recorded with the Doppler sample volume on the left ventricular side of the aortic valve either in an anteriorly angulated four-chamber view or in an apical long axis view. The normal smooth "envelope" of flow with dense signals along the outer edge and few velocity signals within the curve are seen. Again, the baseline and scale are adjusted to prevent aliasing and allow accurate measurements. *B,* Aortic flow velocity is recorded from an apical approach using continuous wave (CW) Doppler. This velocity tracing includes signals from the entire length of the ultrasound beam so that the velocity curve is filled in by lower velocities proximal to the valve. The aortic closing click is seen. In diastole, the relatively broad CW beam intersects the left ventricular inflow curve (*arrow*).

☐ There is only a small increase in velocity between the LV outflow tract and ascending aorta in normal individuals (see Chapter 11).

☐ The CW Doppler recordings of aortic, mitral, and tricuspid regurgitation provide data on the severity of regurgitation (based on the density of the signal) and the transvalvular hemodynamics (based on the time velocity curve).

☐ Color flow Doppler from the apical approach is helpful for evaluation of jet direction and for visualization of proximal jet geometry (vena contracta and proximal isovelocity surface area [PISA]) for mitral regurgitation.

☐ Apical color Doppler of aortic regurgitation shows jet direction but is not helpful for quantitating severity because of the wide beam width at the depth of the aortic valve.

Step 8: Subcostal Window

■ The subcostal window provides:
☐ An alternate acoustic window for evaluation of LV and RV systolic function (Fig. 2–28)
☐ An optimal angle to evaluate the interatrial septum
☐ Estimation of RA pressure based on the size and respiratory variation in the inferior vena cava (Fig. 2–29)
☐ Pulsed Doppler evaluation of hepatic vein flow (right atrial inflow) and proximal abdominal aortic flow, when clinically indicated (Fig. 2–30)

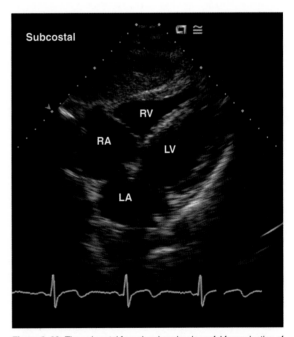

Figure 2–28 The subcostal four-chamber view is useful for evaluation of right and left ventricular function. This view also is best for evaluation of the atrial septum because the ultrasound beam is perpendicular to the septum from this transducer position.

Key points:

☐ Estimation of RA pressure is a standard part of the examination used to calculate pulmonary systolic pressure.

☐ Atrial septal defects often are best visualized on imaging and with color Doppler using a low Nyquist setting from the subcostal window.

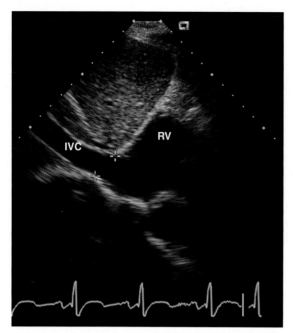

Figure 2–29 The inferior vena cava (*IVC*) is examined from the subcostal view, with the size and respiratory variation used to estimate right atrial pressure, as discussed in Chapter 6.

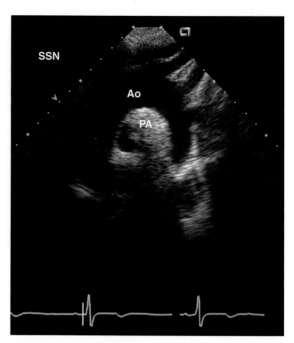

Figure 2–31 The suprasternal notch view showing the ascending aorta (*Ao*), arch, and descending thoracic aorta. A small segment of the right pulmonary artery (*PA*) is seen in cross section.

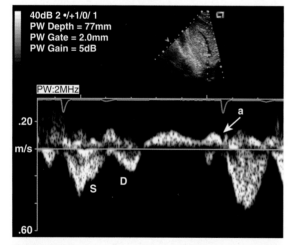

Figure 2–30 Hepatic vein flow can be recorded from the subcostal view to evaluate right atrial filling when tricuspid regurgitation or pericardial disease is of concern. *a,* Atrial reversal; *D,* diastolic fillings; *S,* systolic filling.

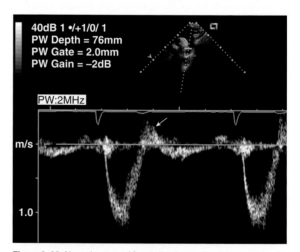

Figure 2–32 Normal pattern of flow in the descending thoracic aorta with antegrade flow in systole, brief early diastolic flow reversal (*arrow*) due to aortic recoil and coronary blood flow, a small amount of antegrade flow in mid-diastole, and slight reversal just before the next cardiac cycle.

❐ Hepatic vein flow patterns are helpful for detection of severe tricuspid regurgitation and for evaluation of pericardial disease.

❐ Descending aortic holodiastolic flow reversal is seen with severe aortic regurgitation.

Step 9: Suprasternal Notch Window

■ The suprasternal notch window is a standard part of the examination of patients with diseases of the aortic valve or aorta.

■ The suprasternal notch window provides:
  ❐ Images of the aortic arch and proximal descending thoracic aorta (Fig. 2–31)
  ❐ Pulsed and CW Doppler evaluation of descending aortic flow, when clinically indicated (Fig. 2–32)
  ❐ A parallel intercept angle with the aortic velocity in some patients with native or prosthetic aortic valve disease

Key points:

❐ Aortic disease, such as aortic dissection, may be visualized from this window.

❐ An increased systolic velocity with persistent antegrade flow in diastole is seen with an aortic coarctation.

❐ Holodiastolic flow reversal in the descending aorta suggests significant aortic valve regurgitation.

Step 10: The Echo Report

■ The Echo Report (Fig. 2–33) consists of four sections:

❐ Clinical data
❐ Measurements
❐ Echo findings
❐ Conclusions (with recommendations)

SAMPLE ECHO REPORT

Name _____ Date of Study _____
Age: 45 years   Sex: M
Indication: Systolic murmur on auscultation
Cardiac medications: None
Clinical history: Chest pain on exertion, systolic murmur, no prior cardiac procedures
Blood pressure: 118/68 mm Hg   Heart rate: 60 bpm   Rhythm: NSR
Sonographer: BGS   Image quality: Excellent

MEASUREMENTS

	Dimensions (cm)	Normal values (men)
LV Chamber		
End-systole	3.2	≤4.0
End-diastole	5.4	4.2 – 5.9
Wall thickness (diastole)	0.8	≤1.0
2D Ejection fraction	65% (estimate)	>55%
Left atrium	3.6	3.0 – 4.0
Aortic root	2.9	≤3.7

DOPPLER FLOWS

	Regurgitation	Velocity, (m/s)	
Aortic valve		Ao	1.0
		A	1.4
Mitral valve	Trace	A	0.4
Pulmonary valve	Trace		
Tricuspid valve	Mild	TR-Jet	2.3

		Normal Values
RA pressure estimate (mm Hg)	5	0-5
PA pressure estimate (mm Hg)	26	20-30

Findings:

Left ventricle: Wall thickness, internal dimension and systolic function are normal with an estimated ejection fraction of 65%. There are no resting regional wall motion abnormalities.

Left atrium: Size is normal.

Aortic valve: Trileaflet with normal systolic opening and no regurgitation.

Aortic root: Normal dimensions with normal contours of the sinuses of Valsalva.

Mitral valve: Normal anatomy and motion with no stenosis and only physiologic regurgitation.

PA pressures: Estimated pulmonary systolic pressure is normal at 21-26 mm Hg, based on the velocity in the TR jet and the size and respiratory variation of the inferior vena cava.

Right heart: Right ventricular size and systolic function are normal. Tricuspid and pulmonic valves show normal anatomy and Doppler flows. Right atrial size is normal.

Pericardium: No effusion.

Conclusions:

1. Normal valve anatomy and function.
2. Normal left ventricle with an estimated ejection fraction of 65%.
3. Normal pulmonary pressures and right heart.

Given these findings, the murmur appreciated on physical examination most likely is a benign flow murmur. Endocarditis prophylaxis is not indicated. Although resting left ventricular regional function is normal, coronary disease cannot be excluded on a resting study. If there is concern that chest pain may be due to coronary disease, a stress study should be considered.   Signed: _____ MD

Figure 2–33 Sample echo report

Key points:

❏ The clinical data section includes the reason for the study, pertinent history and physical examination findings, cardiac medications, and blood pressure.

❏ Standard measurements are indicated in Table 2–2; additional measurements are taken as clinically indicated.

❏ The findings section documents what views and flow were recorded and describes any abnormal and key normal findings.

❏ The conclusions indicate the major diagnosis, associated findings, and pertinent negative findings (depending on the indication for the study).

❏ When clinically appropriate, specific recommendations are made. These include:
  ❏ The need (or lack of need) for endocarditis prophylaxis
  ❏ Recommendations for cardiology evaluation and periodic follow-up

❏ Serious unexpected findings are communicated promptly directly to the referring physician.

❏ When data are not definitive, the findings are described along with a differential diagnosis to explain these findings.

❏ Additional diagnostic approaches are recommended as appropriate.

TABLE 2–2

REFERENCE VALUES FOR ECHOCARDIOGRAPHIC CHAMBER QUANTIFICATION

CHAMBER	MEASUREMENT	NORMAL RANGE (women)	NORMAL RANGE (men)	UNITS
Left ventricle				
	Diastolic diameter	3.9-5.3	4.2-5.9	cm
	(indexed to BSA)	2.4-3.2	2.2-3.1	cm/m^2
	(indexed to height)	2.5-3.2	2.4-3.3	cm/m
	Diastolic volume	56-104	67-155	mL
	(indexed to BSA)	35-75	35-75	mL/m^2
	Systolic volume	19-49	22-58	mL
	(indexed to BSA)	12-30	12-30	mL/m^2
	Ejection fraction	≥55%	≥55%	
	Septal wall thickness	0.6-0.9	0.6-1.0	cm
	Posterior wall thickness	0.6-0.9	0.6-1.0	cm
	LV mass (2D method)	66-150	96-200	g
	(indexed to BSA)	44-88	50-102	g/m^2
	Relative wall thickness	0.22-0.42	0.24-0.42	
Left atrium	AP diameter	2.7-3.8	3.0-4.0	cm
	(indexed to BSA)	1.5-2.3	1.5-2.3	cm/m^2
	LA area	≤20	≤20	cm^2
	LA volume	22-52	18-58	mL
	(indexed to BSA)	22 ± 6	22 ± 6	mL/m^2
Right ventricle	Mid RV diastolic diameter	2.7-3.3	2.7-3.3	cm
	RV diastolic area (A4C)	11-28	11-28	cm^2
	RV systolic area (A4C)	7.5-16	7.5-16	cm^2
	Fractional area change	32-60%	32-60%	
	Tricuspid annular excursion	>1.5	>1.5	cm
Right atrium	RA dimension (A4C)	2.9-4.5	2.9-4.5	cm
	(indexed to BSA)	1.7-2.5	1.7-2.5	cm/m^2

2D, *Two-dimensional;* A4C, *apical four-chamber view;* AP, *anterior-posterior diameter in long axis view;* BSA, *body surface area;* LV, *left ventricular;* RA, *right atrial;* RV, *right ventricular.*

Abstracted from Lang RM, Bierig M, Devereux RB, et al. J Am Soc Echo *18:1440-1463, 2005.*

NOTES

SELF-ASSESSMENT QUESTIONS

QUESTION 1

Identify the structures numbered in Figure 2–34.

1.
2.
3.
4.
5.
6.

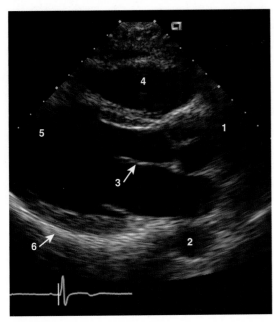

Figure 2–34

QUESTION 2

List four things that would improve the Doppler display shown in Figure 2–35.

1.
2.
3.
4.

Figure 2–35

QUESTION 3

Measure as many of the following dimensions from the 2D images and M-mode tracings shown in Figures 2–36A and B as possible:

LV end-systolic and end-diastolic
    dimension: _____
LV wall thickness: _____
Aortic root diameter: _____
Left atrial anterior-posterior
    dimension: _____

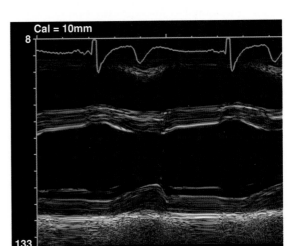

A

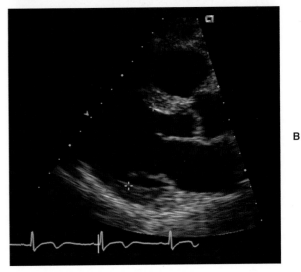

B

Figure 2–36

QUESTION 4

In a 23-year-old asymptomatic man referred for echocardiography for evaluation of a murmur, mitral valve anatomy is normal but mitral regurgitation is detected with a vena contracta width of 2 mm and a faint holosystolic signal on CW Doppler.

The most appropriate comment regarding this finding in the echo report is:

A. Normal finding.
B. Endocarditis prophylaxis is indicated.
C. Additional evaluation with quantitation of regurgitant orifice area is needed.
D. Recommend repeat echocardiogram in 1 year.
E. Transesophageal echocardiography should be considered.

QUESTION 5

The CW Doppler velocity curve shown in Figure 2–37 is consistent with:

A. Mild aortic regurgitation
B. Severe aortic regurgitation
C. Normal pulmonary pressures
D. Severe pulmonary hypertension
E. Mild mitral stenosis
F. Severe mitral stenosis

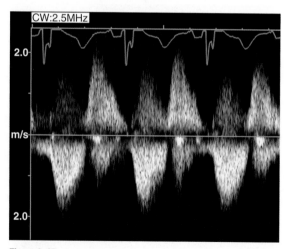

Figure 2–37

QUESTION 6

What is the structure indicated by the arrow in Figure 2–38?

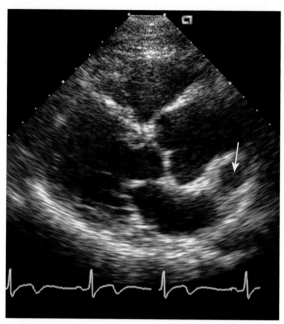

Figure 2–38

ANSWERS

ANSWER 1

This parasternal long axis view shows the aortic root (1) which consists of the sinuses of Valsalva, sinotubular junction and proximal ascending aorta, and the descending thoracic aorta (2) seen in cross section posterior to the left atrium. The mitral leaflet is open in mid-diastole with the anterior mitral leaflet (3) and posterior leaflet easily seen. The right ventricular outflow tract (4) is anterior to the left ventricle and appears normal size in this image. The left ventricular chamber (5) is seen in long axis, a view that is useful for measurement of septal and posterior wall thickness and LV internal dimension at end-diastole (as in this image) and at end-systole. The pericardium (6) is the brightest echo in the image, lying immediately posterior to the LV epicardium.

ANSWER 2

This is a CW Doppler recording of tricuspid regurgitant velocity. For recording Doppler velocity data, the velocity range should be adjusted so the velocity signal fits within, but nearly fills, the velocity range. If needed, the baseline is shifted to ensure the maximum velocity is clearly seen without signal aliasing. For a high velocity, relatively weak strength signal, like this tricuspid regurgitation jet velocity, the signal-to-noise ratio will be improved by increasing the "wall" or high pass filters to eliminate the low velocity but high intensity signals caused by motion of the valve leaflets and myocardium. Then the gain should be increased until background noise is evident and then decreased to just below that point. The gray scale shown is optimal for Doppler velocity measurements as most of the validation of this approach was done with gray scale spectral displays. Use of color displays may result in a denser appearance of low intensity noise signals, resulting in overestimation of blood flow velocity.

ANSWER 3:

LV end-systolic and end-diastolic dimension: 3.4/4.8 cm

LV wall thickness: septum, 0.9 cm; posterior wall, 0.8 cm

Aortic root diameter: 2.9 cm (at sinuses of Valsalva)

Left atrial anterior-posterior dimension: 3.4 cm

M-mode measurements of wall thickness for the interventricular septum (IVS) and posterior

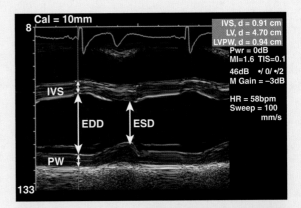

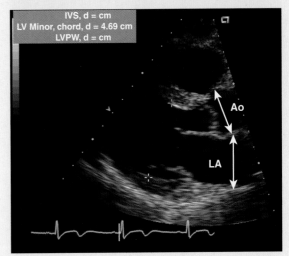

Figure 2–39

wall (PW) and the end diastolic dimension (EDD) are measured at the onset of the QRS complex from leading edge to leading edge as shown. The posterior wall endocardium is the steepest continuous line and often has a brighter chordal structure or trabeculation overlying the endocardium, as in this case. The end systolic dimension (ESD) is measure at the maximum posterior motion of the septum. M-mode also can be used to measure aortic root diameter at end diastole and left atrial dimension at end-systole. These measurements also can be made from 2D images, which allow measurement of the aorta at multiple sites and ensures a perpendicular left atrial measurement.

ANSWER 4: A

This patient has a normal mitral valve with a physiologic (mild) amount of valve regurgitation as evidenced by a narrow vena contracta and weak CW Doppler signal (see Chapter 12). With a diligent search, small amounts of mitral, tricuspid, and pulmonic regurgitation are seen in 70% to 80% of normal adults. When valve anatomy is normal, this degree of regurgitation is not associated with adverse clinical outcomes, does not mandate endocarditis prophylaxis, and should be considered a normal finding. Further evaluation with quantitation of regurgitation, sequential studies, or transesophageal echocardiography (TEE) would be considered only if valve anatomy or motion were abnormal or if image quality was too poor to determine whether regurgitation was more than mild. Aortic regurgitation, even mild, is uncommonly (about 5%) seen in normal individuals, so the presence of aortic regurgitation should prompt careful evaluation of aortic valve and root anatomy.

ANSWER 5: C

This Doppler signal was recorded with CW Doppler because the area within the Doppler curve is "filled in" by the multiple velocities encountered along the length of the ultrasound beam. In systole, there is an ejection-type flow signal (i.e., the flow starts after the QRS and ends before the end of the T wave, with a peak in mid-systole) with a peak velocity of about 1 m/s, suggesting this is antegrade flow across a semilunar (aortic or pulmonic) valve. The diastolic velocity rises quickly in early diastole with a steep deceleration slope consistent with severe semilunar valve regurgitation. The signal of mitral stenosis would be lower in velocity, it would show an A velocity (the ECG shows sinus rhythm), and the flow in systole caused by mitral regurgitation would be

longer in duration. If this was aortic regurgitation, the diastolic velocity of regurgitation would be higher, reflecting the higher pressure difference between the aorta and left ventricle in diastole. Thus this is a recording of flow across the pulmonic valve in a patient with severe pulmonic regurgitation. The low velocity of the pulmonary regurgitant signal at end-diastole indicates there is only a slight pressure difference between the right ventricle and pulmonary artery in diastole. Thus pulmonary pressure is normal. If severe pulmonary hypertension were present, the velocity of the pulmonic regurgitation would be higher.

ANSWER 6: Right pulmonary artery

This parasternal long axis image shows the right pulmonary artery in cross section posterior to the ascending aorta and superior to the left atrium. The right pulmonary artery is often not seen in this view, because acoustic access from the transthoracic parasternal window does not always extend this far superiorly. In the same long axis view on transesophageal echocardiography, the right pulmonary artery is typically seen. The right pulmonary artery also is seen on transthoracic imaging from the suprasternal notch window inferior to the aortic arch. Visualization of the left pulmonary artery is more difficult but can be achieved from the suprasternal approach by rotating to a short axis view of the arch and then rotating the image plane slightly laterally. From the transthoracic parasternal short axis view, the proximal segments of both right and left pulmonary arteries may be seen at the bifurcation of the main pulmonary artery.

NOTES

3 Transesophageal Echocardiography

THE ECHO EXAM: BASIC TRANSESOPHAGEAL EXAM

PROBE POSITION	VIEW		FOCUS ON
High esophageal Set depth to include LV apex	0°	Four-chamber	LV size and function (septum and lateral walls)
			RV size and systolic function
			LA and RA size, pulmonary veins
			Withdraw probe to see LA appendage
			Mitral and tricuspid valves
			Angulate anteriorly to see aortic valve
	~60°	Two-chamber	LV size and function (inferior and anterior walls)
			LA and LA appendage
			Mitral valve
	~120°	Long axis	LV size and function (anterior septum and posterior walls)
			LA size
			Mitral and aortic valves
			Withdraw probe to see ascending aorta
High esophageal Decrease depth to optimize valves	~120°	Long axis	Mitral valve anatomy and function
			Color Doppler for mitral regurgitation
			Antegrade mitral flow with pulsed Doppler
			Aortic valve anatomy and color flow
	~60°	Two-chamber	Mitral valve anatomy and function
			Color Doppler for mitral regurgitation
			LA appendage imaging and Doppler flow
	0°	Four-chamber	Mitral valve anatomy and function
			Color Doppler for mitral regurgitation
			Aortic valve (angulate anteriorly to "five-chamber" view) for anatomy and color flow
			Atrial septum
Transgastric	0°	Short axis	LV wall motion, wall thickness, chamber dimensions
			RV size and function
	90°	Long axis	LV and mitral valve
			Turn medially to image RV and tricuspid valve
Transgastric apical	0°	Four-chamber	Useful for antegrade aortic flow but may still be nonparallel intercept angle
Transgastric to high esophageal	0°	Short axis descending aorta	Image aorta from the diaphragm to aortic arch

LA, *Left atrium;* LV, *left ventricle;* RA, *right atrium;* RV, *right ventricle.*

STEP-BY-STEP APPROACH

Step 1: Clinical Data

■ In addition to the indication for the study and the cardiac history, clinical data establishing the safety of the transesophageal echocardiography (TEE) procedure are needed.

■ The risk of the TEE procedure is related both to conscious sedation and esophageal intubation.

■ Informed consent is obtained before the procedure.

Key points:

❏ Informed consent includes a description of the procedure with explanation of the expected benefits and potential risks.

❏ Complications serious enough to interrupt the procedure occur in less than 1% of cases, and the reported mortality rate is less than 1 in 10,000.

❏ Significant esophageal disease, excessive bleeding risk, and tenuous respiratory status are contraindications to TEE.

❏ The risk of hemodynamic compromise and respiratory depression are assessed using standard preanesthesia protocols and risk levels.

❏ Risk is higher in patients with impaired respiratory status or a history of sleep apnea.

❏ Patients typically have no oral intake for at least 6 hours before the procedure, except in emergencies.

❏ In anticoagulated patients, the level of anticoagulation is checked before the TEE to ensure it is in the therapeutic range.

Step 2: Transesophageal Echocardiography Protocol

■ The conscious sedation standards at each institution apply to TEE procedures.

■ Typically this includes having a skilled health care provider monitor level of consciousness, blood pressure, electrocardiogram (ECG), and arterial oxygen saturation.

■ Oral suction is used to clear secretions and maintain an open airway.

■ The study is optimally performed with a physician to manipulate the probe and direct the examination, a cardiac sonographer to optimize image quality and record data, and a nurse to monitor the patient.

Key points:

❏ Endocarditis prophylaxis is not routinely recommended for TEE.

❏ Adequate local anesthesia of the pharynx improves patient comfort and tolerance.

❏ The specific choice and dose of pharmacologic agents for sedation are based on institutional protocols.

❏ The TEE probe is inserted via a bite block using ultrasound gel for lubrication and to provide acoustic coupling between the ultrasound transducer on the probe and the wall of the esophagus.

❏ The TEE is advanced and angulated, with rotation of the image plane, to obtain diagnostic images in standard tomographic views.

❏ All the health care providers involved in the procedure use universal precautions to prevent exposure to body fluids.

Step 3: Basic Examination Principles

■ Although the TEE study is directed toward answering the clinical question, a systemic complete examination is recorded unless precluded by the clinical situation.

■ Standard tomographic planes are used to evaluate cardiac chambers and valves.

Key points:

❏ In unstable patients, the examination should focus on the key diagnostic issues first, with additional recordings as tolerance and time allow.

❏ Each cardiac structure is evaluated in at least two orthogonal views or, ideally, using a rotational scan of the structure.

❏ Transducer frequency, depth, and zoom are adjusted to optimize visualization of each structure.

❏ With color Doppler, frame rate is optimized by decreasing depth and sector width to focus on the flow of interest.

❏ Only one to two beats of each view are recorded so that the examiner can move quickly through the examination sequence. The total intubation time for a complete TEE ranges from less than 10 minutes for a relatively normal study to up to 30 minutes for complex examinations.

Step 4: Imaging Sequence

■ The basic imaging sequence suggested in the Echo Exam table at the beginning of the chapter is organized by probe position, as this is the most efficient approach to examination in most cases.

■ The imaging sequence is adjusted to focus on the key issues in unstable patients.

■ This step-by-step approach describes the evaluation of each anatomic structure. This evaluation often is incorporated into the standard exam sequence shown in the Echo Exam table at the beginning of the chapter.

Key points:

- ❏ The probe position is constrained by the position of the esophagus, so optimal views are not always possible. The terms "advance" and "withdraw" refer to the vertical motion of the probe in the esophagus and stomach. The term "turn" refers to manual rotation of the entire probe toward the patient's right or left side (Fig. 3–1).
- ❏ The terms "bending" and "extension" refer to motion of the tip of the probe in a plane parallel to the long axis of the probe, controlled by a large dial at the base of the probe (Fig. 3–2).

- ❏ The term "rotation" refers to the electronic movement of the image plane in a circular fashion, controlled by a button on the probe and displayed as an angle on the image (Fig. 3–3).
- ❏ The exact degree of rotation needed for a specific view varies from patient to patient depending on the relationship between the heart and esophagus. The values given here are a starting point; image planes are adjusted based on cardiac anatomy, not specific rotation angle.
- ❏ If a specific view or flow is difficult to obtain, continue with the examination and return to this view later in the study.
- ❏ The specific views and flows recorded depend on the clinical indication and the findings of the study.
- ❏ Although modification of the exam sequence often is necessary, the examiner should quickly review a checklist of the recorded data before removing the probe to ensure a complete exam.

Step 5: Left Ventricle

- ▪ The left ventricle (LV) is evaluated in the high esophageal four-chamber, two-chamber, and long axis views.
- ▪ Additional views of the LV include the transgastric short axis view and the transgastric apical view.

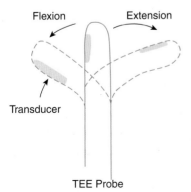

Figure 3–1 The transesophageal multiplane transducer is at the tip of a steerable probe. The probe motion is controlled by the dials, with the rotational angle of the image plane adjusted with a button.

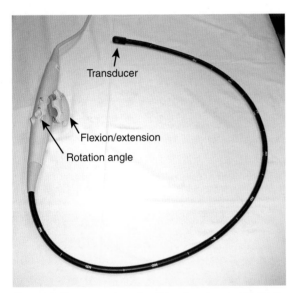

Figure 3–2 The tip of the probe can be extended or flexed to obtain standard image planes.

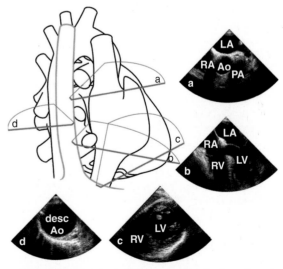

Figure 3–3 Diagram showing the transesophageal echocardiography transducer locations for the four standard imaging views: basal (*a*), four-chamber (*b*), transgastric (*c*), and aortic (*d*). Ao, Aorta; *desc Ao*, descending aorta; *LA*, left atrium; *LV*, left ventricle; *PA*, pulmonary artery; *RA*, right atrium; *RV*, right ventricle. From Burwash IG and Chan KL: Transesophageal echocardiography. In Otto CM (ed): *The Practice of Clinical Echocardiography*, 3rd ed., Philadelphia, Elsevier, 2007, p. 7.

Key points:

❏ The starting point for a TEE is a four-chamber view recorded from a high esophageal position (0-degree rotation) at maximum depth to show the entire LV. Typically the probe is extended to include as much of the apex as possible (Fig. 3–4).

❏ With the probe centered behind the left atrium and with the left ventricular apex in the center of the image, the image plane is rotated to about 60 degrees to obtain a two-chamber view and then rotated further to about 120 degrees for a long axis view (Figs. 3–5 and 3–6).

❏ The transducer position, angulation, and the exact degree of rotation are adjusted to optimize each view.

❏ Regional ventricular function is evaluated as follows:

  1. Lateral and inferior septal walls in the four-chamber view
  2. Anterior and inferior walls in the two-chamber view
  3. Anterior septum and the inferior-lateral wall in the long axis view

❏ Ejection fraction is estimated from these three views. If a quantitative ejection fraction is needed, the biplane approach is used tracing endocardial borders at end-diastole and end-systole in the four-chamber and two-chamber views.

❏ The left ventricular apex often is foreshortened on TEE, even with careful positioning, resulting in underestimation of LV volumes.

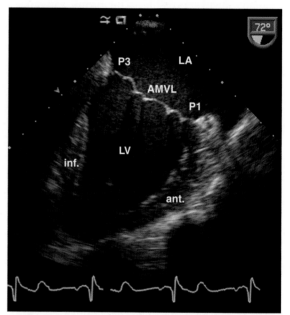

Figure 3–5 With the left ventricular apex centered in the image plane at 0 degrees, the angle is adjusted to about 60 degrees to obtain a two-chamber view, with the anterior and inferior left ventricular walls. The lateral (*P1*) and medial (*P3*) scallops of the posterior mitral leaflet and the central segment of the anterior leaflet (*AMVL*) are typically seen in this view.

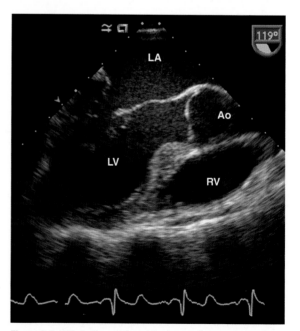

Figure 3–6 With further rotation of the image plane to about 120 degrees, a long axis view is obtained with the aortic valve and ascending aorta (*Ao*) and the inferior-lateral (posterior) and anterior septal walls of the left ventricle.

Figure 3–4 In the 0-degree position with the transducer located posterior to the left atrium, the probe tip is flexed or extended to obtain a four-chamber view. The apparent apex in this view often is part of the anterior wall, as it may not be possible to adjust the image plane to intersect the true apex.

❐ An apical left ventricular thrombus may be missed, as the apex is in the far field of the TEE image; transthoracic imaging is more sensitive for detection of apical thrombus.

Step 6: Left Atrium and Atrial Septum

■ The body of the left atrium (LA) is evaluated in the high esophageal four-chamber, two-chamber, and long axis views.

■ The LA appendage is imaged in at least two orthogonal planes at 0 and 90 degrees.

■ The pulmonary veins are identified using two-dimensional (2D) and color Doppler imaging most easily in the 0-degree image plane, although views at 90 degrees also may be helpful.

Key points:

❐ Images of the LA are recorded at a shallow depth to focus on the structure of interest.

❐ The atrial septum is best examined by centering the septum in the image plane in the four-chamber view and then slowly rotating the image plane, keeping the septum centered, from 0 to 120 degrees (Fig. 3–7).

❐ The atrial appendage is imaged using a high frequency transducer, zoom mode, and a narrow sector to improve image resolution (Fig. 3–8).

❐ Flow in the atrial appendage is recorded with a pulsed Doppler sample volume about 1 cm from the mouth of the appendage (Figs. 3–9 and 3–10).

❐ The left superior pulmonary vein is usually easily visualized and is located adjacent to the atrial appendage and enters the atrium with flow parallel to the ultrasound beam. The left inferior pulmonary vein, seen by advancing

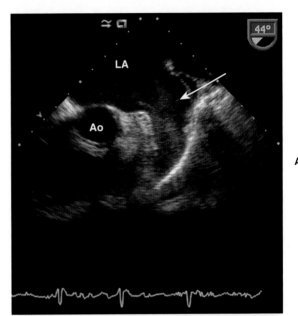

A

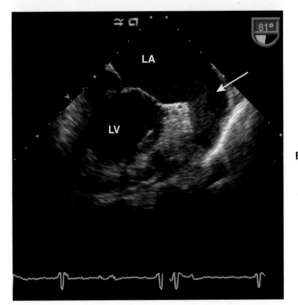

B

Figure 3–8 Two views of the left atrial appendage at 40 (*A*) and 80 (*B*) degrees rotation. The typical crescent shape of the appendage is seen, as is the normal ridge (*arrow*) between the left atrial appendage and left superior pulmonary view. In this patient with a dilated cardiomyopathy and atrial fibrillation, spontaneous contrast (*arrows*) is seen in the appendage, consistent with a low flow state.

Figure 3–7 The atrial septum is examined by centering the septum in the image plane at 0 degrees rotation and then slowly rotating the image plane to 120 degrees. The thin fossa ovalis (between *arrows*) is easily seen on this image.

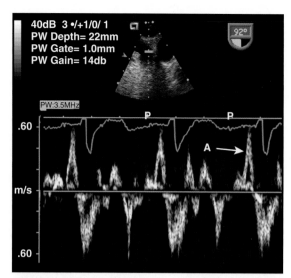

Figure 3–9 Doppler flow patterns in the atrial appendage are recorded with the sample volume in the appendage about 1 cm from the entrance into the left atrium. In this patient in sinus rhythm, the normal antegrade flow with atrial (*A*) contraction has a velocity greater than 0.4 m/s after the ECG P-wave is seen (*arrow*).

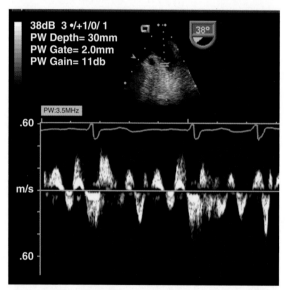

Figure 3–10 Atrial appendage flow in this patient in atrial fibrillation shows a rapid, irregular low velocity flow pattern.

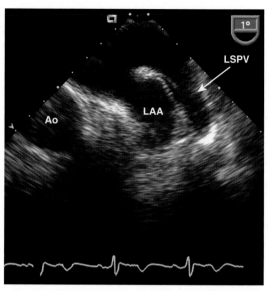

Figure 3–11 From the standard four-chamber view at 0 degrees, the left atrial appendage (*LAA*) and left superior pulmonary vein (*LSPV*) are visualized by moving the transducer up in the esophagus and flexing the probe tip. There often is a normal prominent ridge, seen as a rounded mass in this view, between the atrial appendage and pulmonary vein.

the probe a few centimeters, enters the atrium at a perpendicular angle, relative to the ultrasound beam (Fig. 3–11).

❑ Pulmonary vein flow is recorded with pulsed Doppler in one or more pulmonary veins, depending on the clinical indication for the study.

❑ The right pulmonary veins are imaged in the 0-degree plane by turning the probe toward the patient's right side. Again the superior vein enters the atrium at a parallel angle; the inferior vein is seen by advancing the probe and enters at a perpendicular angle (Fig. 3–12).

❑ Color flow Doppler enhances identification of the pulmonary veins. An orthogonal view

at 90 to 120 degrees also may be helpful, turning the probe rightward for the right pulmonary veins (Fig. 3–13) and leftward for the left pulmonary veins (Fig. 3–14).

Step 7: Mitral Valve

■ The mitral valve is evaluated starting in the four-chamber view; the image plane is then slowly rotated to 120 degrees (long axis view), keeping the valve centered in the image.

■ Additional views of the mitral valve include the transgastric short axis and two-chamber views.

Key points:

■ The image depth is adjusted to just fit the mitral valve on the image. Transducer frequency, harmonic imaging, and gain are adjusted to improve the image (Fig. 3–15).

■ The mitral valve is first evaluated with 2D imaging alone to focus on the details of valve anatomy.

❑ A second rotational scan is performed using color Doppler to evaluate for mitral regurgitation. Regurgitation is evaluated based on measurement of the vena contracta, evaluation of pulmonary venous flow pattern, the continuous wave (CW) Doppler signal, and quantitative parameters as discussed in Chapter 12 (Fig. 3–16).

❑ The transgastric view of the mitral valve offers improved visualization of the subvalvular apparatus, although concurrent evaluation by transthoracic imaging also may be needed (Fig. 3–17).

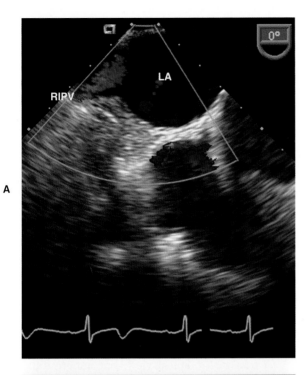

A

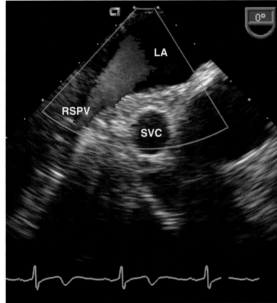

B

Figure 3–12 The right pulmonary veins are identified in the 0-degree image plane by turning the transducer toward the patient's right side. The right inferior pulmonary view (*RIPV, A*) is seen with color Doppler entering the left atrium at a relatively perpendicular angle to the ultrasound beam. The probe is withdrawn 1 to 2 cm to visualize the right superior pulmonary vein (*RSPV, B*), which enters the atrium relatively parallel to the ultrasound beam direction. *SVC,* Superior vena cava.

Step 8: Aortic Valve and Ascending Aorta

- The aortic valve and proximal ascending aorta are evaluated in standard long and short axis views.
- Aortic regurgitation is evaluated by color Doppler in high esophageal views.

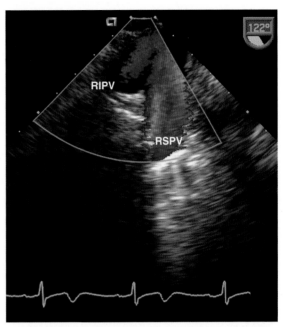

Figure 3–13 The right pulmonary veins also can be imaged in the orthogonal plane by rotating the image plane to a longitudinal view, with the right superior pulmonary vein (*RSPV*) on the right and the right inferior pulmonary vein (*RIPV*) on the left.

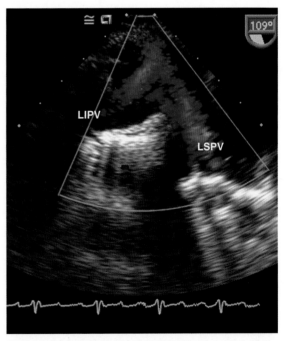

Figure 3–14 Longitudinal view of the left pulmonary veins with the transducer turned toward the patient's left side. In this image, superior structures are to the right of the image and inferior structures to the left. As for the right pulmonary veins, the left inferior pulmonary vein (*LIPV*) enters the atrium at a perpendicular angle to the ultrasound beam, whereas the left superior pulmonary vein (*LSPV*) enters with the flow direction parallel to the ultrasound beam.

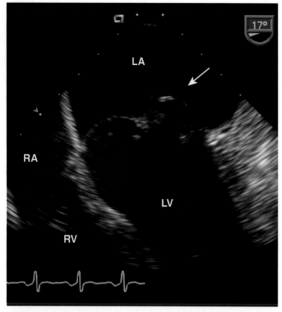

Figure 3–15 The mitral valve is imaged starting at 0 degrees rotation with the valve centered in the image plane and the depth adjusted to focus on the valve. The image plane is then slowly rotated, keeping the mitral valve centered, to examine the entire valve apparatus. In this patient, prolapse of the central (P2) segment of the posterior leaflet is best seen at 17 degrees rotation.

Key points:

❏ The aortic valve is best seen in the long axis view (at about 120 degrees) and in a short axis view of the valve (at about 30 to 50 degrees rotation), using a shallow depth, high frequency transducer, zoom mode, and a narrow 2D sector (Figs. 3–18 and 3–19).

❏ From the standard long axis view, the TEE probe is turned rightward and leftward to see the medial and lateral aspects of the valve. The probe also is withdrawn higher in the esophagus to see as much of the ascending aorta as possible.

❏ From the short axis view, the probe is slowly advanced and withdrawn to visualize the areas immediately inferior and superior to the valve plane.

❏ Aortic regurgitation can be evaluated by color Doppler, with measurement of vena contracta, although precise quantitation of regurgitant severity is difficult on TEE (Fig. 3–20).

❏ CW Doppler of aortic antegrade and retrograde flow sometimes can be recorded from a transgastric apical view, but underestimation of velocity is likely due to a nonparallel intercept angle between the ultrasound beam and flow signal (Fig. 3–21).

❏ Transthoracic imaging often provides more precise quantitation of valve stenosis and regurgitation.

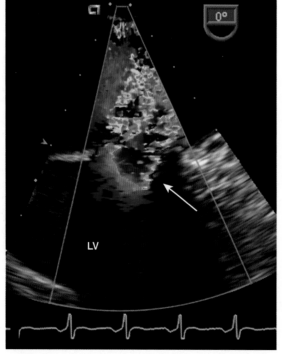

A

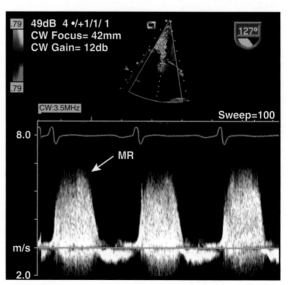

B

Figure 3–16 *A,* Color Doppler is used to identify the presence of mitral regurgitation and to evaluate severity based on vena contracta width (*arrow*) and by the proximal isovelocity surface area (PISA) approach (see Chapter 12). *B,* The continuous wave Doppler velocity curve also is useful for confirming the identity and evaluating severity of regurgitation.

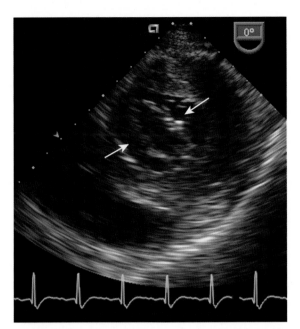

Figure 3–17 From the transgastric short axis view of the left ventricle, the transducer is withdrawn about 1 cm to obtain a short axis view of the mitral valve with the anterior leaflet (AL) and posterior leaflet (PL) seen.

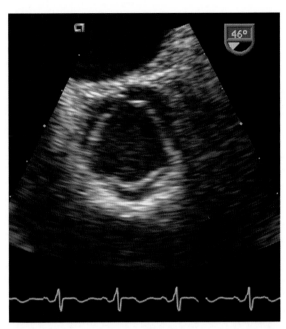

Figure 3–19 The short axis view of the aortic valve is obtained by centering the valve in the image in the long axis image and then rotating the image plane to about 45 degrees. This zoomed image shows the three valve leaflets open in systole.

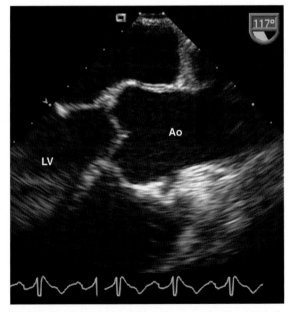

Figure 3–18 A long axis view of the aortic valve and aortic root typically is obtained at about 120 degrees rotation. The exact rotation angle needed varies among patients; the image plane is adjusted to the standard image plane based on anatomy, not a specific rotation angle.

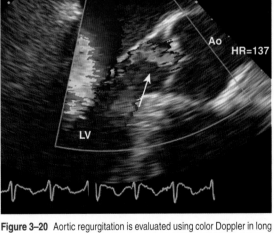

Figure 3–20 Aortic regurgitation is evaluated using color Doppler in long and short axis images. Regurgitant severity is evaluated by measurement of vena contracta width in the long axis view. This example shows a narrow jet (*arrow*), consistent with mild regurgitation.

Step 9: Coronary Arteries

■ The left main coronary artery is easily seen in the short axis view of the aortic valve (Fig. 3–22).

■ The right coronary artery may be seen in a long axis view of the ascending aorta or in the short axis view of the aortic valve but more difficult to visualize.

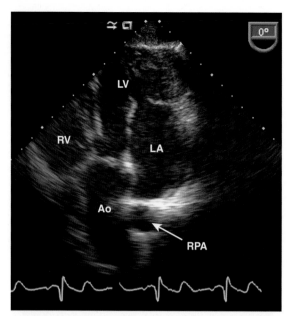

Figure 3–21 From a deep transgastric position, an anteriorly angulated four-chamber view is obtained by flexion of the probe tip. This image plane does not pass through the true left ventricular apex with obvious foreshortening of the left ventricle (*LV*) in this image. The ascending aorta (*Ao*) and right pulmonary artery (*RPA*) are seen.

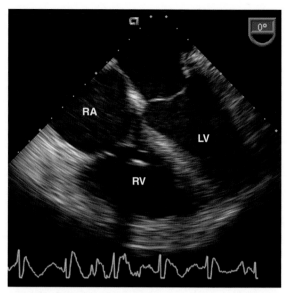

Figure 3–23 The right ventricle (*RV*) is seen in the four-chamber view, but it often is helpful to turn the transducer toward the right ventricle to focus on right ventricular size and systolic function. This patient has moderate RV dilation and systolic dysfunction. Rotation of the image plane allows evaluation of the right ventricular outflow tract in the short axis view at the aortic valve level.

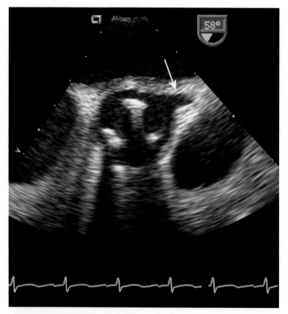

Figure 3–22 The left coronary artery is seen by moving the image plane slightly superior to the aortic valve short axis image plane. In this patient, the three stents of a tissue aortic valve prosthesis are seen at the same level as the left main coronary artery ostium (*arrow*).

Key points:

❑ The left main coronary artery is slightly superior to the aortic valve plane.

❑ Visualization of the coronary ostium is enhanced by using a high frequency transducer and zoom mode.

❑ The bifurcation of the left main into the left anterior descending and circumflex coronary arteries is frequently visualized, but the more distal vessel is not seen in most patients.

❑ Identification of the coronary ostium is most important in adolescents and young adults with exertional symptoms and in patients with prior aortic root surgery with coronary reimplantation.

Step 10: Right Ventricle and Tricuspid Valve

■ The right ventricle (RV) and tricuspid valve are evaluated in the high esophageal four-chamber and right ventricular inflow views (Fig. 3–23).

■ Additional views of the RV and tricuspid valve include the transgastric short axis view and right ventricular inflow views.

Key points:

❑ In the initial TEE four-chamber images, right ventricular size and systolic function are evaluated.

❑ The RV also is seen in the short axis view by starting at the aortic valve level and slowly advancing the transducer to see the tricuspid valve and RV.

❑ From the transgastric short axis view, the image plane is rotated to 90 degrees and the probe is turned rightward to obtain a view of the right atrium, tricuspid valve, and RV,

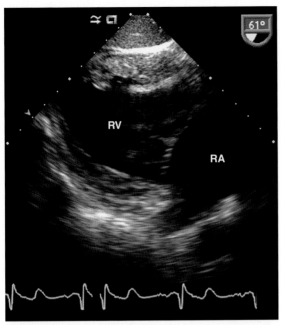

Figure 3–24 From the transgastric short axis view, the image plane is rotated to between 60 and 90 degrees. From the two-chamber view of the left ventricle, the probe is turned toward the patient's right side to obtain this view of the right atrium (*RA*), tricuspid valve, and right ventricle (*RV*).

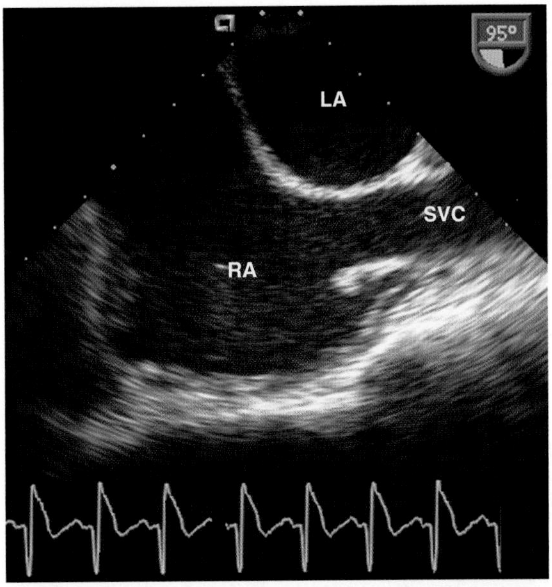

Figure 3–25 A long axis view of the right atrium (*RA*) is obtained with the image plane rotated to 90 degrees and the transducer turned toward the patient's right side. The superior vena cava (*SVC*) enters the atrium near the trabeculated atrial appendage. When the transducer is advanced in the esophagus, the entrance of the inferior vena cava into the atrium also may be seen in this view.

similar to a transthoracic right ventricular inflow view (Fig. 3–24).

- ❒ Tricuspid valve anatomy and motion and color Doppler tricuspid regurgitation are evaluated in each of these views.
- ❒ A CW Doppler recording of tricuspid regurgitant jet velocity may be obtained from the esophageal four-chamber or short axis view, although underestimation of velocity due to a poor intercept angle is possible.

Step 11: Right Atrium

- ■ The right atrium (RA) is evaluated in the high esophageal four-chamber view and in the 90 degree view of the right atrium (Fig. 3–25).
- ■ Additional views of the RA include a low atrial view, at the level of the coronary sinus, and the transgastric two-chamber view of the right heart.

Key points:

- ❒ The RA is visualized by rotating the image plane to 90 degrees and turning the probe rightward to obtain a longitudinal view of the RA, including the entrances of the superior and inferior vena cava.
- ❒ The trabeculated right atrial appendage may be seen adjacent to the entry of the superior vena cava into the atrium

- ❒ The inferior vena cava (IVC) can be evaluated by advancing the probe slowly toward the gastroesophageal junction.
- ❒ The central hepatic vein enters the IVC at a perpendicular angle, allowing Doppler recording of hepatic vein flow, when indicated.
- ❒ From the standard four-chamber plane at 0 degrees, the probe is advanced to obtain a low atrial view at the junction of the coronary sinus with the RA. The size and flow characteristics of the coronary sinus can be evaluated in this view, when needed.

Step 12: Pulmonary Valve and Pulmonary Artery

- ■ The pulmonary valve and pulmonary artery are visualized in a very high esophageal view in the 0 degree image plane or in a 90 degree image plane with the transducer turned toward the left (right ventricular outflow view; Fig. 3–26).
- ■ Images of the pulmonic valve may be suboptimal because the valve is in the far field of the image and as it may be obscured by the air-filled bronchus at this level of the esophagus.

Key points:

- ❒ The pulmonic valve also may be visualized in the transgastric short axis view.

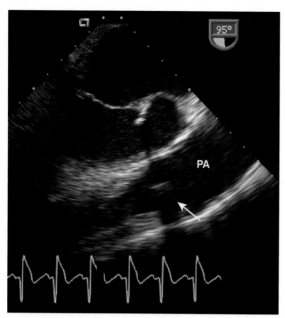

Figure 3–26 With the transducer in the high esophageal position, the pulmonary artery (*PA*) is seen with the image plane rotated to 90 degrees and the transducer turned slightly toward the patient's left side. The anteriorly located pulmonic valve (*arrow*) is relatively distant from the transducer, so image quality often is suboptimal.

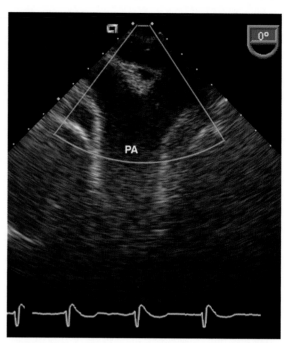

Figure 3–27 The main pulmonary artery (*PA*) and pulmonary artery bifurcation seen in a very high transesophageal view. This probe position may not be well tolerated in some patients, and this image cannot be obtained in all patients.

❐ Doppler flow in the pulmonary artery can be recorded from the high esophageal position.
❐ Evaluation of pulmonic regurgitation with color Doppler is performed in the right ventricular outflow view. However, transthoracic imaging of the pulmonic valve often provides more accurate data.
❐ The pulmonary artery bifurcation and proximal right and left pulmonary arteries may be seen in a high esophageal view, but visualization of more distal pulmonary arteries is rarely possible (Fig. 3–27).
❐ Cardiac magnetic resonance (MR) imaging provides an alternate approach for evaluation of the pulmonic valve and pulmonary artery.

Step 13: Descending Aorta and Aortic Arch

■ The descending aorta is evaluated in a short axis view, starting at the transgastric level, by turning the probe leftward to identify the vessel and then slowly withdrawing the probe to visualize each segment of the descending thoracic aorta (Fig. 3–28).
■ Once the probe reaches the level of the aortic arch, the image plane is turned rightward and the probe extended to visualize the arch and ascending aorta.

Key points:

❐ Between the segment of the ascending aorta visualized in the high esophageal long axis

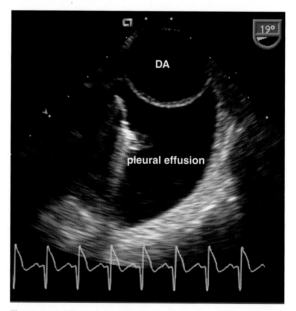

Figure 3–28 With the transducer turned toward the patient's left side, the descending thoracic aorta (*DA*) is imaged in cross-section. This patient also has a pleural effusion.

view and the aortic arch, there is a segment of the ascending aorta that may be missed on TEE imaging.
❐ In addition to short axis images of the descending aorta, the image plane may be rotated to 90 degrees to provide a longitudinal view of the extent of disease. However, the

short axis view should be used to ensure the medial and lateral aspects of the aorta are examined, which would be missed in a single longitudinal image plane.

❑ Normal structures adjacent to the aorta (connective tissue, lymph nodes) should not be mistaken for aortic pathology.

Step 14: The Transesophageal Echocardiography Report

■ The TEE report provides a systematic summary of the findings by anatomic structure.

■ The study includes the diagnostic implications of the findings, notes any limitations of the study, and suggests further evaluation as appropriate.

Key points:

❑ The TEE report includes evaluation of:
  ❑ Left ventricular size and function
  ❑ Right ventricular size and function
  ❑ Left atrial and atrial appendage anatomy and evidence for thrombus
  ❑ Anatomy of the interatrial septum and location of the four pulmonary veins
  ❑ Aortic, mitral, tricuspid, and pulmonic valve anatomy and function
  ❑ Abnormalities of the ascending aorta, descending aorta, or aortic arch
❑ Integration of the data to provide a specific diagnosis (such as "these findings are diagnostic for endocarditis") is provided whenever possible.
❑ Any unresolved clinical issues and areas of uncertainty are identified and specific approaches to resolving these issues are recommended.
❑ The TEE report also includes the details of the procedure, including informed consent, patient monitoring, medications, and any procedural complications.

NOTES

SELF-ASSESSMENT QUESTIONS

QUESTION 1

The left atrial appendage images in Figures 3–29A through D were recorded in patients undergoing TEE-guided cardioversion for atrial fibrillation. The images were recorded using a 7-MHz transducer with depth adjusted (A) and zoom mode (B through D) to focus on the atrial appendage. For each image, chose the best description of the findings from the following choices. Each answer may be used once, more than once, or not at all.

1. Myxoma
2. Ultrasound artifact
3. Trabeculation
4. Thrombus
5. Spontaneous contrast

A _____
B _____
C _____
D _____

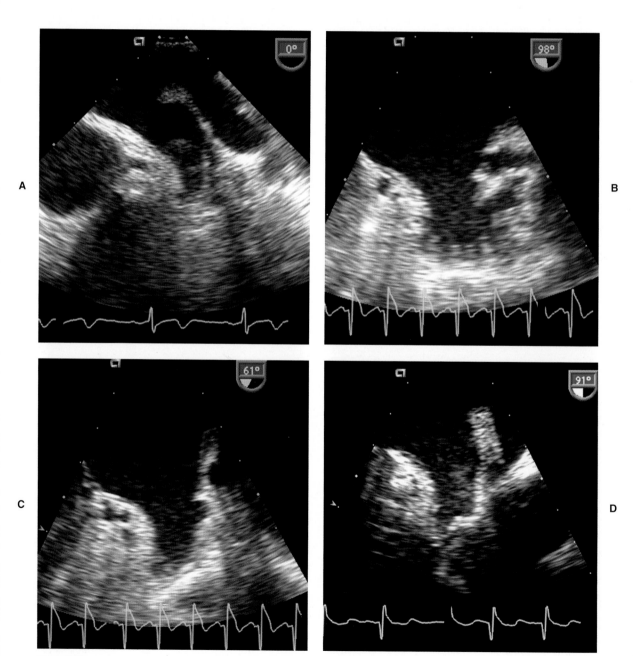

Figure 3–29

QUESTION 2

The pulsed Doppler recording of atrial append-age flow shown in Figure 3–30 is most consistent with:

    A. Normal sinus rhythm
    B. Atrial fibrillation
    C. Atrial flutter
    D. Atrioventricular dissociation
    E. Supraventricular tachycardia

QUESTION 3

The TEE image in Figure 3–31 shows:

    A. Secundum atrial septal defect
    B. Lipomatous hypertrophy of the atrial septum
    C. Atrial myxoma
    D. Aortic root calcification
    E. Right atrial enlargement

QUESTION 4

The images in Figures 3–32A and B were recorded during a TEE study in a 56-year-old man. The most likely diagnosis is:

    A. Mitral valve prolapse
    B. Aortic dissection
    C. Ventricular septal defect
    D. Patent foramen ovale
    E. Aortic to atrial fistula

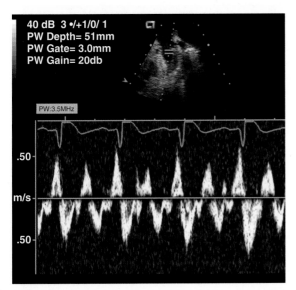

Figure 3–30

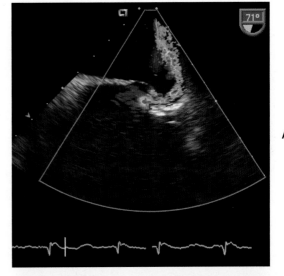

A

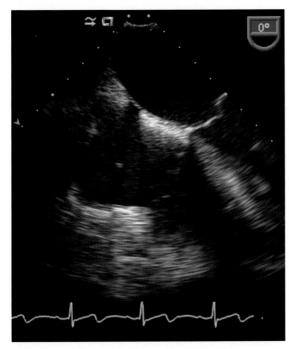

Figure 3–31

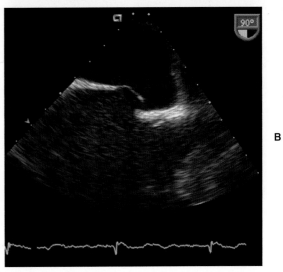

B

Figure 3–32

QUESTION 5

What structure is the arrow in Figures 3–33*A* and *B* pointing at?

_____

QUESTION 6

The flow signal in Figure 3–34 was obtained from the transgastric apical view in a patient with calcific aortic valve disease. The echo report should indicate that aortic stenosis severity is:

A. Mild
B. Moderate
C. Severe
D. Undetermined

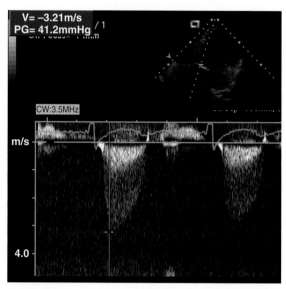

Figure 3–34

A

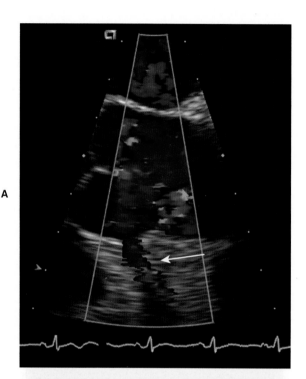

B

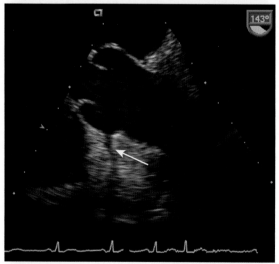

Figure 3–33

ANSWERS

ANSWER 1

Figure 3–29*A* shows an ultrasound artifact with an area of ill-defined echoes in the center of the appendage due to reverberations from the ridge between the left superior pulmonary vein and left atrial appendage. This common artifact is recognized based on the artifact being exactly twice the distance from the transducer as the ridge causing the artifact, and by resolution of the finding with adjustment of transducer position to move the ridge out of the ultrasound path. The image was recorded without zoom mode to show the relative distances of the artifact and origin of the reverberation from the transducer.

Figure 3–29*B* shows prominent trabeculation of a convoluted left atrial appendage. The trabeculations appear as ridges attached to the atrial wall; they are the same echogenicity as the wall and they move with the wall. Most atrial appendages have a simpler curved triangular shape, but some are multilobed, as in this case.

Figure 3–29*C* also shows a small trabeculation at the tip of the appendage, which is distinguished from thrombus by careful imaging in multiple views. This image is from the same patient as Figure 3–29*B*.

Figure 3–29*D* shows spontaneous contrast consistent with a low flow state. In real time, swirling motion of these intracavity echoes is seen.

ANSWER 2: C

The ECG shows a regular ventricular rhythm at a rate of 150 beats per minute, and the appendage flow shows a prominent contraction velocity of about 0.4 m/s at a regular rate of about 300 per minute. These findings are most consistent with atrial flutter with 2:1 atrioventricular conduction. Although the atrial contraction before each QRS might be mistaken for normal atrial contraction, the rate is too fast for normal sinus rhythm. The second atrial contraction with each beat also indicates this is not a normal rhythm. Atrial fibrillation is characterized by lower velocity, irregular atrial contraction. With atrioventricular dissociation, a normal atrial contraction pattern would be seen that did not correspond to the ventricular QRS complexes. A supraventricular tachycardia typically occurs at a faster rate and has only one atrial contraction for each QRS (unless concurrent atrioventricular block is present).

ANSWER 3: B

In this high TEE view at 0 degrees rotation, the four-chamber image has been turned toward the patient's right side and depth decreased to focus on the interatrial septum. As expected with normal atrial anatomy, there is a thin area in the region of the fossa ovalis; however, the septum appear intact, with no visible defect in this view. There is also increased echogenicity and thickening of the rest of the atrial septum, consistent with lipomatous hypertrophy. This normal variant typically spares the fossa ovalis, as seen here. An atrial myxoma protrudes in the right, or more often left, atrial chamber. Aortic root abnormalities may be seen in this view due to the proximity of the aortic root in the elevational plane and the width of the ultrasound beam but are not seen in this case. Although the left atrium is enlarged in this elderly patient, right atrial size is normal.

ANSWER 4: D

This is a longitudinal view of the atrial septum with the superior vena cava on the right side of the image. The fossa ovalis region of the atrial septum is thin and is bowed from right atrium toward left atrium, consistent with a transient increase in right atrial pressure during a Valsalva maneuver. Color Doppler shows right to left flow in the typical location of a patent foramen ovale. Although an eccentric mitral regurgitant jet looks similar, the valve leaflets are thicker than the atrial septum, and the flow shown in this image is diastolic (time indicated by the discontinuity in the ECG tracing, not the white line). A ventricular septal defect would be through the thicker ventricular septum with predominant systolic flow. Flow in an aortic to atrial fistula would be high velocity continuous flow and would originate in the aorta, which is not seen in this image.

ANSWER 5: Right coronary artery

This is a long axis view of the aortic root, which can be identified by the open aortic valve leaflets on the systolic 2D image and the curvature of the sinuses of Valsalva. In this view, the right coronary cusp is more anterior, with the right coronary artery arising from this cusp. The posterior cusp usually is the noncoronary cusp in this view.

The left coronary cusp and left main coronary artery are best seen in a short axis view just above the aortic leaflet image plane. The color Doppler image confirms diastolic flow (the timing is at the break in the ECG tracing) consistent with coronary flow, ensuring this is a true structure (not an echo drop-out artifact) on the 2D images. Additional confirmation of the identify of the right coronary artery could be obtained by pulsed Doppler recording to show the typical low velocity diastolic flow signal.

ANSWER 6: D

Evaluation of aortic stenosis severity on TEE is problematic because accurate velocity measurement depends on a parallel alignment between the ultrasound beam and direction of blood flow. The constraints on transducer position imposed by the TEE approach often result in a nonparallel intercept angle, leading to underestimation of velocity. In this case, the maximum velocity of 3.2 m/s may significantly underestimate stenosis severity. The most appropriate conclusion on the echo report is that aortic stenosis is undetermined; it is at least moderate, but evaluation by transthoracic Doppler is needed.

NOTES

4 Advanced Echocardiographic Modalities

THE ECHO EXAM

STRESS ECHOCARDIOGRAPHY

CONTRAST ECHOCARDIOGRAPHY

THREE-DIMENSIONAL ECHOCARDIOGRAPHY

INTRACARDIAC ECHOCARDIOGRAPHY

INTRAVASCULAR ULTRASOUND

HAND-HELD ECHOCARDIOGRAPHY

SELF-ASSESSMENT QUESTIONS

THE ECHO EXAM: ADVANCED ECHOCARDIOGRAPHIC MODALITIES

MODALITY	INSTRUMENTATION	INDICATIONS	SPECIAL TRAINING
Intraoperative TEE	Transesophageal echo in the OR	Monitoring ventricular function Evaluation of valve repair and other complex procedures	Anesthesiologists with training in echocardiography
Stress echo	Digital cine loop image acquisition Exercise or pharmacologic stress	Suspected or known coronary disease Myocardial viability Valve and structural heart disease	Performance, risks, and interpretation of stress studies
Contrast echo	Microbubbles for right or left heart contrast	Detection of patent foramen ovale LV endocardial definition	Intravenous administration of contrast agents
3D echo	Volumetric or 2D image acquisition Various display formats	Congenital heart disease Rapid acquisition for LV regional function	Image acquisition and analysis
Intracardiac echo (ICE)	5-10 MHz catheter like intracardiac probe	Interventional procedures (ASD closure) EP procedures	Invasive cardiology training and experience
Intravascular ultrasound (IVUS)	20-40 MHz intracoronary catheter	Degree of coronary narrowing and plaque morphology	Interventional cardiology training
Hand-held ultrasound	Small, inexpensive ultrasound instruments	Beside evaluation by physician for pericardial effusion, LV global and regional function	At least level 1 echo training

2D, *Two-dimensional;* 3D, *three-dimensional;* ASD, *atrial septal defect;* EP, *electrophysiology;* LV, *left ventricular;* OR, *operating room;* TEE, *transesophageal echocardiography.*

STRESS ECHOCARDIOGRAPHY (SEE CHAPTER 8)

■ Physiologic abnormalities may be evident only when there is an increased cardiovascular demand.

■ Cardiac workload can be increased with exercise or pharmacologic agents.

■ Echocardiographic imaging before and immediately after (or during) stress is termed "stress echocardiography."

Key points:

❐ Exercise duration, heart rate, and blood pressure response to exercise; electrocardiogram (ECG) changes; and symptoms are all important components of the stress echocardiographic study.

❐ The choice of exercise versus pharmacologic stress depends on the patient's ability to exercise and the specific clinical indication.

❐ Stress echocardiography most often is used for patients with coronary artery disease to:

  ❐ Confirm the presence of coronary artery disease

  ❐ Assess the location and severity of myocardial ischemia

  ❐ Evaluate cardiac risk after revascularization

  ❐ Identify viable myocardium (using a low dose dobutamine stress protocol)

❐ Stress echocardiography evaluates the functional effects of coronary disease but does not provide direct visualization of coronary anatomy (Fig. 4–1).

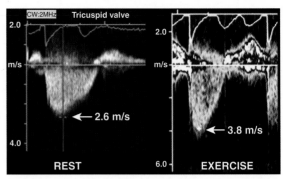

Figure 4–2 Stress echocardiography to evaluate pulmonary systolic pressure in a patient with rheumatic mitral stenosis. The tricuspid regurgitant jet, recorded with continuous wave Doppler, increased from 2.6 m/s at rest to 3.8 m/s after exercise, corresponding to a rise in pulmonary pressure from 32 mm Hg to 63 mm Hg, which is abnormal and is an indication for mitral valvotomy when moderate to severe stenosis is present.

❐ Stress echocardiography also is useful for evaluation of:

  ❐ Valve hemodynamics when aortic stenosis is accompanied by left ventricular (LV) dysfunction

  ❐ Pulmonary pressures with exercise in mitral valve disease (Fig. 4–2)

  ❐ Dynamic outflow obstruction with hypertrophic cardiomyopathy

  ❐ Aortic coarctation gradients

CONTRAST ECHOCARDIOGRAPHY

■ Intravenous injection of microbubbles to opacify the cardiac chambers or evaluate myocardial perfusion is called "contrast echocardiography."

■ Agitated saline contrast opacifies the right heart and is used for detection of right to left intracardiac shunting based on the appearance of contrast in the left heart.

■ Smaller microbubbles (1-5 μm diameter) transverse the pulmonary vasculature, allowing left heart chamber and myocardial opacification.

Key points:

❐ The most common use of right-sided contrast is to detect a patent foramen ovale, either on transthoracic or transesophageal imaging (Fig. 4–3).

❐ Left heart contrast typically is used to enhance left ventricular endocardial border detection when transthoracic image quality is suboptimal (Fig. 4–4).

❐ Available left heart contrast agents in the United States include Definity (Bristol Myers Squibb) and Optison (GE Healthcare).

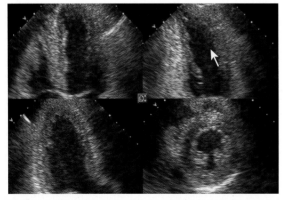

Figure 4–1 Stress echocardiography image display: A quad screen cine loop format is used to show the left ventricle in apical four-chamber (*upper left*), two-chamber (*upper right*), long axis (*lower left*), and parasternal short axis (*lower right*) views. The same views are recorded at peak stress (with dobutamine) or immediately after stress (with treadmill exercise). The baseline and stress images are matched and placed side by side to facilitate recognition of changes in wall motion.

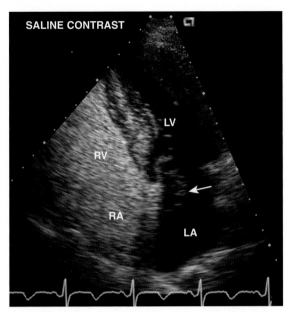

Figure 4–3 Intravenous injection of agitated saline provides opacification of the right heart chambers. A small amount of contrast is seen in the left atrium (*LA, arrow*), consistent with the presence of patent foramen ovale.

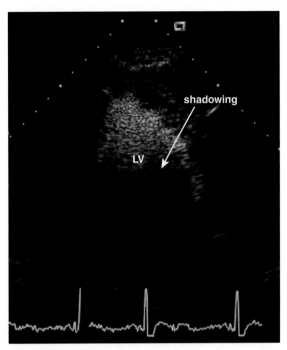

Figure 4–5 Shadowing of the left ventricle (*LV*) by contrast in the apex is seen. Apical shadowing occurs when the volume or rate of contrast injection is too high.

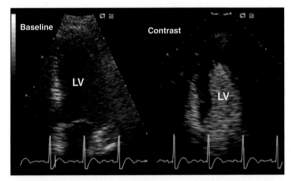

Figure 4–4 In this patient with suboptimal endocardial definition in the apical four-chamber view, intravenous injection of a left heart contrast agent (Definity) opacifies the left ventricle (*LV*), providing improved evaluation of ventricular systolic function.

❏ Instrument settings to optimize left heart contrast images include:
  ❏ A decrease in power output (to a mechanical index of about 0.5)
  ❏ A lower transducer frequency
  ❏ An increase in overall gain and dynamic range
  ❏ Focal depth at the mid- or near-field of the image
❏ When microbubble density is too high, excessive apical contrast results in shadowing of the rest of the ventricle (Fig. 4–5).
❏ A low microbubble density or high mechanical index results in a swirling appearance with inadequate LV opacification (Fig. 4–6).

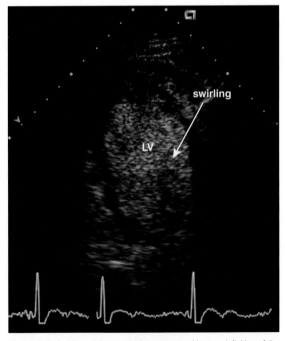

Figure 4–6 Swirling of the ventricular contrast, with poor definition of the endocardium, is seen when the volume of contrast is too low or when the mechanical index is too high, which results in destruction of microbubbles.

❏ Assessment of myocardial perfusion by contrast echocardiography is not widely used for clinical diagnosis, although there is ongoing development of this approach.

THREE-DIMENSIONAL ECHOCARDIOGRAPHY

- Echocardiographic data can be acquired in a three-dimensional (3D) format by:
  - ❏ Integrating data from multiple two-dimensional (2D) images of known spatial location
  - ❏ Use of a transducer that acquires a volume of echocardiographic data
  - ❏ Use of a transducer that simultaneously records more than one 2D image plane
  - ❏ Reconstruction of borders traced on 2D images in a 3D image format
- 3D echocardiography facilitates recognition of complex intracardiac spatial relationships.

Key points:

- ❏ Several types of 3D systems are available, with instrumentation specific to each approach.
- ❏ Most clinical echocardiography laboratories continue to use 2D echocardiography as the primary diagnostic approach.
- ❏ Proposed clinical applications of 3D echocardiography include:
  - ❏ A surgical view of the mitral valve in patients with mitral prolapse, facilitating surgical repair
  - ❏ Evaluation of mitral valve anatomy before and after balloon valvotomy (Fig. 4–7)
  - ❏ More complete visualization of the interatrial septum in patients undergoing percutaneous closure of an atrial septal defect
  - ❏ Evaluation of complex congenital heart disease
  - ❏ More accurate measurement of ventricular volumes and ejection fraction

- ❏ Research applications of 3D echocardiography include:
  - ❏ Studies on the mechanisms of functional mitral regurgitation
  - ❏ Evaluation of regional myocardial function
  - ❏ Changes in the size, shape, and function of the left and right ventricle with pressure or volume overload

INTRACARDIAC ECHOCARDIOGRAPHY

- Intracardiac echocardiography (ICE) is performed in the cardiac catheterization or electrophysiology laboratory using a small transducer (5-10 MHz) on the tip of a catheter.
- ICE imaging is used to guide percutaneous interventions and complex electrophysiology procedures.

Key points:

- ❏ ICE typically is performed by the physician doing the invasive procedure.
- ❏ Manipulation of the transducer-tipped catheter requires considerable experience in intracardiac procedures.
- ❏ Images are obtained primarily from the right atrium, allowing evaluation of the:
  - ❏ Interatrial septum
  - ❏ Left atrium, atrial appendage, and pulmonary veins
  - ❏ Mitral valve and base of the left ventricle
  - ❏ Tricuspid valve and right ventricle (Fig. 4–8)

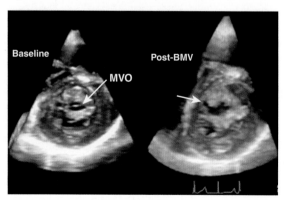

Figure 4–7 A real time three-dimensional echocardiographic image of rheumatic mitral stenosis showing the ovale-shaped mitral valve orifice (*MVO*) in diastole in a short axis orientation "looking" from the apex toward the mitral valve. After balloon mitral valvotomy (*BMV*), the medial commissure (*arrow*) shows improved opening. *Images courtesy of Ed Gill, MD.*

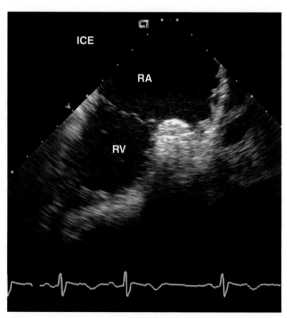

Figure 4–8 Intracardiac echocardiography (*ICE*) with the catheter-tip transducer located in the right atrium (*RA*). The trabeculated right atrial appendage, tricuspid valve, and right ventricle (*RV*) are seen.

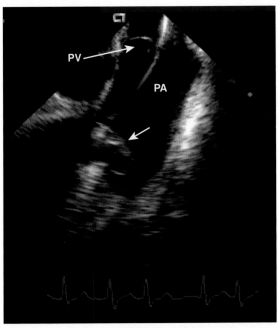

Figure 4–9 Intracardiac echocardiography (ICE) used to guide the position of a biopsy catheter. The ICE transducer is in the right ventricular outflow tract. The biopsy catheter crosses the pulmonic valve (*PV*) with its tip attached to the mass (*arrow*) at the pulmonary artery (*PA*) bifurcation.

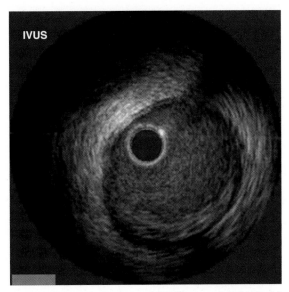

Figure 4–10 Intravascular ultrasound (IVUS) image recorded in the left anterior descending artery. The ultrasound catheter is the dark circle in the vessel lumen. With this high frequency transducer, the blood appears light grey, with a denser crescent of tissue in the vessel due to atherosclerosis. *Image courtesy of Justin Strote, MD.*

❏ ICE is used to guide procedures such as:
  ❏ Atrial septal defect closure
  ❏ Patent foramen ovale closure
  ❏ Arrhythmia ablation procedures
  ❏ Other complex percutaneous procedures (Fig. 4–9)
❏ Some procedures, such as balloon mitral valvuloplasty, can be monitored either by intracardiac, transesophageal, or transthoracic imaging.

INTRAVASCULAR ULTRASOUND

■ Intravascular ultrasound (IVUS) uses a high frequency transducer (20-40 MHz) on an intracoronary catheter to visualize coronary artery atheroma.
■ IVUS allows assessment of the length, severity, and composition of the atherosclerotic plaque (Fig. 4–10).

Key points:
❏ IVUS typically is performed by the interventional cardiologist as part of a coronary intervention.

❏ The image depth is about 2-3 cm.
❏ A small dedicated ultrasound system is used for image acquisition, recording, and analysis.

HAND-HELD ECHOCARDIOGRAPHY

■ The bedside use of small portable ultrasound systems is called "hand-held echocardiography."
■ The capability of portable instruments ranges from simple 2D imaging to the full range of functions of a larger ultrasound system.

Key points:
❏ Appropriate education and training is essential for the appropriate use of hand-held echocardiography.
❏ The most widely used applications of hand-held echocardiography are:
  ❏ Evaluation for pericardial effusion
  ❏ Evaluation of ventricular global and regional systolic function
❏ Cardiologists also use hand-held echocardiography for interim evaluation of patients with complex cardiac disease.

NOTES

SELF-ASSESSMENT QUESTIONS

QUESTION 1

A 68-year-old man is referred for stress echocardiography to evaluate for coronary artery disease prior to elective knee replacement. He has cardiac risk factors of hypertension and hypercholesterolemia. His ECG shows a left bundle branch block. Based on this evaluation, you recommend:

A. No stress test
B. Treadmill ECG stress test
C. Bicycle echocardiographic stress test
D. Dobutamine echocardiography stress test
E. Coronary angiography

QUESTION 2

Transthoracic images of the left ventricle are suboptimal in an obese 62-year-old woman referred for baseline measurement of left ventricular ejection fraction prior to cardiotoxic chemotherapy. The next best step in diagnosis is:

A. Intravenous agitated saline
B. Left heart contrast
C. Transesophageal echocardiography
D. Left ventricular angiography
E. Radionuclide angiography

For each of the clinical issues indicated in Questions 3-7, choose the best initial approach to diagnosis from the following list. Each answer may be used once, more than once, or not at all.

A. Transthoracic echocardiography
B. Transesophageal echocardiography
C. Agitated saline contrast
D. Left heart contrast
E. Stress echocardiography
F. 3D echocardiography
G. Intracardiac ultrasound
H. Intravascular ultrasound

QUESTION 3

Evaluation of prosthetic mitral regurgitation

QUESTION 4

Detection of patent foramen ovale

QUESTION 5

Detection of coronary artery disease

QUESTION 6

Monitoring of percutaneous atrial septal defect closure

QUESTION 7

Evaluation for possible pericardial effusion

QUESTION 8

The aortic root is seen in three different echocardiographic images (Figs. 4–11, 4–12, and 4–13). Match each of these long axis views of the aorta with the ultrasound modality used for image acquisition. Each answer may be used once, more than once, or not at all.

A. Transthoracic
B. Transesophageal
C. 3D imaging
D. Intracardiac
E. Intravascular

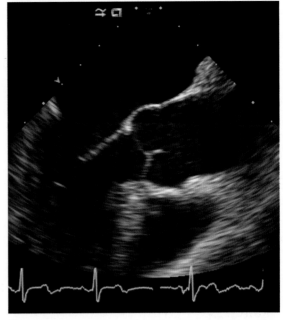

Figure 4–12

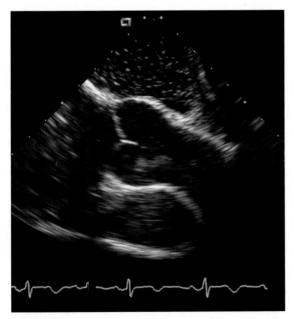

Figure 4–11

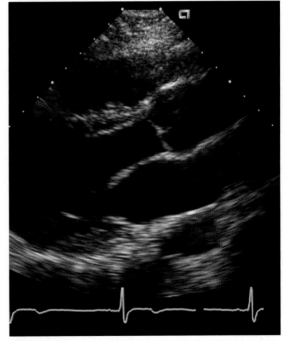

Figure 4–13

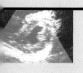

ANSWERS

ANSWER 1: D

This patient has a high pretest likelihood of coronary artery disease based on the presence of cardiac risk factors of age, gender, hypertension, and hypercholesterolemia, so a preoperative evaluation for coronary disease is appropriate. Treadmill and bicycle exercise are likely to be difficult to perform or will result in an inadequate stress level, based on his need for a knee replacement. Dobutamine stress echocardiography is the most appropriate way to evaluate for possible coronary disease in this patient. Stress testing usually is performed before consideration of coronary angiography due to the risks and costs of the invasive angiographic approach.

ANSWER 2: B

A baseline quantitative measurement of left ventricular ejection fraction is needed in patients undergoing cardiotoxic chemotherapy to ensure the safety of the therapy and for comparison with repeat studies after each chemotherapy cycle. Contrast enhancement of endocardial borders using a contrast agent that traverses the pulmonary bed is the most appropriate next step in evaluation because the patient is already undergoing an echocardiographic examination. Saline contrast would only opacify the right heart and thus would not be helpful for this indication. Alternate approaches to evaluation of ventricular function include transesophageal echocardiography (TEE) and left ventricular angiography, but these would be appropriate only if less invasive approaches were not diagnostic. Radionuclide angiography is a reasonable approach to quantitation of LV ejection fraction and is the standard test for this indication at some centers. If evaluation of ventricular function is not possible even after use of left heart contrast, radionuclide angiography would be the best next test.

ANSWER 3: B

Evaluation of prosthetic mitral regurgitation on transthoracic echocardiography is limited by shadowing and reverberations that obscure the left atrium from both apical and parasternal windows. Transesophageal echocardiography provides a view of the left atrial side of the valve so that valve regurgitation can be reliably detected and evaluated.

ANSWER 4: C

Detection of a patent foramen ovale is based on the demonstration of passage of right-sided saline contrast from the right atrium into the left atrium. The patent foramen ovale works like a flap-valve; at rest there may be no shunt because left atrial pressure holds the septal layers in the closed position. However, if right atrial pressure is transiently increased, with a Valsalva maneuver or cough, the flap valve opens and contrast in the right atrium crosses the septum to be seen in the left atrium. In patients with atrial enlargement or with a chronically elevated right atrial pressure, the septal layers may be stretched apart, resulting in shunting even at rest.

ANSWER 5: E

Resting left ventricular global and regional function often is normal at rest, even when significant coronary artery disease is present. However, an increase in cardiac oxygen demand, for example with exercise or pharmacologic stress, results in myocardial ischemia in regions supplied by narrowed coronary arteries; even though myocardial oxygen supply is adequate at rest, blood flow cannot be increased enough to meet tissue needs with stress. Myocardial ischemia leads to a prompt reduction in endocardial motion and wall thickening. Detection of these wall motion abnormalities with stress, which resolve with rest, is the basis of echocardiographic diagnosis of coronary artery disease.

ANSWER 6: G

Percutaneous atrial septal defect closure is monitored by intracardiac echocardiography, because this approach provides detailed images of the atrial septum, allowing optimal positioning of the closure device, and because the imaging catheter can be manipulated by the interventional cardiologist, along with the catheters used for the procedure itself.

ANSWER 7: A

The most appropriate initial approach to evaluation for a possible pericardial effusion is transthoracic echocardiography, either with a standard or hand-held ultrasound system.

ANSWER 8

These images were acquired using intracardiac (see Fig. 4–11), TEE (see Fig. 4–12), and transthoracic (TTE) (see Fig. 4–13) echocardiography. All are shown in the standard echocardiographic display format with the transducer at the top of the image, at the narrow point of the sector. In the TTE image (see Fig. 4–13), the right ventricular (RV) outflow tract is between the transducer and aorta, with the left atrium more distal from the transducer. The left atrium is seen to empty into the left ventricle via the mitral valve. On the TEE image (see Fig. 4–12), the left atrium is between the transducer and aortic root with the RV outflow tract more distally. Thus the TEE and TTE views are very similar, with the only difference being the transducer position. Identification of structures on the intracardiac image is more challenging because the view is not in a standard image plane. The transducer is *in* the right atrium, so that part of the right atrium (with some saline contrast present) is interposed between the transducer and aortic root. The RV outflow tract is more distal, as on a TEE image. Although a small segment of left ventricle is seen adjacent to the aortic valve, the linear structure extending from the posterior aortic root is the atrial septum, not the mitral valve leaflet, in this oblique image plane.

NOTES

5 Clinical Indications

THE ECHO EXAM

BASIC PRINCIPLES
- Understand the Accuracy of Echocardiography for the Specific Diagnosis
- Integrate the Clinical Data and the Echocardiographic Findings
- Recommend Additional Diagnostic Testing as Appropriate

DIAGNOSTIC THINKING FOR THE ECHOCARDIOGRAPHER

ECHOCARDIOGRAPHY FOR COMMON CLINICAL SIGNS AND SYMPTOMS
- Murmur
- Chest Pain
- Heart Failure or Dyspnea
- Palpitations
- Embolic Event
- Fever/Bacteremia

SELF-ASSESSMENT QUESTIONS

THE ECHO EXAM: INDICATIONS FOR ECHOCARDIOGRAPHY

CLINICAL DIAGNOSIS	KEY ECHO FINDINGS	LIMITATIONS OF ECHO	ALTERNATE APPROACHES
Valvular Heart Disease			
Valve stenosis	Etiology of stenosis, valve anatomy Transvalvular ΔP, valve area Chamber enlargement and hypertrophy LV and RV systolic function Associated valvular regurgitation	Possible underestimation of stenosis severity Possible coexisting coronary artery disease	Cardiac cath MRI
Valve regurgitation	Mechanism and etiology of regurgitation Severity of regurgitation Chamber enlargement LV and RV systolic function PA pressure estimate	TEE may be needed to evaluate mitral regurgitant severity and valve anatomy (esp. before MV repair)	Cardiac cath MRI
Prosthetic valve function	Evidence for stenosis Detection of regurgitation Chamber enlargement Ventricular function PA pressure estimate	Imaging prosthetic valves is limited by shadowing and reverberations TEE is needed for suspected prosthetic MR due to "masking" of the left atrium on TTE	Cardiac cath
Endocarditis	Detection of vegetations (TTE sensitivity, 70-85%) Presence and degree of valve dysfunction Chamber enlargement and function Detection of abscess Possible prognostic implications	TEE is more sensitive for detection of vegetations (>90%) A definite diagnosis of endocarditis also depends on bacteriologic criteria TEE is more sensitive for abscess detection	Blood cultures and clinical findings also are diagnostic criteria for endocarditis

2D, *Two-dimensional;* 3D, *three-dimensional;* A2C, *apical two-chamber;* Angio, *angiography;* AR, *aortic regurgitation;* AS, *aortic stenosis;* CAD, *coronary artery disease;* Cath, *catheterization;* CT, *computed tomography;* EF, *ejection fraction;* ETT, *exercise treadmill test;* HOCM, *hypertrophic obstructive cardiomyopathy;* LA, *left atrial;* LV, *left ventricular;* LVEDP, *left ventricular end-diastolic pressure;* LVOT, *left ventricular outflow tract;* MR, *mitral regurgitation;* MRI, *magnetic resonance imaging;* MV, *mitral valve;* ΔP, *pressure gradient;* PA, *pulmonary artery;* PE, *pericardial effusion;* PET, *position emission tomography;* PLAX, *parasternal long axis;* PSAX, *parasternal short axis;* RV, *right ventricular;* SC, *subcostal;* SSN, *suprasternal notch;* TEE, *transesophageal echocardiography;* TR, *tricuspid regurgitation;* TTE, *transthoracic echocardiography;* VSD, *ventricular septal defect.*

Continued

THE ECHO EXAM: INDICATIONS FOR ECHOCARDIOGRAPHY—cont'd

CLINICAL DIAGNOSIS	KEY ECHO FINDINGS	LIMITATIONS OF ECHO	ALTERNATE APPROACHES
Coronary Artery Disease			

Acute myocardial infarction	Segmental wall motion abnormality reflects "myocardium at risk"
	Global LV function (EF)
	Complications:
	  Acute MR vs. VSD
	  Pericarditis
	  LV thrombus, aneurysm
	  RV infarct
		Coronary artery anatomy itself not directly visualized	Coronary angio
			Radionuclide LV angio
			Cardiac cath

Angina	Global and segmental LV systolic function Exclude other causes of angina (e.g., AS, HOCM)	Resting wall motion may be normal despite significant CAD Stress echo needed to induce ischemia and wall motion abnormality	Coronary angio Stress thallium ETT
Prerevascularization/ postrevascularization	Assess wall thickening and endocardial motion at baseline Improvement in segmental function post-procedure	Dobutamine stress and/or contrast echo needed to detect viable but nonfunctioning myocardium	MRI PET Thallium ETT Contrast echocardiography
End-stage ischemic disease	Overall LV systolic function (EF) PA pressures Associated MR LV thrombus RV systolic function		Coronary angio Radionuclide EF
Cardiomyopathy			
Dilated	Chamber dilation (all four) LV and RV systolic function (qualitative and EF) Coexisting atrioventricular valve regurgitation PA systolic pressure LV thrombus	Indirect measures of LVEDP Accurate EF may be difficult if image quality is poor	Radionuclide EF LV and RV angiography
Restrictive	LV wall thickness LV systolic function LV diastolic function PA systolic pressure	Must be distinguished from constrictive pericarditis	Cardiac cath with direct, simultaneous RV and LV pressure measurement after volume loading
Hypertrophic	Pattern and extent of LV hypertrophy Dynamic LVOT obstruction (imaging and Doppler) Coexisting MR Diastolic LV dysfunction		
Hypertension	LV wall thickness and chamber dimensions LV mass LV systolic function Aortic root dilation, AR		
Pericardial Disease	Pericardial thickening Detection, size, and location of PE 2D signs of tamponade physiology Doppler signs of tamponade physiology	Diagnosis of tamponade is a hemodynamic and clinical diagnosis Constrictive pericarditis is a difficult diagnosis Not all patients with pericarditis have an effusion	Intracardiac pressure measurements for tamponade or constriction MRI or CT to detect pericardial thickening

2D, *Two-dimensional;* 3D, *three-dimensional;* A2C, *apical two-chamber;* Angio, *angiography;* AR, *aortic regurgitation;* AS, *aortic stenosis;* CAD, *coronary artery disease;* Cath, *catheterization;* CT, *computed tomography;* EF, *ejection fraction;* ETT, *exercise treadmill test;* HOCM, *hypertrophic obstructive cardiomyopathy;* LA, *left atrial;* LV, *left ventricular;* LVEDP, *left ventricular end-diastolic pressure;* LVOT, *left ventricular outflow tract;* MR, *mitral regurgitation;* MRI, *magnetic resonance imaging;* MV, *mitral valve;* ΔP, *pressure gradient;* PA, *pulmonary artery;* PE, *pericardial effusion;* PET, *position emission tomography;* PLAX, *parasternal long axis;* PSAX, *parasternal short axis;* RV, *right ventricular;* SC, *subcostal;* SSN, *suprasternal notch;* TEE, *transesophageal echocardiography;* TR, *tricuspid regurgitation;* TTE, *transthoracic echocardiography;* VSD, *ventricular septal defect.*

THE ECHO EXAM: INDICATIONS FOR ECHOCARDIOGRAPHY —cont'd

CLINICAL DIAGNOSIS	KEY ECHO FINDINGS	LIMITATIONS OF ECHO	ALTERNATE APPROACHES
Aortic Disease			
Aortic root dilation	Etiology of aortic dilation Accurate aortic root diameter measurements Anatomy of sinuses of Valsalva (esp. Marfan's syndrome) Associated aortic regurgitation	May not visualize entire ascending aorta	CT MRI Aortography
Aortic dissection	2D images of ascending aorta (PLAX, PSAX), aortic arch (SSN), descending thoracic (A2C), and proximal abdominal (SC) aorta Imaging of dissection "flap" Associated aortic regurgitation Ventricular function	TEE is more sensitive (97%) and specific (100%) Cannot assess distal vascular beds	Aortography CT MRI TEE
Cardiac Masses			
LV thrombus	High sensitivity and specificity for diagnosis of LV thrombus Suspect with apical wall motion abnormality or diffuse LV systolic dysfunction	Technical artifacts can be misleading 5 MHz or higher frequency transducer and angulated apical views needed	LV thrombus may not be recognized on radionuclide or contrast angiography
LA thrombus	Low sensitivity for detection of LA thrombus, although specificity is high Suspect with LA enlargement, MV disease	TEE is needed to detect LA thrombus reliably	TEE
Cardiac tumors	Size, location, and physiologic consequences of tumor mass	Extracardiac involvement not clearly seen Cannot distinguish benign from malignant, or tumor from thrombus	TEE CT MRI (with cardiac gating) Intracardiac echo
Pulmonary Hypertension	Estimate of PA pressure Evidence of left-sided heart disease to account for increased PA pressures RV size and systolic function (corpulmonale) Associated TR	Indirect PA pressure measurement Unable to determine pulmonary vascular resistance accurately	Cardiac cath
Congenital Heart Disease	Detection and assessment of anatomic abnormalities Quantitation of physiologic abnormalities Chamber enlargement Ventricular function	No direct intracardiac pressure measurements Complicated anatomy may be difficult to evaluate if image quality is poor (TEE helpful)	MRI Cardiac cath TEE 3D Echo

BASIC PRINCIPLES

■ The diagnostic value of echocardiography for a specific diagnosis depends both on the accuracy of the echocardiographic data and on integration with other clinical information.

■ The framework for echocardiographic data acquisition and reporting is a structured diagnostic approach to the question posed by the requesting physician.

Key points:

❏ The echocardiographic study seeks to provide the appropriate data for clinical decision making depending on the patient's symptoms, signs, and known diagnoses.

- ❏ The list of possible diagnoses that might explain the clinical findings, called the differential diagnosis, is mentally constructed at the beginning of the echocardiographic study.
- ❏ As the study proceeds, some diagnoses are excluded, whereas others may be suggested by specific findings.
- ❏ Pertinent positive data include the abnormal echocardiographic findings.
- ❏ Pertinent negative data include normal echocardiographic findings that help narrow the differential diagnosis.

Step 1: Understand the Accuracy of Echocardiography for the Specific Diagnosis

- ■ The clinical value of echocardiography depends on the certainty with which a specific diagnosis can be confirmed or excluded (Fig. 5–1).
- ■ Sensitivity is the percentage of patients with the diagnosis correctly identified by echocardiography.
- ■ Specificity is the percentage of patients without the diagnosis correctly identified by echocardiography.
- ■ Positive predictive value (PPV) is the percentage of patients with a positive echocardiogram who actually have the diagnosis.
- ■ Negative predictive value (NPV) is the percentage of patients with a negative echocardiogram who actually do not have the diagnosis.

Key points:

- ❏ In a patient with the diagnosis, a positive test is a true positive (TP) and a negative test is a false negative (FN).
- ❏ In a patient without the diagnosis, a negative test is a true negative (TN) and a positive test is a false positive (FP).

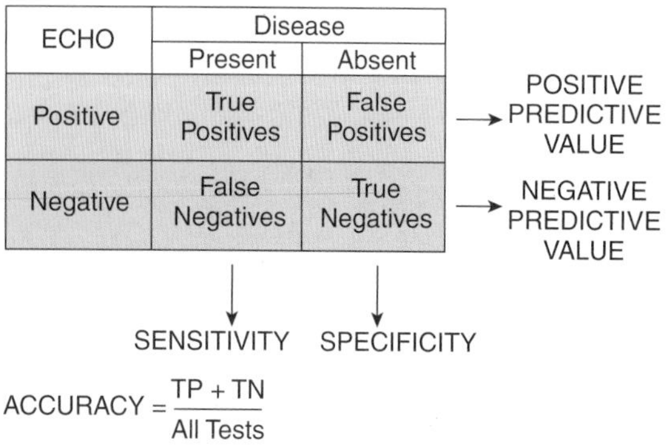

ACCURACY $= \dfrac{TP + TN}{All\ Tests}$

Figure 5–1 Sensitivity and specificity in comparison with positive and negative predictive value. Predictive values depend on the prevalence of disease in the population. *TP,* True positives; *TN,* true negatives. *From Otto CM: Textbook of Clinical Echocardiography, 3rd ed. Philadelphia: Elsevier, 2004.*

- ❏ Sensitivity = TP/(TP + FN)
- ❏ Specificity = TN/(TN + FP)
- ❏ PPV = TP/(TP + FP)
- ❏ NPV = TN/(TN + FN)
- ❏ Accuracy indicates what proportion of all studies indicated a correct diagnosis.
- ❏ The positive predictive value of a test depends on the prevalence of disease in addition to sensitivity and specificity.

Step 2: Integrate the Clinical Data and the Echocardiographic Findings (Fig. 5–2)

- ■ Bayesian analysis calculates the likelihood of a diagnosis based on both the echocardiographic results and the pretest likelihood of disease.
- ■ The threshold approach to clinical decision making indicates that diagnostic testing, such as echocardiography, is most helpful in patients in whom the results will change the subsequent therapy or diagnostic strategy.

Key points:

- ❏ The pretest likelihood of disease is the probability of disease before echocardiography is done—for example, consideration of cardiac risk factors and symptoms in a patient scheduled for stress echocardiography provides an estimate of the probability of coronary artery disease.
- ❏ Echocardiography is most helpful when the pretest likelihood of disease is intermediate and echocardiography has a high accuracy for the diagnosis.
- ❏ When the pretest likelihood of disease is very low, an abnormal echocardiographic finding often is a false positive result.
- ❏ Conversely, when the pretest likelihood of disease is very high, the failure to demonstrate the disease on echocardiography often is a false negative.
- ❏ With the threshold approach, the upper threshold is the point at which the risk of the test is higher than the risk of treating the patient—for example, additional diagnostic testing should not delay surgical intervention for an acute ascending aortic dissection.
- ❏ The lower threshold for transthoracic echocardiography occurs only with a very low probability of disease; the major potential adverse effect is a false positive result leading to further inappropriate testing or therapy.

Step 3: Recommend Additional Diagnostic Testing as Appropriate

- ■ The interpretation of the echocardiogram lists the pertinent positive and negative findings along with any confirmed diagnoses.

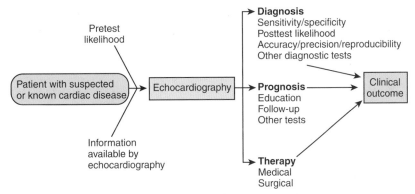

Figure 5–2 Flowchart illustrating the impact of echocardiographic results on diagnosis, prognosis, and therapy. The effects of echocardiography on clinical outcome are the best measure of the usefulness of the test result. *From Otto CM: Textbook of Clinical Echocardiography, 3rd ed. Philadelphia: Elsevier, 2004.*

■ The differential diagnosis of equivocal findings is indicated and appropriate additional diagnostic testing is recommended when the echocardiographic results are not diagnostic.

Key points:

❏ Echocardiography provides qualitative and quantitative information on cardiac structure and function and often provides a definitive diagnosis.

❏ Positive findings are more helpful than negative findings; for example, a dissection flap seen on transthoracic echocardiography is diagnostic for a dissection, but its absence does not exclude this possibility.

❏ A noncardiac cause for symptoms is likely when the echocardiogram is normal.

❏ The echocardiographer often needs to assist in choosing the optimal diagnostic approach (e.g., transthoracic or transesophageal echocardiography, stress echocardiography, contrast study) based on the indication for the study.

❏ Additional diagnostic studies, with either another echocardiographic modality or an alternate imaging approach, are recommended after review of the echocardiographic exam.

DIAGNOSTIC THINKING FOR THE ECHOCARDIOGRAPHER

■ The echocardiographer needs:
❏ Clinical data to estimate the pretest likelihood of disease before starting the exam
❏ An understanding of pertinent positive and negative findings for each clinical indication
❏ Knowledge of the accuracy of echocardiography for each diagnosis
❏ Ability to integrate the echocardiographic findings with the clinical data.

■ The Echo Exam table at the beginning of the chapter summarizes the approach by anatomic diagnosis.

■ Examples of the approach to common clinical indications for echocardiography are discussed in the following sections.

ECHOCARDIOGRAPHY FOR COMMON CLINICAL SIGNS AND SYMPTOMS

Murmur

■ The echocardiographic differential diagnosis for a murmur is based on an anatomic approach with evaluation of all four valves and a search for an intracardiac shunt (Fig. 5–3).

■ Most patients referred to echocardiography for a murmur on auscultation have a benign flow murmur.

Key points:

❏ The echocardiography request form may not specify the type of murmur (e.g., systolic or diastolic), so a systemic echocardiographic exam is essential.

❏ Normal physiologic regurgitation rarely accounts for an audible murmur.

❏ The most common pathologic causes for a murmur in adults are aortic valve stenosis and mitral valve regurgitation.

❏ Murmurs typically are caused by high velocity intracardiac flows (e.g., aortic stenosis or mitral regurgitation), because low velocity flows (e.g., tricuspid regurgitation with normal pulmonary pressures) are not usually audible with a stethoscope.

❏ Congenital heart disease may first be diagnosed in an adult based on finding a murmur. In patients with an atrial septal defect, the murmur is due to increased pulmonary blood flow volume, not to flow across the atrial septum.

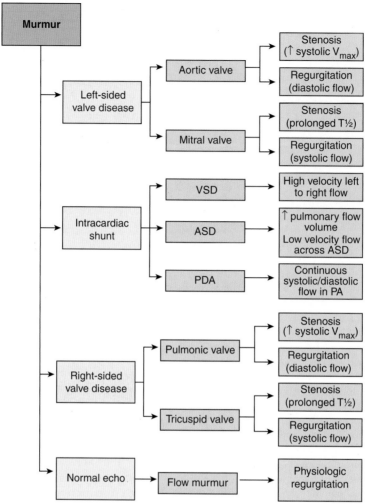

Figure 5–3 Flow chart for the echocardiographic differential diagnosis of a murmur. The flowchart is arranged by anatomy because the echocardiographer often is not provided information about the type of murmur or other clinical findings. The basic echocardiographic examination includes measurement of antegrade flows and evaluation for regurgitation of all four valves. Additional evaluation for murmur includes careful interrogation of flow in the pulmonary artery to detect a patent ductus arteriosus or increased flow due to an atrial septal defect. Flow in the septal region is examined with color and CW Doppler to exclude a ventricular septal defect. Normal physiologic amounts of mitral and tricuspid regurgitation are not audible and do not explain the presence of a murmur. *ASD,* Atrial septal defect; *PDA,* patent ductus arteriosus; *T½,* pressure half time; V_{max}, maximum antegrade velocity; *VSD,* ventricular septal defect.

Chest Pain

- The echocardiographic differential diagnosis for chest pain is based on the major clinical diagnoses that are of immediate clinical concern (Fig. 5–4).
- When the echocardiogram does not establish a diagnosis, further evaluation may be needed emergently.

Key points:

- ❏ Acute chest pain is a medical emergency because the differential diagnosis includes acute coronary syndromes and aortic dissection, both of which require immediate treatment.

- ❏ An abnormal echocardiographic finding, such as anterior wall hypokinesis, may prompt further diagnostic and therapeutic interventions—for example, coronary angiography.
- ❏ Even when the transthoracic echocardiogram is normal, further evaluation may be needed—for example, transesophageal echocardiography or chest computed tomography (CT) in a patient with suspected aortic dissection.
- ❏ Normal resting wall motion does not exclude the possibility of significant coronary artery disease. Wall motion is abnormal only after infarction or with ongoing ischemia—for

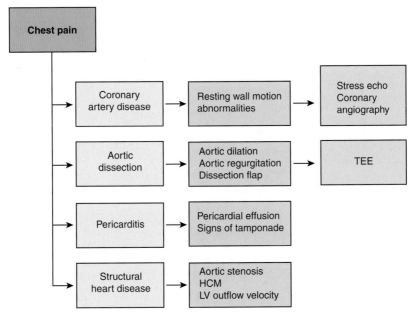

Figure 5–4 Echocardiographic approach to evaluation of chest pain. The primary goal in the acute setting is to exclude life-threatening conditions, such as an acute coronary syndrome or acute aortic dissection. With both acute and chronic chest pain, further diagnostic evaluation often is needed. *HCM,* hypertrophic cardiomyopathy; *LV,* left ventricular; *TEE,* transesophageal echocardiography.

example, with unstable angina or on stress testing.

❏ The presence of a pericardial effusion is consistent with pericarditis, although not all patients with pericarditis have an effusion.

❏ In a patient with aortic dissection, pericardial fluid may be caused by rupture of the aorta into the pericardial space.

❏ With significant left ventricular (LV) outflow obstruction, the increase in LV myocardial wall stress and oxygen demand results in angina-type chest pain.

Heart Failure or Dyspnea

■ Symptoms of dyspnea, edema, and decreased exercise tolerance are nonspecific, with a wide differential diagnosis including cardiac and noncardiac conditions.

■ Heart failure, defined as the inability of the heart to supply adequate blood flow at a normal filling pressure, is the clinical consequence of several types of heart disease (Fig. 5–5).

Key points:

❏ Left ventricular systolic dysfunction may be caused by a cardiomyopathy, coronary disease with prior infarction, long-standing valvular heart disease, or congenital heart disease.

❏ Diastolic dysfunction typically accompanies systolic dysfunction; predominant diastolic dysfunction is seen with hypertensive heart disease, hypertrophic cardiomyopathy, and infiltrative myocardial disease.

❏ Constrictive pericarditis often presents as right heart failure, with ascites and peripheral edema.

❏ Heart failure occurs in patients with valvular heart disease, even when LV function is normal, due to obstruction of blood flow (e.g., mitral stenosis) or elevated pulmonary diastolic pressure (e.g., mitral regurgitation).

❏ Pulmonary hypertension caused by left-sided heart disease, pulmonary vascular disease, or underlying lung disease leads to right heart failure with a dilated hypokinetic right ventricle, sometimes called "cor pulmonale."

❏ Heart failure in patients with congenital heart disease may be caused by ventricular dysfunction, obstructive or regurgitant lesions, or intracardiac shunts.

❏ When heart failure is present with a normal echocardiographic study, noncardiac causes for the patient's symptoms should be considered.

Palpitations

■ Palpitations are the patient's awareness of a forceful, rapid, or irregular heart rhythm.

■ The primary approach to evaluation of palpitations is electrocardiogram (ECG) monitoring or stress testing.

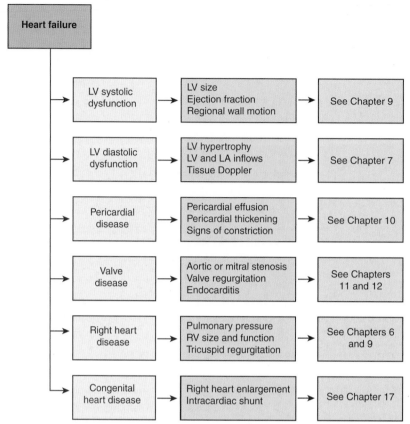

Figure 5–5 Echocardiographic approach to the patient referred for "heart failure." A systemic echocardiographic study will include the two-dimensional views and Doppler flows to identify each of these possible diagnoses. In addition, the sonographer should mentally "check off" each of these conditions as the exam progresses to ensure that the entire differential diagnosis is considered. If the echocardiographic study is normal, a noncardiac cause of symptoms is likely. *LA,* Left atrial; *LV,* left ventricular; *RV,* right ventricular.

■ Echocardiography allows evaluation of any underlying anatomic abnormalities associated with the cardiac arrhythmia.

Key points:
❑ Echocardiography typically is normal in patients with a supraventricular arrhythmia and no prior cardiac history.
❑ Conditions associated with supraventricular arrhythmias include:
   ❑ Ebstein's anomaly in patients with preexcitation syndromes
   ❑ Prior surgery for congenital heart disease
❑ Atrial fibrillation often is associated with hypertensive heart disease, mitral valve disease, and LV systolic dysfunction.
❑ The prevalence of atrial fibrillation increases with age (present in about 4% of people older than 60 years).
❑ Left atrial thrombi are associated with atrial fibrillation but are not reliably visualized on transthoracic echocardiography; transesophageal imaging is more accurate for diagnosis of atrial thrombi.

❑ Echocardiography often is abnormal in patients with ventricular arrhythmias. Quantitative evaluation of ventricular systolic function is particularly important in these patients.

Embolic Event
■ An intracardiac thrombus or mass may result in a systemic embolic event.
■ Aortic atheroma are present in 20% of patients with an embolic event.
■ The presence of a patent foramen ovale or atrial septal aneurysm has been associated with an increased prevalence of systemic embolic events.

Key points:
❑ A systemic transthoracic examination is the first step in evaluation for a potential cardiac source of embolus, but transesophageal echocardiography (TEE) is a more sensitive diagnostic approach.
❑ Conditions associated with systemic embolic events include:
   ❑ Atrial fibrillation

- ❏ Left atrial thrombus
- ❏ Prosthetic heart valves
- ❏ Valvular vegetations (bacterial or nonbacterial thrombotic endocarditis)
- ❏ Patent foramen ovale
- ❏ Atrial septal aneurysm
- ❏ Aortic atheroma
- ❏ LV thrombus (e.g., after anterior myocardial infarction)
- ❏ Left-sided cardiac tumors (atrial myxoma, valve fibroelastoma)
- ❏ In patients with a systemic embolic event, a cardiac source is the presumptive cause when there is atrial fibrillation, a prosthetic valve, an intracardiac thrombus, or tumor.
- ❏ A cause–effect relationship between the cardiac finding and embolic event is more difficult to establish in individual patients with common conditions, such as a patent foramen ovale or aortic atheroma.
- ❏ Diagnosis of a patent foramen ovale is based on demonstration of right to left shunting at rest or with Valsalva's maneuver, using right heart saline contrast. TEE is more sensitive than transthoracic echocardiography for detection of a patent foramen ovale, which is present in about 30% of normal individuals.

Fever/Bacteremia

- ■ Echocardiography is the primary approach to diagnosis of endocarditis in patients with bacteremia (Fig. 5–6).
- ■ In most patients, transthoracic echocardiography is the initial approach, but TEE is more sensitive for detection of valvular vegetations.
- ■ Complications of endocarditis (abscess, fistula, etc.) are best evaluated by TEE.

Key points:

- ❏ Detection of valvular vegetations is a major criterion for diagnosis of endocarditis.
- ❏ Specificity of transthoracic echocardiography for detection of a vegetation is high (i.e., the finding of a vegetation is diagnostic), but sensitivity is low so that failure to demonstrate a vegetation does not "rule out" the diagnosis.

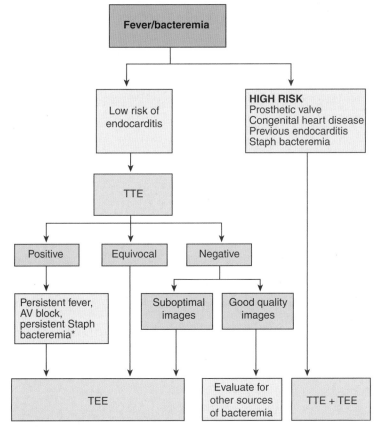

Figure 5–6 Flowchart for a suggested approach to evaluation of patients with fever or bacteremia who are referred for echocardiography. *Or other signs of paravalvular abscess or persistent infection. *AV,* Atrioventricular; *TEE,* transesophageal echocardiography; *TTE,* transthoracic echocardiography. *(Modified from Otto CM: Valvular Heart Disease, 2nd ed. Philadelphia: Elsevier, 2003)*

❑ When bacteremia or other clinical signs of endocarditis are present, TEE is appropriate unless the likelihood of endocarditis is very low and image quality is high on transthoracic imaging.

❑ Both transthoracic and transesophageal echocardiography are appropriate with suspected prosthetic valve endocarditis, because posterior structures are shadowed by the prosthetic valve on transthoracic imaging, whereas anterior structures are shadowed on transesophageal imaging.

❑ Detection of vegetations is enhanced by scanning across the valve, using multiple-image planes, and using nonstandard views, on both transthoracic and transesophageal imaging.

NOTES

SELF-ASSESSMENT QUESTIONS

QUESTION 1

A 36-year-old man with a known bicuspid aortic valve presents with fever and malaise for 2 weeks. His cardiac physical examination is unchanged, with a soft aortic regurgitant murmur and no signs of heart failure. His ECG is remarkable only for LV hypertrophy. Blood cultures are pending. Transthoracic echocardiography shows no valvular vegetations with excellent image quality. The most appropriate management strategy at this point is:

A. Await blood culture results
B. Schedule a repeat echocardiography in 2 weeks
C. Transesophageal echocardiography
D. Stress echocardiography
E. Contrast echocardiography

QUESTION 2

A 24-year-old pregnant woman is referred for evaluation of a murmur. Echocardiography shows normal ventricular size and systolic function. Valve anatomy appears normal on two-dimensional (2D) imaging, but there is trace to mild mitral regurgitation, mild tricuspid regurgitation, and mild pulmonic regurgitation. The antegrade aortic flow velocity is 1.3 m/s, and the pulmonary artery antegrade velocity is 1.2 m/s.

The most likely cause of the murmur appreciated on physical examination is:

A. Mitral regurgitation
B. Aortic stenosis
C. Tricuspid regurgitation
D. Pulmonic stenosis
E. Flow murmur
F. No murmur is present

QUESTION 3

A 28-year-old man is referred for evaluation of a murmur that he says he has had all his life. On echocardiography you find a high velocity (more than 5 m/s) systolic jet of flow using the nonimaging continuous wave Doppler transducer. Aortic and mitral valve anatomy is normal, and left and right ventricular size and systolic function are normal.

The most likely cause of the murmur is:

A. Doppler artifact
B. Aortic stenosis
C. Mitral stenosis
D. Ventricular septal defect
E. Patent ductus arteriosus

QUESTION 4

Echocardiography is requested to evaluate for "heart failure" in a 64-year-old man with a 3-month history of increasing dyspnea on exertion.

Which of the following would *not* explain heart failure symptoms?

A. LV ejection fraction of 32%
B. Mitral valve stenosis
C. Aortic aneurysm
D. Pulmonary artery systolic pressure of 64 mm Hg
E. Constrictive pericarditis

QUESTION 5

A 64-year-old man presents with chest pain that has occurred intermittently over the past 2 days, with more severe pain earlier today that has now resolved. His past medical history is remarkable for a 20-year history of hypertension, current smoking, and an elevated cholesterol level. The electrocardiogram shows ST depression in the inferior leads. Echocardiography is requested and shows a left ventricular ejection fraction of 63% with normal resting wall motion. The aortic root maximum dimension is 3.4 cm with an antegrade aortic flow velocity of 1.1 m/s and trace regurgitation. There is mild posterior mitral leaflet prolapse with mild mitral regurgitation. There is no pericardial effusion.

The most likely cause of chest pain is:

A. Coronary artery disease
B. Aortic dissection
C. Mitral valve prolapse
D. Acute pericarditis
E. Aortic stenosis

ANSWERS

ANSWER 1: A

Patients with a bicuspid aortic valve have a high likelihood of endocarditis, so transthoracic echocardiography certainly was reasonable in this patient with a 2-week history of fevers. However, with excellent image quality and no evidence of valve infection, it is most appropriate to wait for results of the blood cultures before additional diagnostic tests are scheduled. If blood cultures are positive, then it would be reasonable to proceed to transesophageal imaging if the organism is *Staphylococcus aureus* or if there is evidence of persistent infection on antibiotic therapy (persistent fevers, bacteremia, atrioventricular [AV] block). With uncomplicated endocarditis and excellent image quality, a repeat echocardiogram in 2 weeks would be reasonable to monitor the effectiveness of therapy. Stress echocardiography is used to detect ischemic myocardium and would not be helpful in this patient. Contrast echocardiography would obscure, not improve, visualization of valve vegetations.

ANSWER 2: E

A benign flow murmur is present in 80% of pregnant women due to increased cardiac output during pregnancy. The murmur probably originates from increased aortic or pulmonary artery flow volumes, as evidenced by antegrade flow velocities at the upper limits of normal in this patient. Physiologic amounts of valve regurgitation, as in this example, are rarely audible with a stethoscope. Thus, this normal echocardiogram is consistent with a benign flow murmur. A cardiac murmur is the noise heard on cardiac auscultation by an experienced health care provider. A normal echocardiogram does not exclude the presence of a murmur.

ANSWER 3: D

The primary differential diagnosis of a high velocity systolic Doppler signal is aortic stenosis, mitral regurgitation, or a ventricular septal defect. Given normal valve anatomy, the most likely cause of the murmur in this patient is a ventricular septal defect. Further evaluation with color flow imaging would demonstrate the location of the small defect, with high velocity left-to-right flow caused by the much higher left than right ventricular pressure in systole. Adults with a small ventricular septal defect usually are asymptomatic with a loud murmur.

Mitral stenosis results in a diastolic murmur and abnormal diastolic flow across the mitral valve. A patent ductus arteriosus results in a continuous murmur with a corresponding flow signal in the pulmonary artery. Although sometimes a Doppler artifact might be mistaken for a flow signal, the finding of a systolic flow signal in a patient referred for a murmur is likely to be a real finding.

ANSWER 4: C

The differential diagnosis of heart failure includes left ventricular systolic dysfunction (A) and obstructive left-sided valve disease (B). In addition, low output symptoms occur with severe pulmonary hypertension (D) and with constrictive pericarditis (E) because of a small left ventricular stroke volume caused by reduced left ventricular filling volumes. An aortic aneurysm is unlikely to cause heart failure symptoms directly unless there is associated severe aortic valve regurgitation.

ANSWER 5: A

The most likely cause of chest pain in an older male with three other major cardiac risk factors is coronary artery disease. The echocardiogram does not provide any additional information to support this diagnosis but also does not suggest any other likely causes of chest pain. Resting wall motion can be normal in patients with angina between episodes of chest pain because wall motion is abnormal only *during* ischemia or after myocardial infarction. Aortic dissection is a consideration given the history of hypertension, but the aorta is normal at the level of the sinuses and the amount of aortic regurgitation is typical for age. If aortic dissection is suspected based on a more detailed history, a pulse difference between the arms on physical examination, or an abnormal chest radiograph, further evaluation with TEE, chest CT, or cardiac magnetic resonance imaging is needed because transthoracic echocardiography is not sensitive for diagnosis of aortic dissection. Mitral valve prolapse does not cause significant chest pain symptoms. Acute pericarditis is usually associated with ST elevation on ECG, and most patients have at least a small pericardial effusion. Aortic valve stenosis is not present based on imaging of the valve and the normal antegrade velocity.

Left and Right Ventricular Systolic Function

THE ECHO EXAM: SYSTOLIC FUNCTION

Global LV function	Wall thickness
	Internal dimensions/volumes
	dP/dt
	Ejection Fraction
Regional LV function	Segmental wall motion
Global RV function	RV size
	RV systolic function
Pulmonary pressures	Pulmonary systolic pressure
Cardiac output	Stroke volume (SV) and cardiac output (CO)

Example:
A 57-year-old man with a recent inferior myocardial infarction now is hypotensive. Echocardiography shows:

LV wall thickness (diastole)	7 mm
LV end-diastolic dimension	57 mm
LV end-systolic dimension	38 mm
Apical biplane ejection fraction	52%
Time interval between 1 and 3 m/s on MR-Jet	30 msec
Segmental wall motion	Akinesis of basal and mid-LV segments of inferior and infero-lateral walls
RV size	Moderately increased
RV systolic function	Severely decreased
TR-Jet velocity (V_{TR})	2.6 m/s
Inferior vena cava	Normal diameter with inspiratory change < 50%
LV outflow tract diameter ($LVOT_D$)	2.4 cm
LVOT velocity time integral ($VTIL_{VOT}$)	10 cm
Heart rate (HR)	85 bpm

The left ventricle is at the upper limits of normal in size with a mildly reduced ejection fraction and regional wall motion abnormalities consistent with a recent inferior myocardial infarction. Ejection fraction is evaluated qualitatively only when image quality is too poor for tracing endocardial borders for a biplane ejection fraction calculation.

Left ventricular dP/dt is calculated from the time interval between 1 and 3 m/s on the MR jet signal (dt) as:
$$dP/dt = [4(V_2)^2 - 4(V_1)^2]/dt = [4(3)^2 - 4(1)^2]/dt$$
$$= [36 - 4 \text{ mm Hg}]/.030 \text{ s} = 1067 \text{ mm Hg/s}$$
which is at the lower limits of normal (>1000 mm Hg/s).

RV size and systolic function are graded qualitatively. The findings of a moderately dilated RV with severe systolic dysfunction in this patient are consistent with right ventricular infarction accompanying the inferior LV infarction, as the coronary artery that supplies the LV inferior wall also often supplies the RV free wall.

Right atrial pressure is mildly elevated (estimate 10-15 mm Hg) as shown by the < 50% change in the diameter of a nondilated inferior vena cava with respiration.

Pulmonary systolic pressure (PAP) is calculated from the tricuspid regurgitant jet velocity (V_{TR}) and estimate of right atrial pressure (RAP) as:
$$PAP = 4(V_{TR})^2 + RAP = 4(2.6)^2 + 10 = 27 + 10 = 37 \text{ mm Hg}$$
This is consistent with mild pulmonary hypertension.

Cardiac output (CO) is calculated using the LVOT diameter to calculate the circular cross-sectional areas of flow:
$$CSA_{LVOT} = \pi(LVOT_D/2)^2 = 3.14(2.4/2)^2 = 4.5 \text{ cm}^2$$
Stroke volume across the aortic valve (cm^3 = ml), then is:
$$SV_{LVOT} = (CSA_{LVOT} \times VTI_{LVOT}) = 4.5 \text{ cm}^2 \times 10 \text{ cm} = 45 \text{ cm}^3$$
Cardiac output is:
$$CO = SV \times HR = 45 \text{ ml} \times 85 \text{ beats/min} = 3830 \text{ ml/min or } 3.83 \text{ L/min}$$
This low cardiac output is caused by the right ventricular infarction and explains his hypotension.

CO, *Cardiac output;* LV, *left ventricular;* MR-Jet, *mitral regurgitation jet;* RV, *right ventricular;* SV, *stroke volume.*

QUANTITATION OF LEFT AND RIGHT VENTRICULAR SYSTOLIC FUNCTION

PARAMETER	MODALITY	VIEW	RECORDING	MEASUREMENTS
Ejection fraction	2D	Apical four-chamber and two-chamber	Adjust depth, optimize endocardial definition, harmonic imaging, contrast if needed	Careful tracing of endocardial borders at end-diastole and end-systole in both views
dP/dt	CW Doppler	MR jet, usually from apex	Pt positioning and transducer angulation to obtain highest velocity MR jet, decrease velocity scale, increased sweep speed	Time interval between 1 m/s and 3 m/s on Doppler MR velocity curve
PA pressures	CW Doppler	Parasternal and apical	Pt positioning and transducer angulation to obtain highest velocity TR jet	Estimate of RA pressure from size and appearance of IVC
Cardiac output	2D and pulsed Doppler	Parasternal LVOT diameter Apical LVOT velocity time integral	Ultrasound beam perpendicular to LVOT with depth decreased and gain adjusted to see mid-systolic diameter LVOT velocity from ant. angulated A4C view with sample volume just on LV side of aortic valve	LVOT diameter from inner edge to inner edge in mid-systole, adjacent and parallel to aortic valve Trace modal velocity of LVOT spectral Doppler envelope

2D, *Two-dimensional;* A4C, *apical four-chamber;* CW, *continuous wave;* IVC, *inferior vena cava;* LV, *left ventricular;* LVOT, *left ventricular outflow tract;* MR, *mitral regurgitation;* RA, *right atrial;* PA, *pulmonary artery;* Pt, *patient;* TR, *tricuspid regurgitation.*

LEFT VENTRICULAR SYSTOLIC FUNCTION

Step 1: Measure Left Ventricular Size

Left Ventricular Chamber Dimensions

- Two-dimensional (2D)-guided M-mode measurement of left ventricular (LV) minor axis internal dimensions at end-diastole and end-systole are measured when the M-line can be oriented appropriately.
- 2D measurement of LV minor axis internal dimensions are used when the M-line is oblique.

Key points:

- ❏ LV internal dimensions are measured from the parasternal window because the ultrasound beam is perpendicular to the blood–myocardial interface, providing high axial resolution (Fig. 6–1).
- ❏ The parasternal long axis view allows verification that measurements are perpendicular to the long axis of the LV. An oblique angle may not be recognized in short axis views.
- ❏ 2D imaging in long and short axis views is used to ensure the dimension is measured in the minor axis of the ventricle (not at an oblique angle, which would overestimate size; Fig. 6–2).
- ❏ The rapid sampling rate of M-mode (compared with the slow frame rate of 2D imaging) provides more accurate identification of the endocardial borders (Fig. 6–3).
- ❏ End-diastolic measurements are made at the onset of the QRS complex; end-systolic mea-

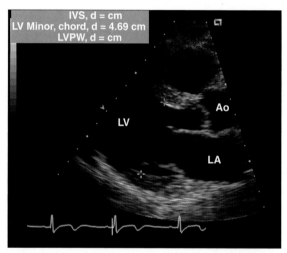

IVS, d = cm
LV Minor, chord, d = 4.69 cm
LVPW, d = cm

Ao
LV
LA

Figure 6–1 Parasternal long axis view showing two-dimensional measurement of left ventricular internal dimension at end-diastole (onset of the QRS) from the septal endocardium to the posterior wall endocardium at the level of the mitral valve chords. This minor axis dimension is measured perpendicular to the long axis of the left ventricle (*LV*).

surements are made at the minimum chamber size, just before aortic valve closure.
- ❏ Measurements are made from the leading edge of the septal endocardium to the leading edge of the posterior LV wall.
- ❏ The posterior LV wall is identified on M-mode as the steepest most continuous line. Identification of the endocardial border on 2D images is less reliable (Fig. 6–4).
- ❏ Measurements of LV internal dimensions and wall thickness are made at the level of the mitral valve chords.

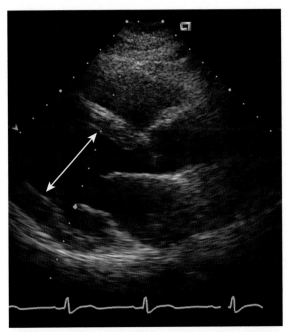

Figure 6–2 Parasternal long axis view showing that an M-mode measurement of left ventricular dimensions, along the dotted line, would overestimate ventricular size because the sample line is oblique compared with the minor axis dimension, shown by the arrows.

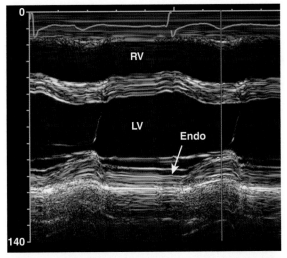

Figure 6–3 When the M-mode beam can be aligned perpendicular to the long axis of the left ventricle (LV), based on two-dimensional long and short axis views, the advantage of the M-mode recording is a high temporal sampling rate. The rapid motion of the septal and posterior wall endocardium allows precise measurements. The endocardium typically is the most continuous line with the steepest slope in systole. Measurement of the end-systolic dimension (maximum posterior motion of the septum, or minimal LV dimension) is shown.

Left Ventricular Chamber Volumes

- Endocardial borders are traced in apical four-chamber and two-chamber views at end-diastole and end-systole (Fig. 6–5).
- Volumes are calculated by the ultrasound system using the biplane method of disks.

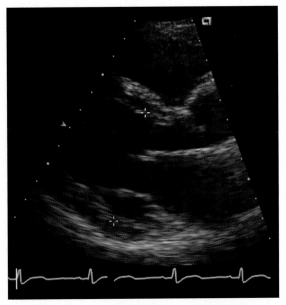

Figure 6–4 Identification of the posterior wall endocardium on a still frame end-diastolic two-dimensional image can be difficult, as shown in this example.

- LV end-diastolic and end-systolic volumes are indexed by dividing by body surface area (Table 6–1).

Key points:

- ❏ Care is needed to obtain images from a true apical position; use of a steep left lateral decubitus position with an apical cutout in the stretcher allows optimal transducer positioning.
- ❏ Depth is adjusted so the mitral annulus just fits on the image; gain and processing curves are adjusted to optimize endocardial definition.
- ❏ Left-sided echo contrast enhances recognition of endocardial borders when image quality is poor.
- ❏ End-diastolic tracings are made at the onset of the QRS (first frame on digital systems); end-systole is defined as minimal LV volume and is identified visually by frame-by-frame viewing of the images (Fig. 6–6).
- ❏ Volumes are more reflective of the degree of LV dilation than linear dimensions.
- ❏ The most common limitation of this approach is a foreshortened apical view resulting in underestimation of ventricular volumes (Fig. 6–7).
- ❏ Body surface area may not be the ideal measure of body size but is widely used clinically.

Left Ventricular Wall Thickness

- 2D-guided M-mode measurement of LV septal and posterior wall thickness at end-diastole are made from the parasternal window.

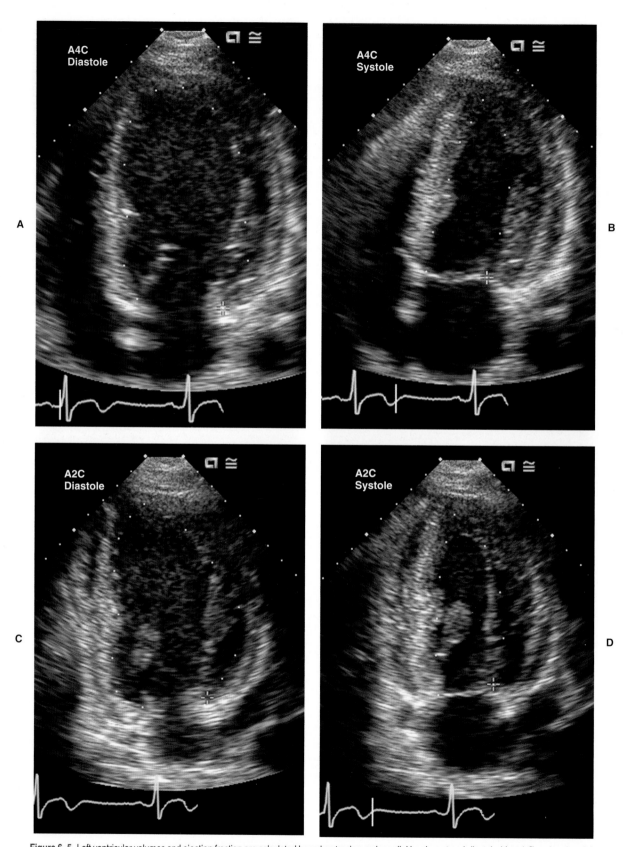

Figure 6–5 Left ventricular volumes and ejection fraction are calculated based on tracing endocardial borders at end-diastole (*A* and *C*) and end-systole (*B* and *D*) in both apical four-chamber (*A* and *B*) and apical two-chamber views (*C* and *D*). Identification of endocardial borders is optimized by playing the cine loop to show endocardial motion.

TABLE 6–1

NORMAL LEFT VENTRICULAR DIMENSIONS AND VOLUMES IN ADULTS

		END-DIASTOLE	END-SYSTOLE	SHORTENING FRACTION	EJECTION FRACTION
Minor axis dimensions (M-mode or 2D)	Women	3.9-5.3 cm		27-45%	
		2.4-3.2 cm/m²		25-43%	
	Men	4.2-5.9 cm			
		2.2-3.1 cm/m²			
Ventricular volumes (2D)	Women	56-104 mL	19-49 mL		≥55%
		35-75 mL/m²	12-30 mL/m²		
	Men	67-155 mL	22-58 mL		≥55%
		35-75 mL/m²	12-30 mL/m²		
Wall thickness	Women	0.6-0.9 cm			
	Men	0.6-1.0 cm			
LV mass	Women	66-150 g			
		44-88 g/m²			
	Men	96-200 g			
		50-102 g/m²			

2D, *Two-dimensional;* LV, *left ventricular.*
Adapted from: Lang RM et al, JASE 18:1440-1463, 2005, and other sources (for end-systolic dimensions).

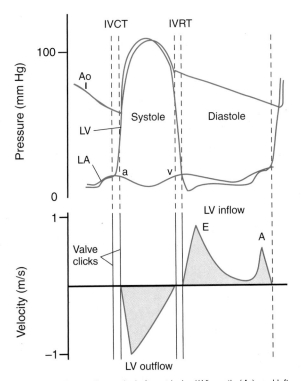

Figure 6–6 The cardiac cycle. Left ventricular (*LV*), aortic (*Ao*), and left atrial (*LA*) pressures are shown with the corresponding Doppler LV outflow and inflow velocity curves. The isovolumic contraction time (*IVCT*) represents the time between mitral valve closure and aortic valve opening, whereas the isovolumic relaxation time (*IVRT*) represents the time between aortic valve closure and mitral valve opening. *From Otto CM: Textbook of Clinical Echocardiography, 3rd ed. Philadelphia: Elsevier, 2004.*

■ 2D measurement of LV wall thickness is used when the M-line is oblique.

Key points:

❏ LV wall thickness is measured from the parasternal window, because the ultrasound beam is perpendicular to the blood–myocardial interface, providing high axial resolution (Fig. 6–8).

❏ The rapid sampling rate of M-mode (compared with the slow frame rate of 2D imaging) provides more accurate identification of the endocardial borders.

❏ Wall thickness of both the septum and posterior wall is measured at the level of the mitral valve chordae at end-diastole.

❏ The septal wall thickness measurement does not include trabeculations on the right ventricular side of the septum and does not mistake the mid-septal stripe for the right-sided endocardium.

❏ The posterior LV wall thickness is measured from the endocardium to the posterior epicardium.

Left Ventricular Mass and Wall Stress

■ LV wall thickness measurements usually are sufficient for clinical care.

■ LV mass and wall stress can be calculated from 2D images and LV pressures, if needed.

Key points:

❏ LV mass is calculated from endocardial and epicardial border tracing in a short axis view at the papillary muscle level and measurement of LV length (Fig. 6–9).

A

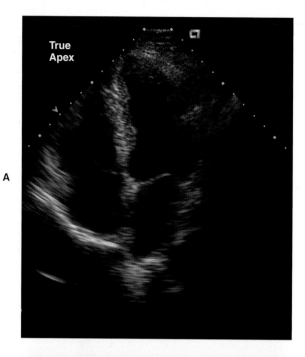

**True
Apex**

B

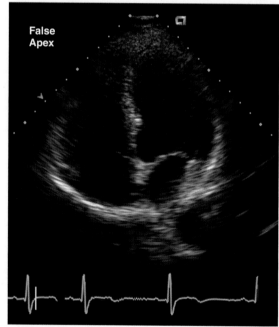

**False
Apex**

Figure 6–7 When the transducer is on the true apex of the left ventricle (LV), the chamber is ellipsoid in shape (*A*), compared with a foreshortened view (*B*), in which the ventricle appears more spherical. LV volumes will be underestimated in a foreshortened view, and apical wall motion abnormalities may be missed.

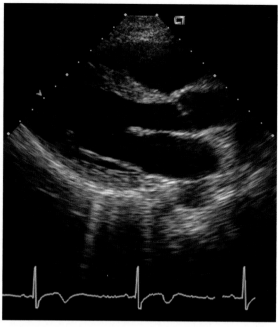

Figure 6–8 Parasternal long axis view for measurement of left ventricular wall thickness. The ultrasound beam is perpendicular to the blood–myocardial interface from this window, allowing accurate identification of the walls.

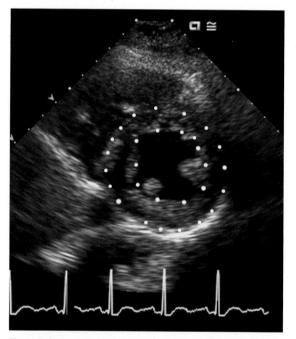

Figure 6–9 To calculate left ventricular (LV) mass, the endocardial and epicardial borders are traced in a parasternal short axis view. This provides a mean wall thickness that is used in the LV mass calculations. In clinical practice, the diagnosis of LV hypertrophy typically is based on a single linear measurement of wall thickness or quantitative assessment in multiple views. Two-dimensional quantitation of LV mass is used mainly for research applications.

- ❐ LV wall stress can be calculated based on tracing LV endocardial and epicardial borders and measuring LV systolic pressure.
- ❐ Wall thickness of both the septum and posterior wall is measured at the level of the mitral valve chordae at end-diastole.
- ❐ LV mass and wall stress calculations are mainly useful for research studies and are rarely needed for clinical decision making.
- ❐ Color Doppler strain rate imaging may be helpful as clinical guidelines are developed. This advanced topic is discussed in other textbooks (see, for example, Otto, *The Practice of Clinical Echocardiography*, 3rd ed.).

Step 2: Measure Left Ventricular Ejection Fraction

- ▪ LV ejection fraction (EF) is visually estimated based on parasternal and apical views.
- ▪ LV EF is quantitated using the apical biplane method by tracing endocardial borders at end-diastole and end-systole in apical four- and two-chamber views (Fig. 6–10).
- ▪ When the visual estimate and measured EF are similar, the measurement is reported; when there is disagreement, the measurement is repeated or only the visual estimate is reported (if image quality precludes accurate border tracing).

Key points:

- ❐ LV EF is visually estimated based on parasternal short axis and apical four-chamber, two-chamber, and long axis views. Estimates by an experienced observer are very reliable.
- ❐ LV EF is calculated from end-diastolic volume (EDV) and end-systolic volume (ESV) as:

$$EF = [(EDV - ESV) / EDV] \times 100\%$$

- ❐ When the visual estimate disagrees with the measured EF, the traced endocardial borders are reviewed to ensure the correct transducer positioning and image planes and accurate identification of the endocardium (Fig. 6–11).
- ❐ When image quality is suboptimal, left-sided contrast may enhance identification of endocardial borders.
- ❐ When quantitation of EF is not needed or is limited by image quality, the visual estimate

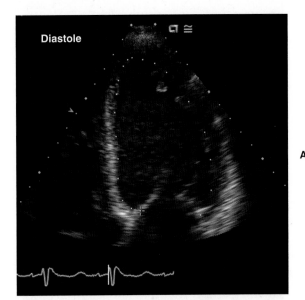

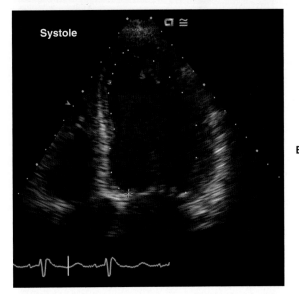

Biplane apical

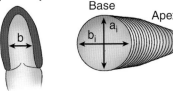

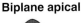

Base   Apex

Figure 6–10 Illustration of the apical biplane formula for left ventricular volume calculations showing the two-dimensional echocardiographic views and measurements on the left and the geometric model on the right. Endocardial borders are traced in apical four-chamber and two-chamber views, which are used to define a series of orthogonal diameters (*a* and *b*). A "Simpson's rule" assumption based on stacked disks is used to calculate volume. *From Otto CM: Textbook of Clinical Echocardiography, 3rd ed. Philadelphia: Elsevier, 2004.*

Figure 6–11 Endocardial borders were retraced by the physician interpreting this study to ensure that the calculated ejection fraction was accurate when the visual estimate appeared different from the initial measurements. The endocardial borders at end-diastole (*A*) and end-systole (*B*) in the apical four-chamber view are shown in this patient with severely reduced systolic function and a calculated ejection fraction of 16%.

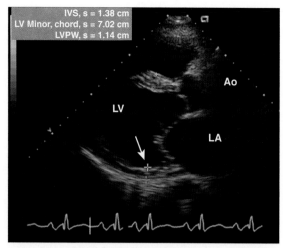
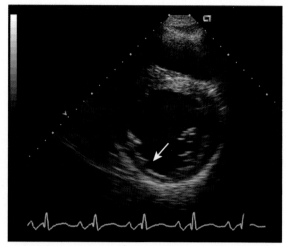

IVS, s = 1.38 cm
LV Minor, chord, s = 7.02 cm
LVPW, s = 1.14 cm

Ao

LV

LA

A

B

Figure 6–12 In these parasternal long axis (A) and short axis (B) views, the inferior and inferior-lateral (or posterior) left ventricular (LV) walls are thin compared with the septum, consistent with a previous inferior myocardial infarction.

is reported, along with a descriptive scale as follows:
Normal (EF > 55%)
Mildly reduced (EF 40-55%)
Moderately reduced (EF 20-40%)
Severely reduced (EF < 20%)

Step 3: Evaluate Regional Ventricular Function

- Regional (or segmental) ventricular function is evaluated as detailed in Chapter 8.
- Wall motion and thickening for each myocardial segment is graded as normal, hypokinetic, or akinetic.
- Any areas of thinning and increased echogenicity (consistent with scar) are noted (Fig. 6–12).

Key points:

- ❏ The presence of wall motion abnormalities in a pattern corresponding to coronary artery perfusion suggests ischemic cardiac disease.
- ❏ In a short axis view, the inferior wall may normally flatten along the diaphragm in diastole (with normal systolic motion); this normal pattern should not be mistaken as a wall motion abnormality.
- ❏ Optimal endocardial definition is needed to evaluate regional function.
- ❏ Wall thickening, as well as endocardial motion, should be evaluated for each myocardial segment.

Step 4: Calculate Left Ventricular Stroke Volume and Cardiac Output

- Stroke volume calculations are not a routine part of every examination but are helpful when ventricular function is abnormal and when

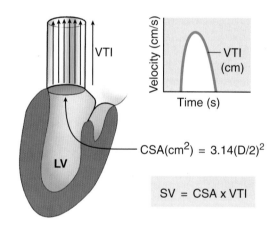

VTI

VTI (cm)

Velocity (cm/s)

Time (s)

$CSA(cm^2) = 3.14(D/2)^2$

LV

$SV = CSA \times VTI$

Figure 6–13 Doppler stroke volume calculation. The cross-sectional area (CSA) of flow is calculated as a circle based on a two-dimensional echo diameter (D) measurement. The length of the cylinder of blood ejected through this cross-sectional area on a single beat is the velocity-time integral (VTI) of the Doppler curve. Stroke volume (SV) then is calculated as CSA × VTI. From Otto CM: Textbook of Clinical Echocardiography, 3rd ed. Philadelphia: Elsevier, 2004.

valve regurgitation or an intracardiac shunt is present.
- Stroke volume (SV in cubic centimeters or milliliters) is the product of the cross-sectional area of flow (CSA in square centimeters) multiplied by the velocity time integral (VTI in centimeters) of flow at that site (Fig. 6–13):

$$SV = CSA \times VTI$$

- Stroke volume can be calculated at any site where diameter and velocity can be measured but most often is measured in the LV outflow tract, just proximal to the aortic valve.

■ Cardiac output (CO in liters per minute) is stroke volume (in milliliters) times heart rate (beats per minute), divided by 1000 ml/L:

$$CO = [SV(ml) \times \text{heart rate (beats/min)}]/ \\ 1000 \ ml/L = L/min$$

Key points:

□ LV outflow tract diameter (D) is measured from a parasternal long axis view in mid-systole, from inner edge to inner edge, immediately adjacent to the base of the aortic valve leaflets (Fig. 6–14).

□ Cross-sectional area is calculated as the area of a circle: $CSA = \pi(\text{radius})^2 = 3.14(D/2)^2$.

□ LV outflow velocity is recorded using pulsed Doppler, with a 2-3 mm sample volume length, from the apical window with the sample volume just proximal to the aortic valve (Fig. 6–15).

□ A visible aortic valve closing (but not opening) click on the Doppler tracing ensures correct sample volume placement.

□ The modal velocity (darkest part of the velocity curve) is traced to obtain the VTI.

□ The VTI represents the "stroke distance" or the length of cylinder of blood ejected by the left ventricle on each beat.

□ A similar approach can be used to calculate stroke volume across the mitral annulus or the pulmonic valve.

□ A normal stroke volume is about 60, and a normal cardiac output is about 5 L/min.

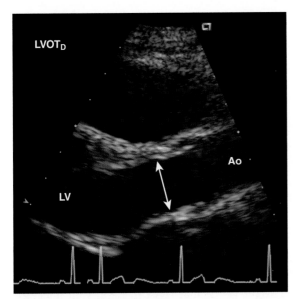

Figure 6–14 Left ventricular (*LV*) outflow tract diameter is measured in a parasternal long axis view (for axial resolution) in mid-systole using zoom mode. The diameter is measured at the base of the open aortic valve leaflets from the inner edge of the septal endocardium to the inner edge of the anterior mitral leaflet, as shown.

Step 5: Calculate Left Ventricular dP/dt

■ The rate of rise of ventricle pressure, or change in pressure (dP) over time (dt), is a load-independent measure of ventricular function.

■ LV dP/dt can be calculated from the rise in velocity of the mitral regurgitant jet (Fig. 6–16).

■ This measurement is useful in select patients with evidence of ventricular dysfunction or with significant mitral regurgitation.

Key points:

□ The time interval (dt) between the points on the mitral regurgitant velocity curve at 1 and 3 m/s is measured in seconds (Fig. 6–17).

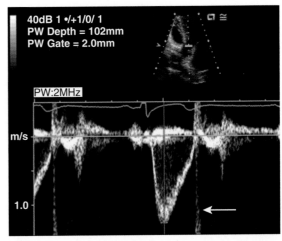

Figure 6–15 The left ventricular outflow velocity curve is recorded from the apical window, so the ultrasound beam is parallel to the direction of flow, with the 2-3 mm sample volume on the left ventricular side of the valve. Appropriate positioning is confirmed by the presence of an aortic valve closing click (arrow) but no opening click. The Doppler curve should show a narrow band of velocities with a clearly defined peak. The velocity time integral is measured by tracing the modal velocity of the systolic flow signal.

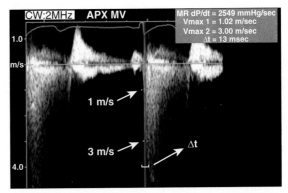

Figure 6–16 The rate of rise of left ventricular pressure in early systole is calculated by measuring the time integral between 1 and 3 m/s on the mitral regurgitant Doppler velocity curve. The pressure difference corresponding to a change in velocity from 1 to 3 m/s (32 mm Hg) is divided by this time in seconds. In this example, the dP/dt is 32 mm Hg divided by 0.013 sec (13 milliseconds), which equals 2549 mm Hg/sec.

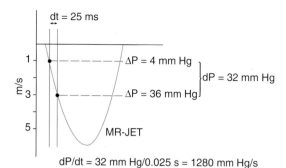

dP/dt = 32 mm Hg/0.025 s = 1280 mm Hg/s

Figure 6–17 Schematic diagram showing measurement of dP/dt from the mitral regurgitation velocity curve. The points where the velocity reaches 1 m/s and 3 m/s are identified and the time interval (*dt*) between these two points is measured as shown. The pressure difference (*dP*) between 1 m/s (4 mm Hg) and 3 m/s (36 mm Hg) is 32 mm Hg, so dP/dt is calculated as shown.

□ The pressure difference (dP) between 1 and 3 m/s, calculated using the Bernoulli equation, is $4(3)^2 - 4(1)^2 = 32$ mm Hg.

□ Thus dP/dt is 32 mm Hg divided by the time interval in seconds.

□ A normal dP/dt is more than 1000 mm Hg/s.

Step 6: Other Measures of Left Ventricular Systolic Function

■ Other signs of LV systolic function that are not independently diagnostic may aid in recognition of abnormal function and prompt quantitative evaluation of ventricular function.

■ These findings include increased E-point septal separation, aortic root anterior–posterior motion, and mitral annular apical motion.

Key points:

□ The distance between the most anterior motion of the mitral leaflet and the most posterior motion of the septum normally is only 0-5 mm. An increased mitral E-point to septal separation occurs with LV dilation or systolic dysfunction, aortic regurgitation, or mitral stenosis. This finding is best appreciated on M-mode tracings (Fig. 6–18).

□ The movement of the aortic root in an anterior–posterior direction on M-mode reflects the filling and emptying of the left atrium, which is confined between the aortic root and spine. A decrease in atrial filling and emptying, for example, with a low forward stroke volume, results in decreased motion of the aortic root (Fig. 6–19).

□ Ventricular contraction occurs along the long axis of the ventricle, in addition to circumferential shortening. The mitral annulus moves apically with longitudinal contraction of the left ventricle, with the magnitude of motion

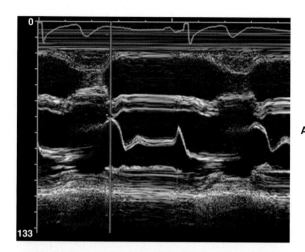

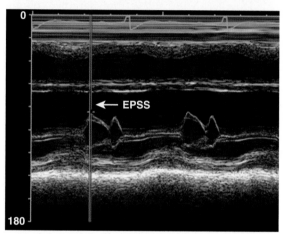

Figure 6–18 The vertical distance between the maximum anterior motion of the mitral leaflet (E-point) and the maximum posterior motion of the septum, or E-point septal separation (*EPSS*), reflects left ventricular (LV) size and systolic function. The normal EPSS is <5 mm. A larger separation indicates LV dilation or systolic dysfunction. The EPSS also is increased with aortic regurgitation due to impingement of the regurgitant jet on the anterior mitral leaflet, and with mitral stenosis, due to restricted motion of the mitral leaflet. Examples of a normal (*A*) and increased (*B*) E-point separation (due to a low LV ejection fraction) are shown.

reflecting ventricular function. Reduced apical motion of the annulus (<8 mm) indicates an ejection fraction of <50% (Fig. 6–20).

RIGHT VENTRICULAR SYSTOLIC FUNCTION

Step 1: Evaluate Right Ventricular Chamber Size and Wall Thickness

■ Right ventricular (RV) size and wall thickness are evaluated from multiple views, including parasternal short axis and RV inflow views, the apical four-chamber view, and the subcostal four-chamber view.

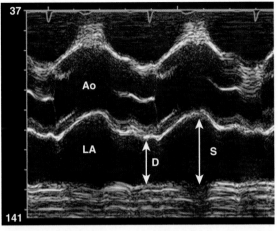
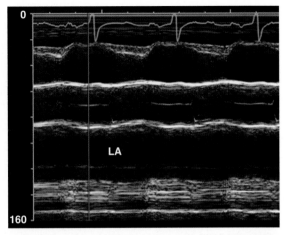

Figure 6–19 Left atrial (*LA*) filling in systole (*S*) results in anterior motion of the aortic root because LA expansion is constrained posteriorly by the spine. An example of normal aortic root motion on M-mode in a patient with normal LA filling and emptying and a normal cardiac output (*A*) is compared with the reduced aortic root motion seen in a patient with severe left ventricular dysfunction (*B*) and reduced LA filling and emptying. Conversely, aortic root motion may be increased when significant mitral regurgitation is present. *D*, Diastole.

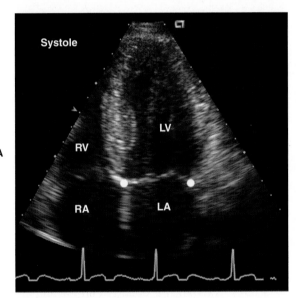
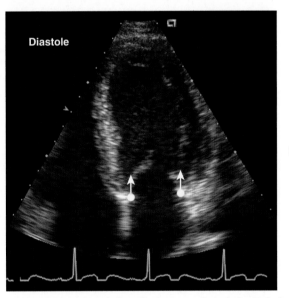

Figure 6–20 The distance the mitral annulus moves toward the left ventricular (*LV*) apex in systole, as indicated by the arrow, reflects the longitudinal shortening of the ventricle. This measurement is similar to the tissue Doppler systolic velocity at the annulus.

■ RV size is graded qualitatively as normal (RV < LV, with the RV apex more basal than the LV apex), mildly enlarged (enlarged but RV < LV), moderately enlarged (RV = LV), and severely enlarged (RV > LV).

■ RV wall thickness is evaluated qualitatively, or free wall thickness can be measured.

Key points (Table 6–2):

❏ The best views for evaluation of RV size are an apical four-chamber view tilted toward the right ventricle and a subcostal four-chamber view (Figs. 6–21*A* and *B*).

❏ RV size may be overestimated if the apical view is foreshortened, if the transducer is medial to the LV apex, or if the free wall of the RV is not well visualized.

❏ The subcostal view provides the most reliable estimate of RV size, because the ultra-

TABLE 6–2

NORMAL RIGHT VENTRICULAR DIMENSIONS IN ADULTS

Mid-RV diameter	2.7-3.3 cm
RV outflow tract diameter	2.5-2.9 cm
RV free wall thickness	<0.5 cm

RV, *Right-ventricular.*
Data from: Lang RM et al, *JASE 18:1440-1463, 2005.*

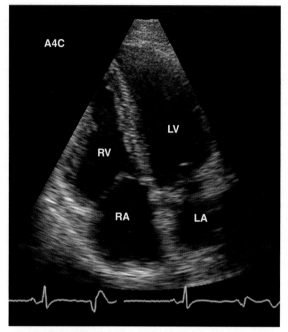 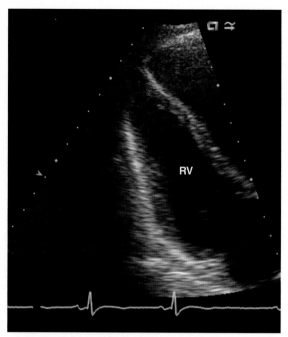

Figure 6–21 Evaluation of right ventricular (*RV*) size and systolic function is performed (*A*) in the apical four-chamber view (note that the transducer is correctly located over the left ventricular [*LV*] apex) and in (*B*) a zoom view with the transducer tilted toward the RV.

sound beam is perpendicular to the RV free wall and ventricular septum.
- ❏ RV hypertrophy is seen when the RV free wall is larger than 5 mm or when the RV wall appears as thick as the LV wall (Fig. 6–22).

Step 2: Examine the Pattern of Ventricular Septal Motion

- ■ Ventricular septal motion is evaluated in 2D parasternal long and short axis images.
- ■ M-mode evaluation of ventricular septal motion may be helpful in some cases.

Key points:

- ❏ With right ventricular volume overload, the ventricular septum is flattened in diastole, but in systole the LV assumes the normal circular configuration (Fig. 6–23).
- ❏ With RV pressure overload, the ventricular septum remains flattened or reversed in systole so that the LV assumes a D-shape in the short axis view (Figs. 6–24 and 6–25).
- ❏ The pattern of ventricular septal motion is also altered by conduction abnormalities, previous cardiac surgery, and pericardial disease.

Step 3: Estimate Right Ventricular Systolic Contraction

- ■ RV systolic function is assessed from multiple views, including parasternal short axis and RV

inflow views, the apical four-chamber view, and the subcostal four-chamber view.
- ■ RV systolic function is graded qualitatively as normal or mildly, moderately, or severely reduced.

Key points:

- ❏ The best views for evaluation of RV systolic function are an apical four-chamber view tilted toward the right ventricle and a subcostal four-chamber view.
- ❏ RV systolic function can be graded in comparison with LV systolic function.
- ❏ If LV systolic function is reduced and the right ventricle looks similar to the left ventricle, the degree of dysfunction is similar.
- ❏ The subcostal view provides the most reliable estimate of RV systolic function, because the ultrasound beam is perpendicular to the RV free wall and ventricular septum.

Step 4: Calculate Pulmonary Systolic Pressure

- ■ Noninvasive calculation of pulmonary systolic pressures is possible in more than 80% of transthoracic echocardiograms.
- ■ The RV–to–right atrial (RA) systolic pressure gradient is calculated from the maximum velocity in the tricuspid regurgitant jet (TR-Jet) using the Bernoulli equation: $\Delta P_{RV-RA} = 4 \ (TR\text{-Jet})^2$ (Fig. 6–26).

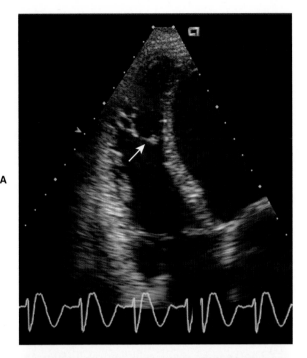

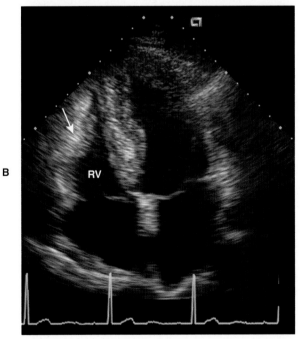

Figure 6–22 The right ventricular (*RV*) free wall normally is thinner than the left ventricular wall, although prominent trabeculations and the moderator band (*arrow*) may be appreciated, as seen in this patient with mild RV dilation (*A*). An increased thickness (*arrow*) of the RV free wall (*B*) is seen in this patient with pulmonary hypertension.

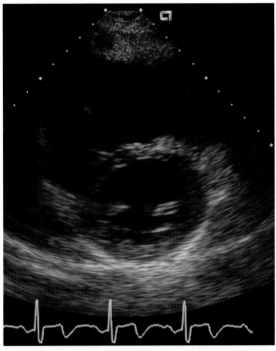

Figure 6–23 With right ventricular volume overload, the right ventricle is enlarged and septal motion is flat in diastole. However, in systole the contour of the septum is normal, as seen here, with a circular shape of the left ventricle in a short axis view.

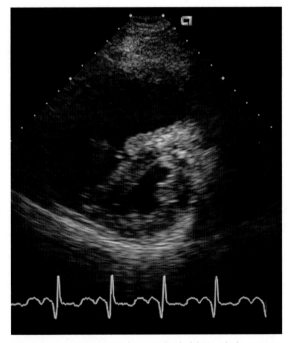

Figure 6–24 In contrast to volume overload, right ventricular pressure overload results in septal flattening in both diastole and in systole, as seen here.

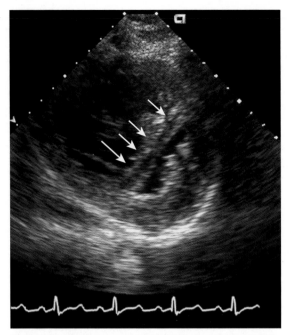

Figure 6–25 With more severe right ventricular pressure overload, the left ventricle appears compressed due to the systolic motion (*arrows*) of the septum toward the left ventricle in systole.

■ Right atrial pressure (RAP), estimated from the size and respiratory variation in the inferior vena cava, is added to this pressure gradient to determine right ventricular systolic pressure (Table 6–3).

Key points:

❑ In the absence of pulmonic valve stenosis, right ventricular and pulmonary systolic pressures are the same.

❑ When pulmonic stenosis is present, pulmonary systolic pressure is calculated by subtracting the RV–to–pulmonary artery gradient from the estimated RV systolic pressure.

❑ A diligent search for the highest tricuspid regurgitant jet velocity includes continuous wave (CW) Doppler recording from parasternal and apical views. The highest signal obtained is the most parallel to jet direction.

❑ Signal strength may be enhanced by repositioning the patient or having the patient hold his or her breath at end expiration or in mid-inspiration.

❑ The Doppler scale, gain, and wall filters are adjusted to show a gray scale spectrum with

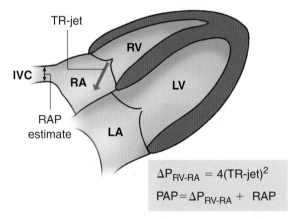

$$\Delta P_{RV\text{-}RA} = 4(TR\text{-jet})^2$$

$$PAP = \Delta P_{RV\text{-}RA} + RAP$$

Figure 6–26 Pulmonary artery pressure (*PAP*) can be calculated noninvasively based on the velocity in the tricuspid regurgitant (*TR*) jet and the respiratory variation in inferior vena cava (*IVC*) size as an estimate of right atrial pressure (*RAP*). *LA*, Left atrium; *LV*, left ventricle; *RA*, right atrium; *RV*, right ventricle. *From Otto CM: Textbook of Clinical Echocardiography, 3rd ed. Philadelphia: Elsevier, 2004.*

TABLE 6–3

ESTIMATION OF RIGHT ATRIAL PRESSURE

IVC	CHANGE WITH RESPIRATION OR "SNIFF"	ESTIMATED RIGHT ATRIAL PRESSURE
Small (<1.5 cm)	Collapse	0-5 mm Hg
Normal (1.5-2.5 cm)	Decrease by >50%	5-10 mm Hg
Normal	Decrease by <50%	10-15 mm Hg
Dilated (>2.5 cm)	Decrease <50%	15-20 mm Hg
Dilated with dilated hepatic veins	No change	>20 mm Hg

From Otto CM: Textbook of Clinical Echocardiography, 3rd ed. Philadelphia: Elsevier, 2004.

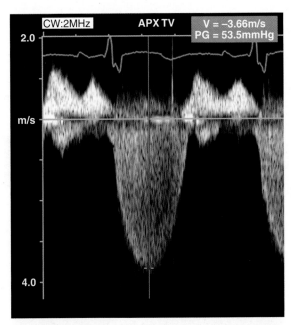

Figure 6–27 Tricuspid regurgitant jet recorded with continuous wave Doppler showing a smooth velocity curve with a dark edge and a well-defined peak velocity. Although these characteristics are consistent with a high signal-to-noise ratio, they do not exclude the possibility of underestimation of velocity caused by a nonparallel intercept angle between the flow direction and Doppler beam.

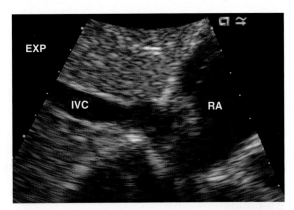

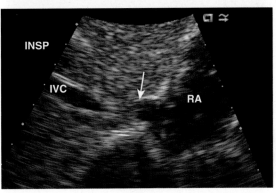

Figure 6–28 Right atrial pressure is estimated from zoom views of the inferior vena cava (*IVC*) from the subcostal window. The size of the inferior vena cava at the caval–right atrial (*RA*) junction during expiration (*EXP, A*; 1.8 cm in this case) and the change in size during inspiration (*INSP, B*) or with a sniff (>50% in this case) indicate the right atrial pressure, as shown in Table 6–3 (5-10 mm Hg in this example).

a dense outer edge and smooth systolic curve (Fig. 6–27).

☐ Estimation of RA pressure from the respiratory variation in the inferior vena cava is only useful in spontaneously breathing patients. In ventilated patients, a measured central venous pressure is used or an estimated range of pulmonary pressures is provided (Fig. 6–28).

NOTES

SELF-ASSESSMENT QUESTIONS

QUESTION 1

In a 62-year-old man with a dilated cardiomyopathy referred for echocardiography, heart rate is 80 bpm with a blood pressure of 100/60 mm Hg. Ventricular volumes, measured by tracing endocardial borders in the apical four-chamber and two-chamber views, were 180 ml in diastole and 120 ml in systole.

Calculate:
LV ejection fraction: _____
LV stroke volume: _____
Cardiac output: _____

QUESTION 2

A schematic of a mitral regurgitant velocity curve on an expanded time scale is shown in Figure 6–29. Calculate the left ventricular dP/dt from this curve.

QUESTION 3

In a patient in the intensive care unit, the LV outflow tract was imaged from a parasternal long axis view with the outflow tract diameter measured at 2.2 cm. The LV outflow tract pulsed Doppler signal from the apical view is shown in Figure 6–30.

Calculate:
Stroke volume: _____
Cardiac output: _____

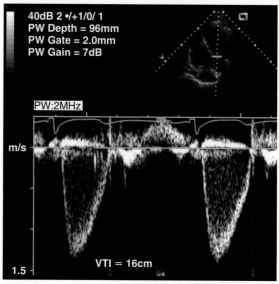

Figure 6–30

QUESTION 4

A 32-year-old woman with primary pulmonary hypertension is referred for follow-up of her pulmonary pressures. In addition to tricuspid regurgitant jet velocity, the following information is needed to estimate pulmonary systolic pressure in this patient:

    A. RV free wall thickness
    B. Mitral regurgitation maximum velocity
    C. Imaging of the inferior vena cava
    D. Hepatic vein flow
    E. Antegrade velocity in the pulmonary artery

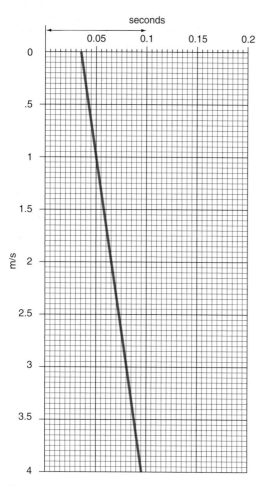

Figure 6–29

QUESTION 5

In a patient with a congenital heart disease, the maximum tricuspid regurgitant velocity is 4.0 m/s, the antegrade velocity in the pulmonary artery is 2.8 m/s, and the inferior vena cava and hepatic veins are dilated with no change in diameter with respiration. The estimated pulmonary systolic pressure is:

    A. >75 mm Hg
    B. 50-75 mm Hg
    C. 25-50 mm Hg
    D. <25 mm Hg
    E. Cannot be determined from this information

QUESTION 6

A 27-year-old woman presents with a 3-week history of a viral upper respiratory infection followed by persistent shortness of breath. Her lungs are found to be congested on examination, and echocardiography is requested. The M-mode tracing from that study, shown in Figure 6–31, is most consistent with:

    A. Mitral valve prolapse
    B. Aortic stenosis
    C. Pericardial effusion
    D. Dilated cardiomyopathy
    E. Severe pulmonary hypertension

QUESTION 7

A quantitative ejection fraction has been requested for an obese patient with poor endocardial definition. Which of the following is most likely to be helpful for improving endocardial definition?

    A. An increased imaging depth
    B. A lower frame rate
    C. Fundamental imaging
    D. A steep left lateral decubitus position
    E. Lower gain settings

QUESTION 8

The M-mode tracing in Figure 6–32 is most consistent with:

    A. Pulmonary hypertension
    B. Atrial septal defect
    C. Left ventricular hypertrophy
    D. Dilated cardiomyopathy
    E. Previous open heart surgery

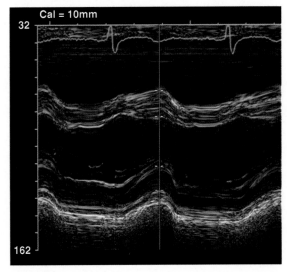

Figure 6–32

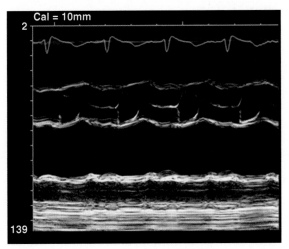

Figure 6–31

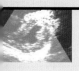

ANSWER 1

The LV stroke volume is end-diastolic volume minus end-systolic volume (180 ml − 120 ml = 60 ml), and ejection fraction is stroke volume divided by end-diastolic volume (60 ml/180 ml = 33%). Cardiac output is stroke volume times heart rate (60 ml × 80 bpm = 4800 ml/min = 4.8 L/min). Despite a low ejection fraction, forward cardiac output is adequate due to compensatory left ventricular dilation.

ANSWER 2

The points on the regurgitant velocity curve corresponding to 1 and 3 m/s are identified, and a vertical line is drawn through each of these points. The time interval between these two lines is 7 small boxes (each 5 ms), or 35 ms, which equals 0.035 seconds. As the mitral regurgitant velocity increased from 1 m/s to 3 m/s, the transmitral pressure increased from 4 to 36 mm Hg, indicating a rise in LV pressure (dP) of 32 mm Hg. The rate of rise in pressure (dP/dt) then is 32 mm Hg divided by 0.035 s, or 900 mm Hg/s. A normal dP/dt is more than 1000 mm Hg/s. Lower values indicate progressively more severe LV systolic dysfunction.

ANSWER 3

The LV outflow tract radius is $\frac{1}{2}$ the diameter, or 1.1 cm. Cross-sectional area (CSA) is calculated as the area of a circle (CSA = πr^2), so CSA is $3.14(1.1)^2 = 3.8$ cm^2 . Stroke volume is CSA times the velocity time integral (16 cm), so stroke volume is 3.8 cm^2 × 16 cm = 61 cm^3 or 61 mL. Cardiac output is stroke volume times heart rate. Heart rate is calculated by dividing 60 seconds/minute by the R-R interval on the ECG (in seconds). In this case, heart rate is 60/0.9 = 67 bpm. Cardiac output is then 4.07 L/min.

ANSWER 4: C

Pulmonary systolic pressure is estimated based on the RV–to–RA systolic pressure difference, calculated from the tricuspid regurgitant jet, using the Bernoulli equation. This pressure difference is added to the estimated RA pressure to determine RV (or pulmonary artery) systolic pressure. RA pressure is estimated from the size and respiratory variation of the inferior vena cava.

Although RV free wall thickness is likely to be increased when pulmonary hypertension is pres-

ent, it does not provide a numerical estimate of pulmonary pressure. The mitral regurgitation velocity reflects the LV to left atrial systolic pressure difference and is not helpful for estimating pulmonary pressures. Hepatic vein flow patterns correspond to the pattern of RA filling and are helpful in evaluation of pericardial and tricuspid valve disease but do not indicate the RA pressure. The antegrade velocity in the pulmonary artery would be important if pulmonary valve stenosis was present, because in this situation the RV–to–pulmonary artery systolic pressure gradient needs to be subtracted from the estimated RV pressure to obtain pulmonary pressures. However, this patient has primary pulmonary hypertension, not congenital heart disease.

ANSWER 5: B

The RV-to-RA pressure difference is $4(4)^2$ or 64 mm Hg. The estimated RA pressure (see Table 6–3) is at least 20 mm Hg, but RV systolic pressure is more than 84 mm Hg. However, there is mild pulmonic stenosis with a maximum gradient of $4(2.8)^2$ or 31 mm Hg. Subtracting the pulmonic valve gradient from the estimated RV systolic pressure indicates a pulmonary systolic pressure of about 53 mm Hg.

ANSWER 6: D

This M-mode tracing of the aortic root and left atrium shows decreased anterior–posterior motion of the aortic root consistent with a low cardiac output. Thus the most likely diagnosis is a dilated cardiomyopathy. The left atrium is mildly enlarged, compared with the size of the aortic root. There is no evidence of mitral valve prolapse as this is a recording of the aortic valve. Aortic stenosis is not present because the thin aortic leaflets show normal systolic opening. The echo-free space posterior to the left atrium is the descending aorta. Although pericardial fluid occasionally extends behind the left atrium, it is more typical to detect pericardial fluid posterior to the left ventricle. No conclusions about pulmonary pressures can be made from this tracing.

ANSWER 7: D

Endocardial definition on echocardiographic imaging is improved with optimal patient positioning. Use of a stretcher with an apical cutout with the patient in a steep left lateral decubitus position provides close contact between the LV apex and the chest wall with improved ultrasound tissue penetration. Instrument settings to optimize endocardial definition include a decreased depth of interrogation, a higher frame rate, use of harmonic (not fundamental) imaging, and adjusting gain, dynamic range, and the time-gain compensation curve to improve the image. The highest transducer frequency with adequate tissue penetration is used. In difficult cases, some echocardiographers find B-color imaging helpful. In many cases, the use of left-sided echo-contrast is needed to evaluate LV systolic function.

ANSWER 8: A

This M-mode tracing at the mid-ventricular level shows "paradoxical" septal motion, defined as systolic motion of the septum anteriorly in the chest, instead of toward the center of the left ventricle.

This tracing is most consistent with RV pressure overload caused by severe pulmonary hypertension. The RV chamber size is markedly increased, the free wall of the RV is increased in thickness (faintly seen at the top of the tracing), the septum thickens and moves anteriorly in systole, and the septum moves toward the LV and is flattened in diastole.

In contrast, with RV volume overload, as with an atrial septal defect, ventricular motion in diastole is also flattened but systolic motion is relatively normal. With LV hypertrophy, LV wall thickness is increased but septal motion is relatively normal. With dilated cardiomyopathy, the LV chamber is dilated and the pattern of septal motion reflects concurrent pulmonary hypertension or RV dysfunction. In patients with previous cardiac surgery, although systolic thickening of the septal myocardium is normal, the septum shifts anteriorly, resulting in "paradoxical" septal motion with the maximum anterior motion of the septum in late systole with the normal diastolic motion of the septum resulting in a very "flat" appearance of septal motion on M-mode recordings.

NOTES

7 Ventricular Diastolic Filling and Function

THE ECHO EXAM

STEP-BY-STEP APPROACH
Measure Left Ventricular Inflow Velocities
Record Left Atrial Inflow
Record Tissue Doppler at the Mitral Annulus
Measure the Isovolumic Relaxation Time
Consider Other Useful Measurements
Integrating the Data

SELF-ASSESSMENT QUESTIONS

THE ECHO EXAM: DIASTOLIC DYSFUNCTION

PARAMETER	PHYSIOLOGIC DESCRIPTOR
Relaxation	$-dP/dt$ or tau
Compliance	dV/dt
Filling Pressure	LV-EDP or LAP or PAWP

ECHO EXAM

LEFT VENTRICULAR INFLOW AT MITRAL LEAFLET TIPS
E = Early diastolic filling velocity (m/s)
A = Filling velocity after atrial contraction (m/s)
DT = Deceleration time (msec)

LV INFLOW AT MITRAL ANNULUS
A_{dur} = duration of atrial filling velocity (msec)

MYOCARDIAL TISSUE DOPPLER AT BASE OF SEPTUM
E_m = Early diastolic filling velocity (m/s)
A_m = Filling velocity after atrial contraction (m/s)

ISOVOLUMIC RELAXATION TIME
IVRT = isovolumic relaxation time (msec)

PULMONARY VENOUS INFLOW
PV_S = Peak systolic velocity
PV_D = Peak diastolic velocity
PV_a = Peak atrial reversal velocity
a_{dur} = Pulmonary vein atrial reversal duration

Example

A 62-year-old man with amyloidosis has an echocardiogram that shows a symmetric increase in wall thickness with an ejection fraction of 52%. The following parameters of diastolic function are recorded:

E velocity	1.1 m/s
A velocity	0.6 m/s
Deceleration time (DT)	160 msec
A_{dur}	130 msec
E_M/A_M ratio	<1
IVRT	40 msec
PV_S/PV_D	<1
PV_a	0.4 m/s
a_{dur}	155

The E/A ratio is > 1, but the E_M/A_M ratio is less than 1, indicating a pattern of pseudo-normalization suggestive of moderate diastolic dysfunction with decreased compliance. Moderate diastolic dysfunction is confirmed by the short IVRT and relatively short deceleration time.

There also is evidence of elevated filling pressures with a PV_a > 0.35 m/s and with the duration of pulmonary vein atrial flow minus the duration of atrial flow at the mitral annulus > 20 msec.

DT, *Time interval from peak velocity to baseline, extrapolated from slope of diastolic deceleration curve;* EDP, *end-diastolic pressure;* IVRT, *isovolumic relaxation time;* LV, *left ventricular;* LAP, *left atrial pressure;* PAWP, *pulmonary artery wedge pressure.*

QUANTITATION OF DIASTOLIC FUNCTION

PARAMETER	MODALITY	VIEW	RECORDING	MEASUREMENTS
LV inflow at leaflet tips	Pulsed Doppler	A4C with 2-3–mm sample volume positioned at mitral leaflet tips	Parallel to flow Normal expiration Low wall filters	E and A peak velocities, DT along outer edge of spectral envelope using linear slope from peak to baseline
LV inflow at annulus	Pulsed Doppler	A4C with 2-mm sample volume at mitral annulus	Parallel to flow Normal expiration Low wall filters	A_{dur}
Myocardial tissue Doppler	Pulsed Doppler	A4C with 2-3–mm sample volume placed within basal segment of septal wall	Very low gain settings Low wall filters Decreased velocity scale	E_M and E_M/A_M
IVRT	Pulsed Doppler	Anteriorly angulated A4C with 2-3–mm sample volume midway between aortic and mitral valves	Clear aortic closing click and clear onset of transmitral flow Low wall filters	IVRT as time interval from middle of aortic closure click to onset of mitral flow
Pulmonary venous inflow	Pulsed Doppler (color to guide location)	Right superior pulmonary vein in A4C view using color flow to visualize flow	2-3–mm sample volume 1-2 cm into pulmonary vein	PV_a, a_{dur}, and relative ratio of S/D

DT, *Deceleration time;* IVRT, *isovolumic relaxation time;* LV, *left ventricular;* S/D, *ratio of pulmonary vein systolic–to–diastolic flow velocities or velocity time integrals.*

CLASSIFICATION OF DIASTOLIC DYSFUNCTION

	NORMAL	MILD	MILD-MODERATE	MODERATE	SEVERE
Pathophysiology		↓ relaxation	↓ relaxation ↑ LV-EDP	↓ relaxation ↓ compliance ↑ LV-EDP	↓ relaxation ↓↓ compliance ↑↑ LV-EDP
E/A ratio	1-2	< 1	< 1	1.0-2.0	> 2.0
E_m/A_m ratio	1-2	< 1	< 1	< 1	> 1
IVRT (msec)	50-100	> 100	Normal	↓	↓
DT (msec)	150-200	> 200	> 200	150-200	< 150
PV_S/PV_D	1	$PV_S > PV_D$	$PV_S > PV_D$	$PV_S < PV_D$	$PV_S < PV_D$
PV_a (m/s)	< 0.35	< 0.35	≥ 0.35	≥ 0.35	≥ 0.35
$a_{dur} - A_{dur}$ (msec)	< 20	< 20	≥ 20	≥ 20	≥ 20 msec

↑, *Increased;* ↓, *decreased;* DT, *deceleration time;* IVRT, *isovolumic relaxation time.*
Modified from Canadian Consensus Guidelines, Rakowki H, et al: J Am Soc Echocadiogr *9:736-760, 1996; Yamada H, et al:* J Am Soc Echocardiogr *15:1238-1244, 2002; and Redfield MM:* JAMA *289:194-202, 2003.*

STEP-BY-STEP APPROACH

Step 1: Measure Left Ventricular Inflow Velocities

- Left ventricular (LV) inflow velocities are recorded at the mitral leaflet tips and at the mitral annulus (Figs. 7–1*A* and *B*).
- Standard measurements are E-velocity and deceleration time and A-velocity and duration (Fig. 7–2).
- The normal pattern of a higher E than A velocity is reversed with impaired early diastolic relaxation, but the pattern may be "pseudo-normalized" with more severe diastolic dysfunction.

Key points:

- ❏ LV inflow velocities are recorded at the mitral leaflet tips (highest velocity signal) in the apical four-chamber view using pulsed Doppler with a sample volume of 2-2.5 mm in length.
- ❏ The Doppler scale, baseline, and gain are adjusted to show a clear velocity curve.
- ❏ Low wall filter settings allow accurate measurements that require identification of where the velocity signal intersects the baseline (Fig. 7–3).
- ❏ Recordings at the leaflet tips are used to measure E and A velocity and deceleration slope. Recordings at the annulus are used to measure A duration.
- ❏ Recording LV inflow at the mitral leaflet tips with the patient performing a Valsalva maneuver results in a decrease in preload. The decrease in preload may unmask impaired relaxation in patients with superimposed elevated filling pressures.

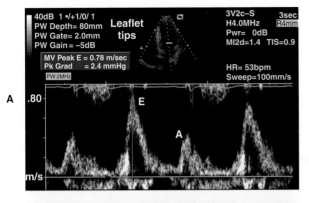

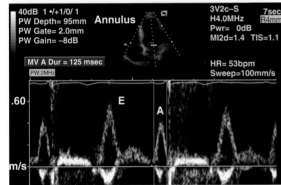

Figure 7–1 Left ventricular inflow velocities recorded using pulsed Doppler with the sample volume at the mitral leaflet tips (A) and at the mitral annulus (B).

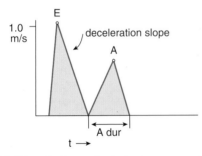

Figure 7–2 Schematic diagram showing basic measurements from the left ventricular inflow curve: the early (E) diastolic peak velocity, the velocity after atrial (A) contraction, the early diastolic deceleration slope, and the duration of the A velocity (from the recording at the annulus).

Step 2: Record Left Atrial Inflow

- Left atrial (LA) inflow velocities are recorded in the right superior pulmonary vein from an apical four-chamber view on transthoracic echocardiography (TTE) or in any pulmonary vein on transesophageal echocardiography (TEE) (Fig. 7–4).

- Standard measurements are peak systolic velocity (PV_S), peak diastolic velocity (PV_D), and the atrial velocity peak (PV_a) and duration (a_{dur}) (Fig. 7–5).

- A $PV_a > 0.35$ m/s and an a_{dur} 20 ms longer than transmitral A-duration indicate an elevated LV end-diastolic pressure.

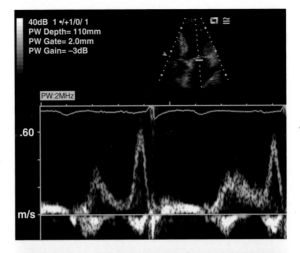

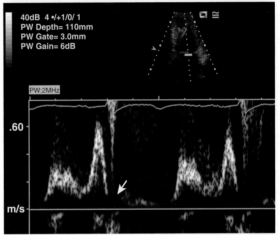

Figure 7–3 Example of left ventricular inflow recorded at the annulus with the wall filters set at a low level (indicated by the first 1 on the top line) to allow accurate timing measurements (A). When the wall filter is inappropriately high (level is set at 4), the intersection of the Doppler signal with the baseline is no longer seen (B).

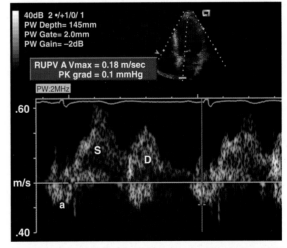

Figure 7–4 Left atrial inflow is recorded with pulsed Doppler in the right superior pulmonary vein from an apical four-chamber approach, in the same patient as Figure 7–1. With atrial contraction, there is a small atrial reversal velocity (a), with a normal pattern of systolic (S) and diastolic (D) inflow into the atrium.

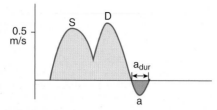

Figure 7–5 Schematic of measurements for pulmonary vein flow showing atrial (*a*) reversal peak and duration and peak systolic (*S*) and diastolic (*D*) filling velocities.

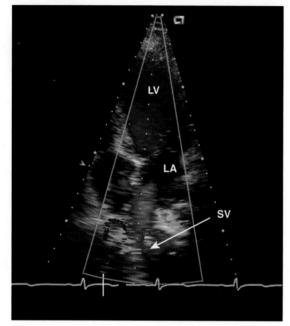

Figure 7–6 Identification of the right superior pulmonary vein from the transthoracic apical four-chamber view may be enhanced with color Doppler imaging. The pulsed Doppler sample volume (*SV, arrow*) is positioned about 1 cm into the pulmonary vein for optimal data quality.

Key points:

❑ LA inflow velocities from the transthoracic approach may be difficult to record because of poor signal strength at the depth of the pulmonary vein.

❑ Color flow imaging may be helpful in locating the pulmonary vein and optimizing sample volume position. The 2 to 3 mm length sample volume should be at least 1 cm distal to the pulmonary vein orifice (Fig. 7–6).

❑ The Doppler scale, baseline, and gain are adjusted to show a clear spectral signal.

❑ Low wall filter settings allow accurate measurements that require identification of where the velocity signal intersects the baseline.

Step 3: Record Tissue Doppler at the Mitral Annulus

■ Tissue Doppler myocardial velocities are recorded at the mitral annulus from a TTE apical approach (Fig. 7–7).

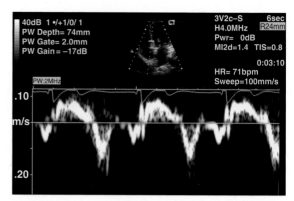

Figure 7–7 Doppler myocardial tissue velocities are recorded at the septal side of the mitral annulus using a small sample volume, with the velocity scale reduced (note that the velocity range is only 0.2 m/s), the wall filters at a low level (setting is 1), and the gain reduced to a very low level (setting is −17 dB).

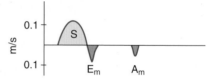

Figure 7–8 Schematic diagram of tissue Doppler measurements. The typical early (*E*) and late (*A*) tissue Doppler velocities are seen in diastole directed away from the transducer (as the ventricle fills). In systole, there is a velocity component toward the transducer corresponding to systolic contraction of the ventricle.

■ Standard measurements are the early myocardial velocity (E_M) and atrial myocardial velocity (A_M) (Fig. 7–8).

■ An E_M to A_M ratio >1.0 is normal, with a reduced ratio indicating impaired early diastolic relaxation.

■ A ratio of the transmitral E velocity to the tissue Doppler E_M velocity >15 predicts an LV end-diastolic pressure >15 mm Hg.

Key points:

❑ In the apical four-chamber view, a small (2 mm) sample volume is positioned in the myocardium about 1 cm from the mitral annulus (Fig. 7–9).

❑ The tissue Doppler instrument settings include a velocity scale of about 0.2 m/s, low gain settings, low velocity scale, and low wall filters.

❑ Tissue Doppler recordings at the septal side of the annulus are more reproducible than signals from the lateral wall (Fig. 7–10).

❑ The E_M and A_M velocities are less dependent on preload than the transmitral flow velocities.

Step 4: Measure the Isovolumic Relaxation Time

■ Pulsed Doppler is used to show the time interval between aortic valve closure and mitral

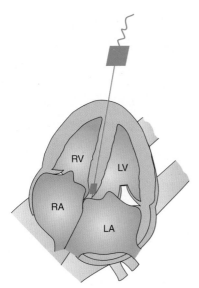

Figure 7–9 Schematic diagram showing position of the sample volume for Doppler tissue velocity recording. In the apical four-chamber view, the sample volume is placed about 1 cm apical to the medial mitral annulus.

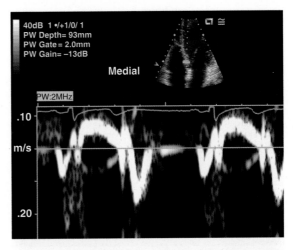

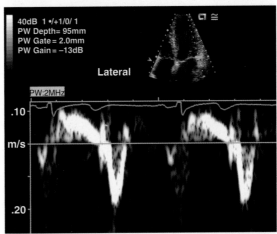

Figure 7–10 Although tissue Doppler velocities can be recorded both from the medial side of the annulus (*A*) and the lateral side (*B*), the medial annular signal tends to be more reliable for evaluation of diastolic dysfunction.

valve opening (the isovolumic relaxation time [IVRT]; Fig. 7–11).

■ The IVRT (normal 50 to 100 ms) is prolonged with impaired relaxation but is shortened with severe diastolic dysfunction and impaired compliance (Fig. 7–12).

Key points:

❏ In an anteriorly angulated four-chamber view, a 2 to 3 mm sample volume is positioned midway between aortic and mitral valves to show both LV ejection and LV filling velocity curves (Fig. 7–13).

❏ The wall filters are set at a low level to identify the end of aortic outflow and onset of mitral inflow at their intersection with the baseline.

❏ The time interval is measured in milliseconds (ms).

Step 5: Consider Other Useful Measurements

■ The diastolic slope of the apical color M-mode recording of LV inflow (the propagation velocity) reflects the rate of LV diastolic relaxation (Fig. 7–14).

■ The rate of decline in velocity of the mitral regurgitant jet at end-systole reflects the early diastolic rate of decline in LV pressure (Fig. 7–15).

Key points:

❏ These additional measures may be helpful in selected cases.

❏ Propagation velocity is measured from an apical view using a narrow sector, a depth that just includes the mitral annulus, with the

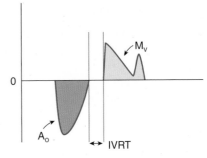

Figure 7–11 The isovolumic relation time is measured from aortic valve closure to mitral valve opening on the Doppler tracing, corresponding to the phase of the cardiac cycle where left ventricular pressure is rapidly declining but left ventricular volume is constant.

aliasing velocity set to 0.5 to 0.7 m/s, at a fast (100 to 200 mm/s) sweep speed.

❏ The early diastolic $-dP/dt$ is measured from the mitral regurgitant continuous wave (CW) Doppler curve by measuring the time interval between 3 and 1 m/s and dividing by 32 mm Hg (analogous to measurement of

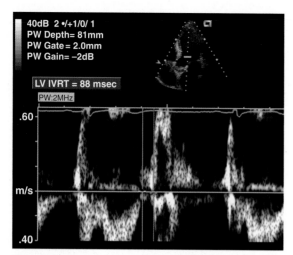

Figure 7–12 Measurement of isovolumic relaxation time (*IVRT*) as the time interval between the end of aortic antegrade flow and the onset of diastolic inflow across the mitral valve. The scale and wall filters have been adjusted to optimize identification of the onset and end of flow, at their intersection with the baseline. A rapid sweep speed (100 mm/s) is used to improve the accuracy of the measurement. In this patient, the IVRT is normal at 88 ms (normal is 50 to 100 ms).

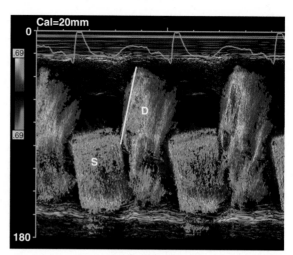

Figure 7–14 Color M-mode propagation velocity. Left ventricular (LV) inflow is recorded from an apical view using a color Doppler M-mode beam aligned along the center of the mitral annulus. Thus the vertical axis indicates distance from the left atrium (at about 160 mm depth on the scale) to the apex (at the top of the scale) with the horizontal axis indicating time, using an electrocardiogram for timing of the cardiac cycle. Flow toward the transducer in diastole represents LV filling with the slope of the edge of this signal (*line*) reflecting the velocity of the movement of blood from the annulus to the apex.

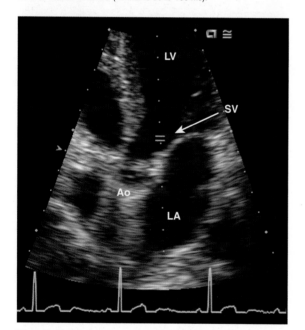

Figure 7–13 Sample volume position for recording the isovolumic relaxation time is shown. In an apical four-chamber view angulated anteriorly to include the aortic (*Ao*) valve, the sample volume (*SV*) is positioned so that it is on the left ventricular (*LV*) side of the anterior mitral leaflet in systole (to record LV outflow) and on the atrial side in diastole (to record LV inflow).

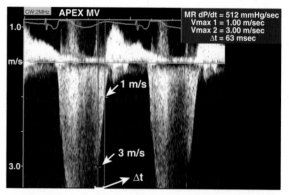

Figure 7–15 The rate of decline in left ventricular pressure (or negative dP/dt) can be measured from the mitral regurgitant jet velocity as velocity decelerates, analogous to measurement of positive dP/dt from the rate of acceleration in velocity. The pressure difference between 1 and 3 m/s (32 mm Hg) is divided by the time interval (Δ*t*, in seconds) measured between these points on the velocity curve at 1 and 3 m/s to give the −dP/dt in mm Hg/s.

+dP/dt from the early systolic part of the mitral regurgitant velocity curve).

Step 6: Integrating the Data

■ Diastolic dysfunction can be detected and graded based on integration of data from the LV filling velocities, LA filling velocities, tissue Doppler, and IVRT.

■ The clinical interpretation of the data also takes several other factors into consideration, including severity of mitral regurgitation, LV systolic function, LV wall thickness, clinical signs, and symptoms.

■ Normal diastolic function (Fig. 7–16):
  ❏ Transmitral flow shows E/A velocity ratio is 1 to 2.
  ❏ The E-deceleration time is 150 to 200 ms.
  ❏ The tissue Doppler E_M/A_M ratio is 1 to 2.
  ❏ The pulmonary vein systolic (S) to diastolic (D) flow ratio is ≥1.
  ❏ The pulmonary vein a velocity is <0.35 m/s, and duration is <20 ms longer than transmitral A duration.

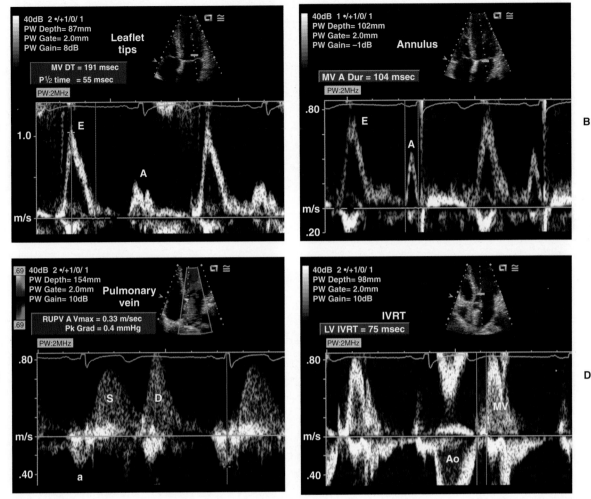

Figure 7–16 An example of normal diastolic function. *A*, The left ventricular inflow curve at the mitral leaflet tips shows a normal E and A velocity with a deceleration time of 191 msec. *B*, Inflow recorded at the annulus shows the duration of the atrial flow curve (104 msec) is the same as the duration of atrial reversal in the pulmonary vein recording (*C*). The pulmonary vein flow also shows normal systolic and diastolic inflow signals. *D*, The isovolumic relaxation time (*IVRT*) is normal at 75 msec.

■ Factors that affect LV diastolic filling, independent of diastolic function:
  ❏ At a higher heart rate (shorter diastolic filling time), the A velocity may be increased as it is superimposed on the E deceleration slope (Fig. 7–17).
  ❏ The transmitral E/A ratio decreases with age, reversing at about 50 years. Similarly, the pulmonary vein diastolic flow declines, so that the systolic to diastolic ratio increases with age.
  ❏ A higher preload increases the transmitral E velocity; hypovolemia results in a lower velocity. During the Valsalva maneuver, E velocity falls because of reduced venous return (Fig. 7–18).
  ❏ Increased transmitral volume flow caused by mitral regurgitation increases the transmitral E velocity.
  ❏ Atrial contractile function affects LV filling, LA filling, and tissue Doppler signals (Fig. 7–19).

■ Mild diastolic dysfunction (impaired relaxation; Fig. 7–20):
  ❏ Impaired relaxation is typical of mild diastolic dysfunction, due, for example, to hypertensive heart disease, ischemic disease, or an early infiltrative cardiomyopathy.
  ❏ The decreased rate of early diastolic filling is associated with a reduced E velocity (reduced E/A ratio), a reduced E_M/A_M ratio on tissue Doppler, reduced pulmonary vein diastolic flow, and a prolonged IVRT.
  ❏ LV filling pressure may be normal with mild diastolic dysfunction; therefore pulmonary vein atrial velocity and duration are normal.

■ Moderate diastolic dysfunction (pseudo-normalization; Fig. 7–21):
  ❏ Relaxation is impaired and LV filling pressures are elevated with moderate diastolic dysfunction—for example, due to dilated, hypertrophic, or restrictive cardiomyopathy.

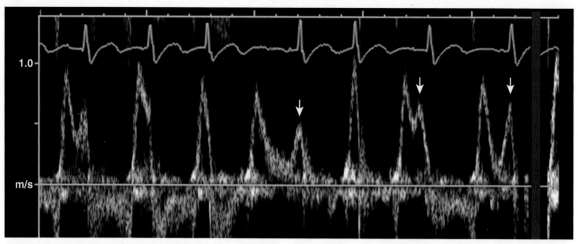

Figure 7–17 The pattern of left ventricular filling across the mitral valve in this patient with a variable R-R interval illustrates the effect of the duration of diastolic filling on the E/A ratio. Notice that the E/A ratio is >1 on the longer R-R interval and the apparent higher A velocities (*arrows*) when the A velocity is superimposed on the E deceleration slope when diastole is shorter. There is fusion of the E and A velocities on the shortest diastolic intervals.

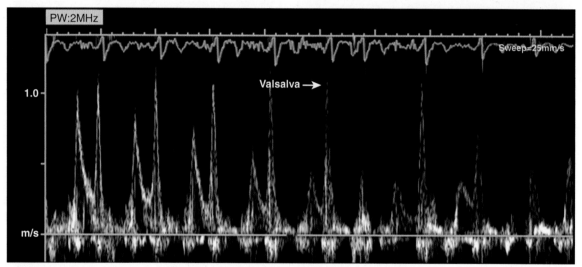

Figure 7–18 Left ventricular inflow recorded at a slow sweep speed during the Valsalva maneuver shows a gradual reduction in E velocity, caused by a relative decrease in left ventricular preload, but no change in A velocity. Thus the E/A ratio is dependent on preload.

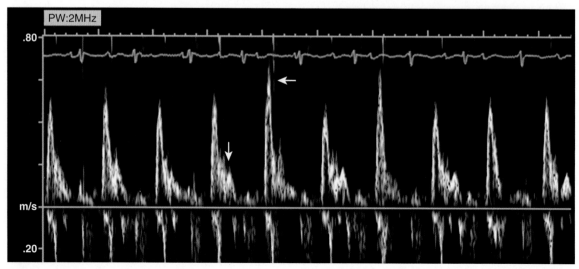

Figure 7–19 In this patient with third-degree atrioventricular block, the height of the E velocity varies with the timing of atrial contraction. When atrial contraction occurs in mid- to late diastole, a separate A velocity is seen (*horizontal arrow*), but when atrial contraction occurs in early diastole, a higher (summated) E velocity is seen (*vertical arrow*).

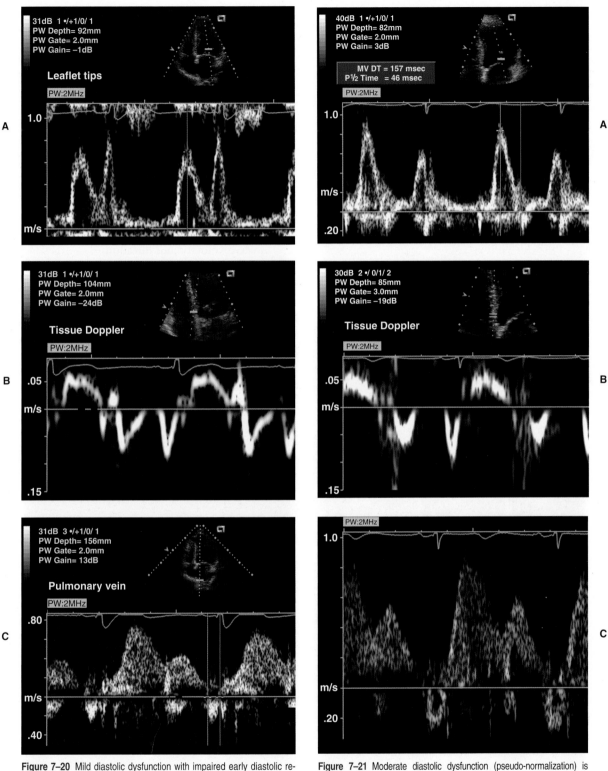

Figure 7–20 Mild diastolic dysfunction with impaired early diastolic relaxation is characterized by (*A*) an E/A ratio of <1 on the left ventricular inflow curve, (*B*) a tissue Doppler early-to-late diastolic velocity ratio of <1, and (*C*) a pulmonary vein flow curve with a reduced diastolic inflow curve but a relatively normal atrial reversal velocity and duration.

Figure 7–21 Moderate diastolic dysfunction (pseudo-normalization) is characterized by (*A*) a mitral inflow curve with an E/A velocity between 1 and 2 but a relatively steep deceleration time (longer than 150 msec) and (*B*) a tissue Doppler E_M/A_M of <1. Typically, the pulmonary vein flow signal shows greater systolic than diastolic flow and a prolonged duration and increased velocity of the atrial reversal. However, in this case the pulmonary venous flow signal (*C*) does not show these features, suggesting the degree of diastolic function falls between mild-moderate and moderate (pseudo-normal), as shown in the classification in the Echo Exam tables.

❒ In addition to the findings seen with mild diastolic dysfunction, there is evidence for elevated filling pressures, including a higher peak (>0.35 m/s) and duration of the pulmonary vein A velocity, an increased E/E_M ratio (>15), and a shortened E velocity deceleration time.

❒ The LV filling velocity shows an apparently normal E/A ratio of 1:2 (pseudo-normal) that is distinguished from a true normal by the tissue Doppler showing an E_M/A_M of <1 and a shortened E velocity deceleration time.

❒ The change in the transmitral flow pattern with Valsalva maneuver also can be used to identify a pseudo-normal transmitral flow pattern–the E velocity decreases with pseudo-normalization.

■ Severe diastolic dysfunction (decreased compliance Fig. 7–22):

❒ Severe diastolic dysfunction is characterized by decreased compliance, in addition to impaired relaxation and an elevated filling pressure.

❒ Decreased compliance means there is a greater increase in LV pressure for a given increase in LV volume compared with a normal ventricle.

❒ Although the E/A ratio is >2 and the E_M/A_M ratio is >1, severe diastolic dysfunction is differentiated from normal by the higher E/A ratio, shorter IVRT, decreased deceleration time (<150 ms), blunted pulmonary vein systolic flow, and increased pulmonary a-wave velocity and duration.

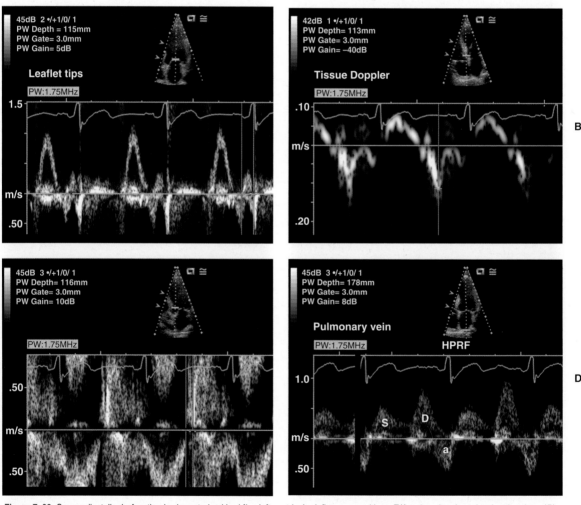

Figure 7–22 Severe diastolic dysfunction is characterized by (A) a left ventricular inflow curve with an E/A >2 and a short deceleration time, (B) a tissue Doppler E_M/A_M >1, (C) a short isovolumic relaxation time, and (D) reduced systolic flow compared with diastolic flow in the pulmonary vein with a pulmonary vein A reversal that is prolonged (>20 msec longer than transmitral A duration) and increased in velocity (≥0.35 m/s).

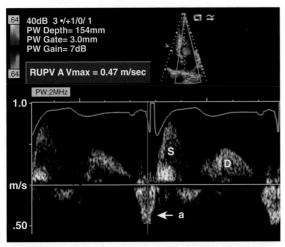

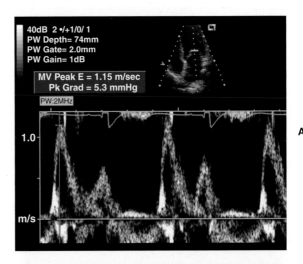

A

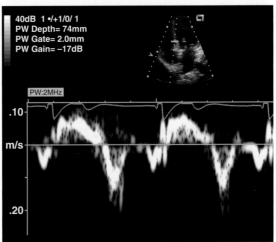

B

Figure 7–23 Pulmonary vein recording in a patient with hypertrophic cardiomyopathy and severe diastolic dysfunction. The diastolic inflow velocity is reduced compared with systolic flow. The atrial reversal duration is prolonged, with an elevated velocity of 0.47 m/s. These findings suggest markedly elevated left ventricular filling pressures.

Figure 7–24 Another marker of an elevated left ventricular filling pressure is a ratio of the transmitral E velocity (*A*) to myocardial tissue Doppler velocity (*B*) >15. In this example, the ratio is 1.15 to 0.15, or 7.7, suggesting normal filling pressures.

- Left atrial pressure estimates:
  - Exact measurement of LA (or LV filling) pressure is not possible with echocardiography, but several parameters suggest significant elevation of LA pressures:
    - Pulmonary vein atrial reversal velocity (PV_a) >0.35 m/s (Fig. 7–23)
    - Pulmonary vein atrial reversal duration (a_{dur}) at least 20 ms longer than transmitral A duration (A_{dur}) recorded at the mitral annulus
    - Ratio of transmitral E velocity to myocardial tissue E_M velocity >15 (Fig. 7–24)
    - Pulmonary venous diastolic flow deceleration time <175 ms
    - E velocity deceleration time <140 ms
    - E/A ratio >2
  - When more than one parameter is consistent with elevated LA pressure, the diagnosis is more certain.

NOTES

SELF-ASSESSMENT QUESTIONS

For Questions 1-9, match each set of Doppler recordings with the most likely diagnosis. Each answer may be used once, more than once, or not at all.

Diagnoses:
- A. Normal diastolic function for age
- B. Impaired early diastolic relaxation (mild diastolic dysfunction)
- C. Pseudo-normalization (moderate diastolic dysfunction)
- D. Decreased diastolic compliance (severe diastolic dysfunction)
- E. Elevated filling pressures
- F. Mitral regurgitation
- G. Atrial fibrillation
- H. Heart block

QUESTION 1

Diagnosis _____

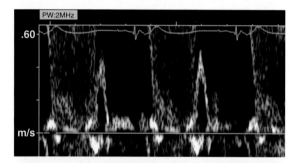

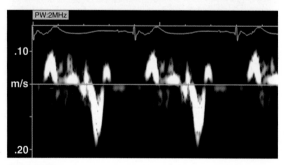

Figure 7–25

QUESTION 2

Diagnosis _____

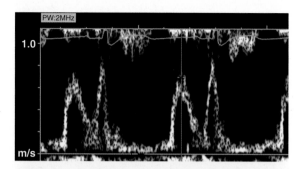

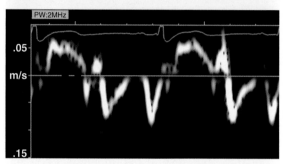

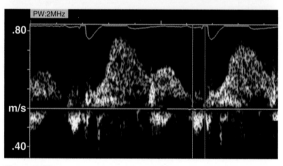

Figure 7–26

QUESTION 3

Diagnosis _____

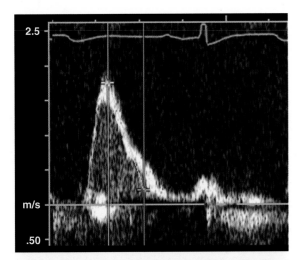

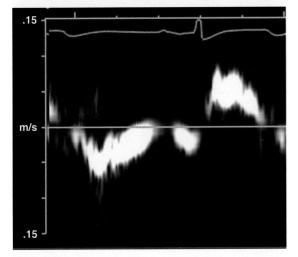

Figure 7–27

QUESTION 4

Diagnosis _____

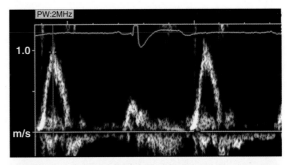

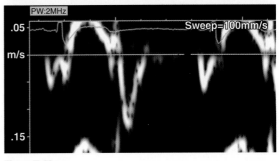

Figure 7–28

QUESTION 5

Diagnosis _____

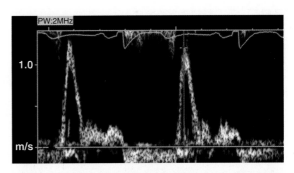

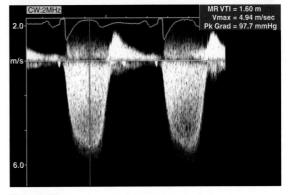

Figure 7–29

QUESTION 6

Diagnosis _____

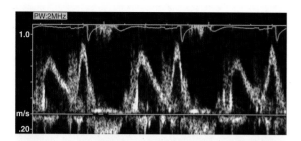

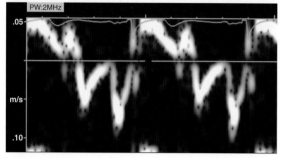

Figure 7–30

QUESTION 7

Diagnosis _____

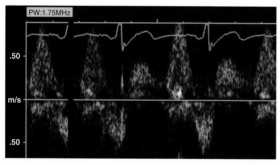

Figure 7–31

QUESTION 8

Diagnosis _____

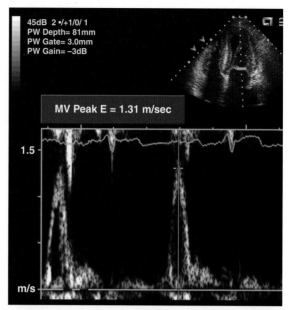

MV Peak E = 1.31 m/sec

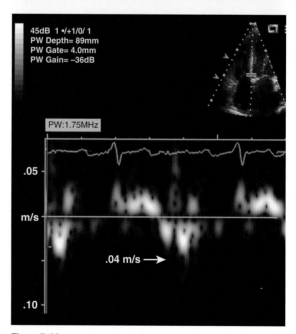

Figure 7–32

QUESTION 9

Diagnosis _____

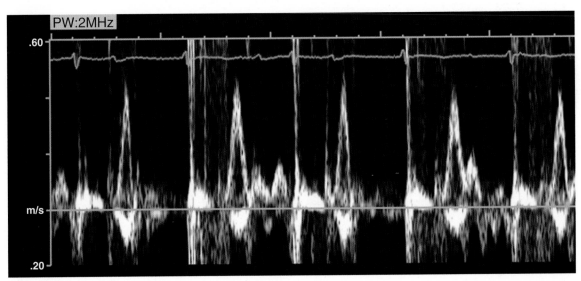

Figure 7–33

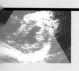

ANSWERS

ANSWER 1: G

This mitral inflow shows an E velocity of 0.5 m/s and no A velocity. This suggests atrial fibrillation. Although a small signal is seen on the electrocardiogram (ECG) where a P wave might be expected, the duration is very short. Atrial fibrillation is associated with an irregular rate, but that may be difficult to appreciate with only two beats recorded and with digital cine-loop images of only one cardiac cycle. The tissue Doppler shows an early diastolic velocity of 0.18 m/s and, again, no visible A velocity. In addition to the relatively normal E_M velocity, the E to E_M velocity ratio is only 0.5:0.18, or 2.7, which does not suggest elevated filling pressures. A longer Doppler recording would be helpful to confirm this is atrial fibrillation.

ANSWER 2: A

These tracings were recorded in a 78-year-old woman with no significant heart disease. Although this flow pattern in a younger patient (younger than 50 years) suggests impaired relaxation, here diastolic filling patterns are typical for patient age. The mitral inflow shows an E/A ratio of <1 with a relatively normal E deceleration time. The tissue Doppler shows about equal early and late diastolic filling velocities with an E/E of about 10. The pulmonary venous flow pattern demonstrates slightly blunted diastolic flow compared with systolic flow, but the atrial reversal is short in duration and low in velocity.

ANSWER 3: D

This mitral inflow curve shows a high E velocity (1.7 m/s) with a relatively normal deceleration time and a very small A velocity. Tissue Doppler shows an E_M that is greater than A_M, but both velocities are low, with an E_M velocity of 0.07 m/s. Thus the E to E_M ratio is 1.7:0.07, or 24. These findings suggest that the mitral inflow pattern is not normal, but instead represents severe diastolic dysfunction with decreased compliance and an elevated filling pressure.

ANSWER 4: A

These left ventricular inflow and tissue Doppler signals were recorded in a young, healthy individual. The LV inflow shows an E/A of more than 1 and a normal deceleration time. The tissue Doppler also shows a normal pattern of early versus late diastolic velocities.

ANSWER 5: F

When significant mitral regurgitation is present, as shown by the CW Doppler regurgitant jet with a dense systolic signal, the transmitral E velocity is higher because of an increased antegrade volume flow rate across the mitral valve in diastole. The A velocity is relatively low compared with this higher E velocity. Evaluation of diastolic function is problematic based on mitral E and A velocities with mitral regurgitation present.

ANSWER 6: B

This figure shows transmitral and tissue Doppler flow signals. These Doppler flows are most consistent with impaired diastolic relaxation (early diastolic dysfunction) with a transmitral E velocity less than A velocity and a slow diastolic deceleration slope. The tissue Doppler signal confirms an E_M less than A_M, again consistent with impaired relaxation. This could be further evaluated with pulmonary vein flows, which are expected to show reduced diastolic inflow compared with systolic inflow.

ANSWER 7: E

This pulmonary vein flow pattern shows a reduced diastolic compared with systolic inflow signal. In addition, the atrial reversal velocity has a long duration and high velocity. An atrial reversal velocity duration at least 20 ms longer than the transmitral A velocity, with a velocity >0.35 m/s, indicate an elevated (>15 mm Hg) left ventricular end-diastolic pressure.

ANSWER 8: D

This patient has both severe diastolic dysfunction (decreased compliance) and elevated filling pressures. The mitral inflow shows an E velocity of 1.3 m/s with a steep deceleration slope and no evident A velocity. The tissue Doppler shows an E_M velocity of 0.04 m/s resulting in an E/E_M ratio of 1.3:0.04, or 32. An E/E_M ratio >15 indicates a left ventricular filling pressure of >15 mm Hg, whereas an E/E_M of <8 is consistent with a normal LV end-diastolic pressure. This

32-year-old woman had acute rejection after heart transplant at the time of this recording. The ECG shows a P wave, but there is no appreciable A velocity on either the mitral inflow or tissue Doppler tracing. It is unclear whether this is the result of severe diastolic dysfunction or of ineffective atrial contraction.

ANSWER 9: H

This transmitral flow Doppler tracing shows an E velocity of about 0.4 m/s in early diastole after each QRS signal. In late diastole, the first beat shows no A velocity, the second beats shows a mid-diastolic signal followed by a 0.1 m/s A velocity, the third beat shows no A velocity, and the fourth beat shows an A velocity right after the E velocity. Also, notice there is some variation in the height and duration of the E velocity. These findings are consistent with complete heart block with an atrial rate of 100 beats per minute and a ventricular rate of 60 beats per minute. In the center of the ECG tracing, find the P waves on either side of the third QRS complex. Using this P-to-P interval as the reference, note that the P waves on the ECG and the A velocities on the Doppler tracing "march out" and have no consistent relationship to the QRS complex. Some of the atrial contractions occur during early diastole (resulting in a higher E velocity), some occur during ventricular systole (resulting in no A velocity because the mitral valve is closed), and others occur in late diastole.

NOTES

8 Ischemic Cardiac Disease

THE ECHO EXAM: ISCHEMIC CARDIAC DISEASE

MYOCARDIAL ISCHEMIA
Stress Echo Modalities
Treadmill exercise
Supine bicycle
Dobutamine

Digital Cine-Loop Views
Short axis mid-cavity
Apical four-chamber
Apical two-chamber
Apical long axis

Interpretation
Exercise duration
Heart rate and blood pressure
Symptoms
Wall motion at rest and with stress
Ejection fraction at rest and with stress

Utility
Diagnosis of coronary artery disease
Severity of disease
    Number of vessels involved
    Extent of myocardium at risk
Overall LV systolic function
Diastolic LV function
Clinical prognosis

ACUTE MYOCARDIAL INFARCTION
Detection of wall motion abnormalities
Evaluation of recurrent chest pain
Assessment of the response to reperfusion
Complications of acute myocardial infarction
    LV systolic dysfunction
    LV thrombus
    Aneurysm formation
    Acute mitral regurgitation
    Ventricular septal defect
    LV rupture (pseudoaneurysm)
    Pericardial effusion

LV PSEUDOANEURYSM
Abrupt transition from normal myocardium to aneurysm
Acute angle between myocardium and aneurysm
Narrow neck
Ratio of neck diameter to aneurysm diameter < 0.5
May be lined with thrombus

END-STAGE ISCHEMIC DISEASE
LV Systolic Dysfunction
Decreased ejection fraction
Decreased dP/dt
Regional pattern may be seen

RV SYSTOLIC DYSFUNCTION
May be present if RV infarction or
    if pulmonary pressures elevated

MITRAL REGURGITATION (MR)
Diverse mechanisms of ischemic MR
    LV dilation and systolic dysfunction
    Regional wall motion abnormality
    Papillary muscle dysfunction or rupture
Quantitate severity (see Chapter 12)

LV ANEURYSM AND THROMBUS FORMATION

STRESS ECHOCARDIOGRAPHY

PARAMETER	MODALITY	VIEW	RECORDING	INTERPRETATION
Resting regional wall motion	2D	PSAX mid-cavity level Apical four-chamber Apical two-chamber Apical long-axis	Depth that includes only LV, optimize endocardial definition, use contrast if needed	Select optimal image from series of digital cine loops for quad-screen cine-loop format
Stress regional wall motion	2D	PSAX mid-cavity level Apical four-chamber Apical two-chamber Apical long-axis	Same depth as baseline, optimize endocardial definition, use contrast if needed	Compare optimal baseline and stress images in same views
Clinical and hemodynamic data		Symptoms Heart rate and rhythm Blood pressure	Continuous during exam, report values at each stage of stress	Maximal work load affects accuracy of echo results for detection of ischemia
LV systolic function	2D Doppler	Ejection fraction dP/dt	See section on systolic function for details	

2D, *Two-dimensional;* LV, *left ventricular;* PSAX, *parasternal short axis.*

REVIEW OF CORONARY ANATOMY AND LEFT VENTRICULAR WALL SEGMENTS

■ Evaluation of coronary artery disease by echocardiography is based on visualization of endocardial motion and wall thickening.
■ For description of regional myocardial function, the left ventricle is divided into segments that correspond to the coronary artery blood supply (Fig. 8–1).
■ Myocardial infarction results in thinning and akinesis of the affected regions. With myocardial ischemia, wall motion may be normal at rest.

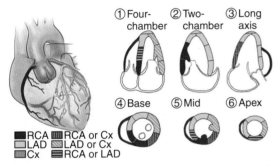

Figure 8–1 Typical coronary artery distribution of blood flow shown in the apical and parasternal short axis views. *Cx,* Circumflex; *LAD,* left anterior descending; *RCA,* right coronary artery. *From Lang RM, Bierig M, Devereux RB, et al: J Am Soc Echocardiogr 18(12):1440-1463, 2005.*

■ The ostia of the right and left main coronary arteries often can be identified, but direct visualization of distal coronary anatomy by echocardiography is limited (Figs. 8–2 and 8–3).

Key points:

❏ The ventricle is divided into basal, mid-ventricular, and apical segments, plus the tip of the apex.
❏ A distal coronary stenosis results in apical abnormalities, a mid-coronary lesion results in mid-ventricular and apical wall motion changes, and proximal coronary disease results in abnormalities that extend from the base to the apex.
❏ In the short axis plane, the ventricle is divided into six segments: anterior, anterior-lateral, inferior-lateral, inferior, inferior-septal, and anterior-septal.
❏ The left anterior descending coronary supplies the entire anterior wall and anterior septum and typically extends to supply the apical segment of the inferior septum and the tip of the apex.
❏ The right coronary artery supplies the basal and mid-ventricular segments of the inferior septum and the entire inferior wall and sometimes supplies the inferior-lateral wall.
❏ The circumflex coronary artery supplies the entire anterior-lateral and inferior-lateral wall.

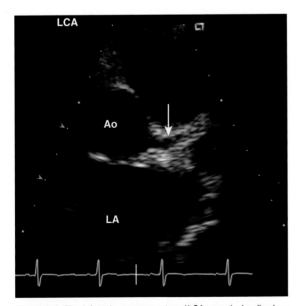

Figure 8–2 The left main coronary artery (*LCA, arrow*) visualized on transthoracic echocardiography arising from the aorta (*Ao*) anterior to the left atrium (*LA*) in a transthoracic parasternal short axis view just above the aortic valve plane.

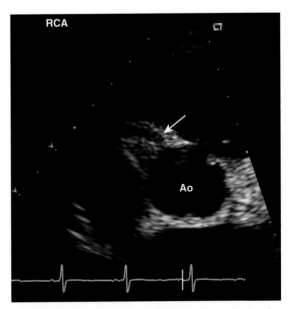

Figure 8–3 The right coronary artery (*RCA, arrow*) is seen in a transthoracic parasternal short axis view arising from the aorta (*Ao*) by slight adjustment of the image plane.

STEP-BY-STEP APPROACH

Stress Echocardiography

Basic Principles

- Left ventricular (LV) global and regional function is normal at rest, even when significant coronary artery disease is present.
- With an increase in myocardial oxygen demand, myocardial ischemia is evidenced by reversible regional hypokinesis or akinesis.
- The basis of stress echocardiography is comparison of images of the left ventricle acquired at rest and after induction of myocardial ischemia, either with exercise or pharmacologic intervention (Figs. 8–4 and 8–5).

Key points:

- ❏ The accuracy of stress echocardiography correlates with the stress load achieved. Typically, the goal is a peak heart rate at least 85% of the patient's maximum predicted heart rate.
- ❏ Comparison of resting and stress images is facilitated by acquiring images in a cine-loop format, gated from the onset of the QRS to include the same number of frames for each image.
- ❏ Because ischemia may be induced with the stress protocol, appropriate medical supervision and monitoring is essential for patient safety and to promptly treat any complications of the procedure.

Step 1: Prepare for the Stress Echo

- The patient is instructed to refrain from taking beta-blocking medications the day before and day of the stress test.

- The reason for the stress study and the patient history are reviewed, followed by a directed physical examination.
- Informed consent is obtained for either exercise or pharmacologic stress echo.
- Patient monitoring includes continuous 12-lead electrocardiography (ECG) monitoring (with a recording at each stress stage) and intermittent blood pressure measurement under the supervision of a qualified medical professional, in a procedure room with resuscitation equipment and medications readily available.
- When needed, an intravenous line is placed for infusion of dobutamine or use of contrast agents.

Key points:

- ❏ Any potential contraindications or risk factors for the stress study are identified and discussed with the referring health care provider before beginning the test.
- ❏ The risks and benefits of the stress echo study are discussed with the patient, in the context of the patient's medical history and cardiac function.
- ❏ Because the cardiac sonographer's attention is focused on image acquisition, patient monitoring typically is performed by an additional health care professional.
- ❏ The rationale for a pharmacologic versus exercise stress is reviewed. Usually, exercise stress

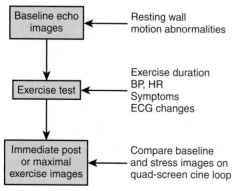

Figure 8–4 Flow chart of treadmill stress echocardiography. *BP,* Blood pressure; *ECG,* electrocardiography; *HR,* heart rate.

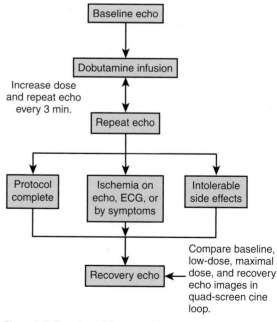

Figure 8–5 Flow chart of the protocol for dobutamine stress echocardiography. *ECG,* Electrocardiography.

is preferred because of the additional information gained regarding hemodynamics and symptoms.

❏ Pharmacologic (usually dobutamine) stress echo is preferred in patients unable to walk on a treadmill or use a supine bicycle due to orthopedic or vascular problems and in some specific patient subgroups, such as patients who have received a heart transplant.

Step 2: Evaluate Regional and Global Left Ventricular Systolic Function at Rest

■ LV global and regional function is evaluated in parasternal long and short axis views and in apical four-chamber, two-chamber, and long axis views (Fig. 8–6).

■ The function for each myocardial segment is graded as hyperdynamic, normal, hypokinetic, akinetic, or dyskinetic based on the degree of endocardial motion and wall thickening (Table 8–1).

■ Overall LV ejection fraction is visually estimated or (preferably) measured using the apical biplane approach.

Key points:

❏ The four standard views (with the long axis view from the apical or parasternal window, whichever is best) are recorded in cine-loop format. A beat with clear definition of endocardial borders and optimal image plane alignment is chosen for each view.

❏ Depth is reduced to maximize LV image size, including the mitral annulus, but not the left atrium. The same depth and sector width is used for the stress images.

❏ If endocardial definition is suboptimal, left-sided echo contrast is used to improve evaluation of regional endocardial motion (Fig. 8–7).

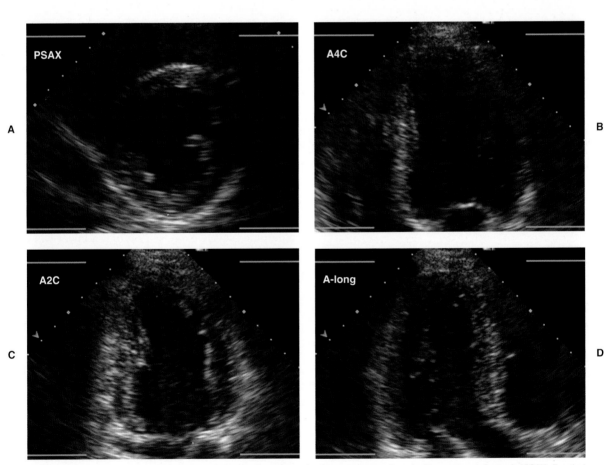

Figure 8–6 Images of the left ventricle are recorded at baseline using a cine-loop quad-screen format, with parasternal short axis (*PSAX, A*), apical 4-chamber (*A4C, B*), apical 2-chamber (*A2C, C*), and apical (or parasternal) long axis (*A-long, D*) views. Several beats are acquired, and the best image saved. The cine loop only includes only systole to allow matching with the stress images. Images are again acquired at peak stress (with dobutamine) or immediately post-stress (with exercise) in the same image planes. The rest and exercise images are then matched by view to allow comparison of the same myocardial segments on side-by-side views. Because a set number of frames are recorded and there is little change in the duration of systole with stress, the rest and exercise images move at the same speed, despite the difference in heart rates.

TABLE 8–1

QUALITATIVE SCALE FOR ASSESSMENT OF SEGMENTAL WALL MOTION ON ECHOCARDIOGRAPHY

SCORE*	WALL MOTION	DEFINITION
1	Normal	Normal endocardial inward motion and wall thickening in systole
2	Hypokinesis	Reduced endocardial motion and wall thickening in systole
3	Akinesis	Absence of inward endocardial motion or wall thickening in systole
4	Dyskinesis	Outward motion or "bulging" of the segment in systole, usually associated with thin, scarred myocardium

*A score of 0 may be used for hyperkinesis, defined as increased endocardial inward motion and wall thickening in systole.

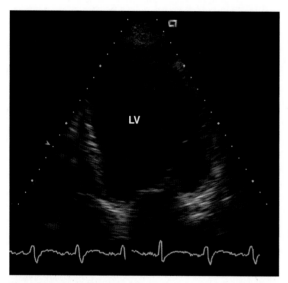
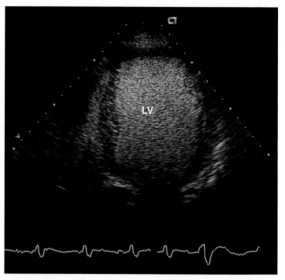

A   **B**

Figure 8–7 When endocardial definition is suboptimal (*A*), echo contrast enhancement is used (*B*) to improve evaluation of regional and global function with stress echocardiography.

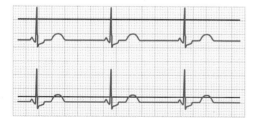

Figure 8–8 *Top,* Schematic of an appropriate electrocardiography (ECG) signal with little noise and a QRS height greater than the T wave, allowing accurate triggering for digital image acquisition and (*bottom*) an example with the T wave equal in height to the QRS signal so that both signals will trigger image acquisition, resulting in very short cine loops that do not include the full cardiac cycle.

❏ The ECG leads and gain are adjusted to show a clear signal with an adequate QRS height for accurate ECG gating (Fig. 8–8).

Step 3: Perform the Stress Protocol

Exercise stress

■ Any standard exercise protocol can be used with ECG and blood pressure monitoring.

■ Upright treadmill exercise provides the highest workload, but images can only be obtained post-exercise, so rapid image acquisition is essential.

■ Supine bicycle exercise provides a lower workload, but images can be acquired during exercise using a dedicated stress-echo stretcher and bicycle.

Key points:

❏ With treadmill exercise, ensuring the patient can rapidly move from the treadmill to the echo stretcher is important.

❏ In addition to echo images, the heart rate and blood pressure response to exercise, patient symptoms, arrhythmias, and ST segment changes are important clinical parameters (Fig. 8–9).

❏ The endpoint for a maximal exercise stress study is when the patient cannot exercise further due to shortness of breath, leg fatigue, or other symptoms.

❏ The exercise test also is stopped for any decline in blood pressure, significant arrhythmias, an excessive increase in blood pressure, or significant ST-segment depression.

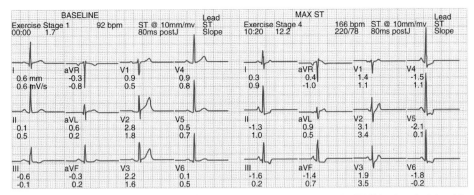

Figure 8–9 Exercise stress echocardiogram, with the 12-lead resting electrocardiography (ECG) leads on the left and the exercise ECG on the right. The numbers below each averaged ECG lead show the amount of ST depression (in mm) and the slope of the ST segment for each lead. In this 42-year-old man with multiple cardiac risk factors and chest pain symptoms, there is a 1.5- to 2-mm flat ST depression in the inferior and lateral leads consistent with myocardial ischemia.

	Normal	Ischemia	Stunned or hibernating	Infarction
Baseline	Normal	Normal	Hypokinetic or akinetic	Hypokinetic or akinetic
Low dose	Normal	Normal	Improved	Hypokinetic or akinetic
High dose	Hyperkinetic	Hypokinetic or akinetic	Hypokinetic or akinetic	Hypokinetic or akinetic

Figure 8–10 Chart of the patterns of wall motion with dobutamine stress echo in ischemic disease.

Dobutamine stress

■ A typical dobutamine stress protocol is to infuse intravenous dobutamine beginning at 5 (if there are resting wall motion abnormalities) or 10 mg/kg/min, with an increase by 10 mg/kg/min every 3 minutes to a maximum dose of 40 mg/kg/min.

■ Atropine in increments of 0.25 mg (maximum 1 mg total) may be added to achieve target heart rate, if needed.

■ The primary endpoint is a heart rate of 85% of maximum predicted heart rate for age.

■ Other endpoints include:
  ❏ Maximum dose allowed by protocol
  ❏ Definite wall motion abnormality in two or more adjacent segments
  ❏ Fall in systolic blood pressure to <100 mm Hg or increase in blood pressure to >200 mm Hg
  ❏ Diastolic blood pressure >120 mm Hg
  ❏ Significant arrhythmia
  ❏ Patient discomfort

Key points:

❏ Careful monitoring of heart rate, blood pressure, ECG, and symptoms is needed.

❏ Maximum predicted heart rate typically is 220 minus the patient's age.

❏ About 10% of patients will have a fall in blood pressure; this does not indicate coronary disease but may necessitate ending the dobutamine infusion.

❏ ST-segment depression with dobutamine is not diagnostically useful. ST segment elevation is rare but is predictive of significant coronary disease.

❏ Both ventricular and atrial arrhythmias may be precipitated by dobutamine and require prompt cessation of dobutamine infusion.

❏ When needed, the effects of dobutamine can be reversed with a rapidly acting intravenous beta-blocker, such as esmolol.

❏ Improvement in wall motion with low dose dobutamine of a myocardial segment that was abnormal at rest is evidence for myocardial viability.

❏ A biphasic response is identified when a myocardial segment that is abnormal at rest shows increased wall thickening after administration of low dose dobutamine (viability) and then worsening of wall motion at high dose (ischemia) (Fig. 8–10).

Step 4: Evaluate Regional and Global Left Ventricular Systolic Function at Peak Heart Rate

- Cine-loop images of the ventricle are acquired at (or immediately after) peak stress using the same four image planes as the baseline images (Fig. 8–11).
- The image depth, sector width, and ECG gating on the stress images are the same as on the baseline images.
- Rest and exercise images are compared side-by-side in the cine-loop format.

Key points:

- ❐ With exercise stress, the images are obtained as quickly as possible after exercise.
- ❐ With pharmacologic stress, images are acquired at each dosage stage, as well as at peak dose and heart rate.

- ❐ If endocardial definition is suboptimal, left-sided echo contrast is used to improve evaluation of regional endocardial motion.
- ❐ Several cine loops are quickly acquired in each view with subsequent selection of the best image to compare to the baseline images.
- ❐ Using ECG gating and the same cine loop length for rest and exercise images results in a similar timing of contraction on both images.
- ❐ The normal response to exercise or dobutamine stress is hyperkinesis of all segments with a decrease in ventricular chamber size (Fig. 8–12).
- ❐ Each myocardial segment is graded as hyperkinetic, normal, hypokinetic, akinetic, or dyskinetic.

Step 5: Monitor Patient Recovery

- The patient is monitored until all symptoms or wall motion abnormalities (if any) resolve and

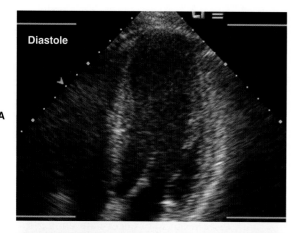

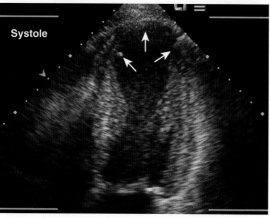

Figure 8–11 Resting myocardial wall motion was normal in this 56-year-old man with exertional chest discomfort. The immediate post-stress images with the apical four-chamber view at end-diastole (*A*) and end-systole (*B*) show akinesis of the apical lateral wall and inferior septum. These findings are consistent with inducible ischemia in the territory of the distal left anterior descending coronary artery.

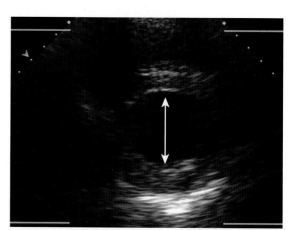

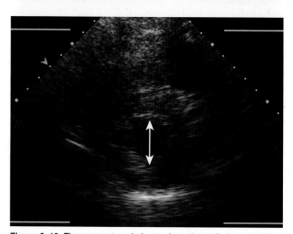

Figure 8–12 These parasternal short axis end-systolic images at rest (*A*) and maximum dose dobutamine (*B*) demonstrate the normal decrease in ventricular size with dobutamine stress.

heart rate has returned to normal (<100 bpm or within 10 bpm of resting heart rate).

■ If symptoms or wall motion abnormalities were seen at peak dose dobutamine, heart rate may be slowed more rapidly with a short-acting beta blocker.

Key points:

❑ Ischemia is reversible, so stress-induced wall motion abnormalities quickly resolve as heart rate declines.

❑ Post-stress images are recorded to document that LV global and regional function has returned to baseline on completion of the study.

❑ If ischemia is induced, as evidenced by chest discomfort or wall motion abnormalities, a short-acting beta-blocker, such as esmolol, is used to reduce heart rate and relieve symptoms.

Step 6: Review and Interpretation of the Stress Study

■ Baseline and stress echocardiographic images are reviewed in a side-by-side cine-loop format using a systemic approach to grading wall motion for each myocardial segment.

■ The stress study interpretation depends on integration of clinical (symptoms, exercise duration), hemodynamic (blood pressure, heart rate), ECG (ST changes and arrhythmias), and echocardiographic data.

Key points:

❑ The stress echo report includes the following minimal elements:
  ❑ Exercise duration or maximum dobutamine/atropine dose
  ❑ Heart rate and blood pressure at baseline and maximum stress
  ❑ ECG ST-segment changes or arrhythmias
  ❑ Symptoms
  ❑ Resting global and regional LV systolic function
  ❑ Global and regional LV systolic function at maximal stress
  ❑ Integration of these data to indicate study quality (images and maximum stress achieved), the likelihood of coronary disease, and the probable affected vessels

❑ The maximum stress achieved is a key element in interpretation; typically the study is considered nondiagnostic unless the maximum heart rate is at least 85% of the maximum predicted heart rate for that patient.

❑ An inducible wall motion abnormality is defined as hypokinesis or akinesis of a segment that was normal at rest. Failure of a normal segment to become hyperkinetic also is evidence of ischemia (Fig. 8–13).

❑ Echocardiographic evidence of an inducible wall motion abnormality in one or more adjacent segments is consistent with coronary artery disease, with the probable affected coronary artery identified from the location of the wall motion abnormality.

❑ With three-vessel coronary disease, instead of a regional wall motion abnormality, the only finding may be the absence of hyperkinesis and failure of ventricular size to decrease appropriately.

❑ Symptoms of chest discomfort accompanied by inducible wall motion abnormalities are consistent with ischemia; symptoms with normal regional function suggest noncardiac chest pain.

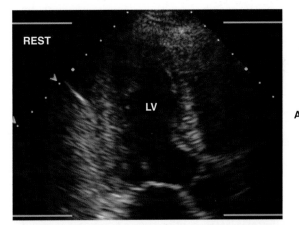

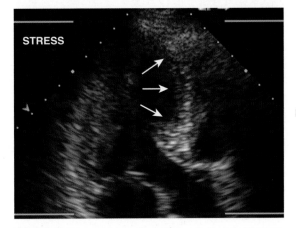

Figure 8–13 Example of inducible ischemia with the apical long axis view. At rest, there is normal wall motion, as seen on this end-systolic image (*A*). With exercise stress, there is akinesis of the mid- and apical segments of the anterior septum (*B, arrows*).

Acute Coronary Syndrome

Basic Principles

- Acute coronary syndrome includes patients with all of the following:
  - ❒ ST-segment elevation myocardial infarction (STEMI)
  - ❒ Non-ST segment elevation myocardial infarction (NSTEMI)
  - ❒ Unstable angina
- Other causes of acute chest pain that require immediate intervention (Table 8–2) are:
  - ❒ Aortic dissection
  - ❒ Pericarditis
  - ❒ Pulmonary embolism

Step 1: Evaluate Regional Ventricular Function

- A regional wall motion abnormality in a patient with chest pain indicates myocardial infarction or ischemia.
- In a patient with prior coronary disease, pre-existing regional dysfunction may be difficult to distinguish from acute dysfunction.
- Regional ventricular function may be normal between episodes of chest pain in patients with unstable angina.

Key points:

- ❒ Echocardiographic evaluation of wall motion is most helpful when the ECG is nondiagnostic; prompt revascularization is appropriate in patients with ST-elevation myocardial infarction.
- ❒ A remote transmural myocardial infarction results in akinesis, myocardial thinning, and increased echogenicity, consistent with scar (Fig. 8–14).
- ❒ However, with a prior non-ST elevation or reperfused myocardial infarction, wall thickness may be relatively normal.

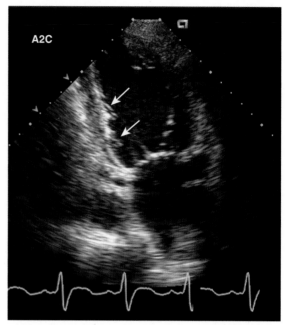

Figure 8–14 The inferior wall is thinned, bright, and akinetic in the two-chamber view in a patient with a prior ST-elevation inferior myocardial infarction.

- ❒ Normal regional myocardial function simultaneous with chest pain symptoms indicates a very low likelihood of an acute coronary syndrome.

Step 2: Estimate or Measure Ejection Fraction

- Evaluation of overall LV systolic function is clinically useful in management of patients with acute chest pain.
- Hospitalization and further evaluation often is needed in patients with a reduced ejection fraction, even when it results from causes other than acute coronary syndrome.

Key points:

- ❒ Measurement of ejection fraction using the apical biplane approach is preferred when endocardial definition is adequate and there are no time constraints (Fig. 8–15).
- ❒ In urgent situations, a visual estimate of ejection fraction based on parasternal short axis and apical four-chamber, two-chamber, and long axis views is appropriate.
- ❒ Left-sided echo contrast may be helpful for definition of both global and regional function when image quality is suboptimal.

Step 3: Consider Alternate Causes of Chest Pain

- Echocardiography may suggest other causes of chest pain when LV function is normal.

TABLE 8–2
MEDICALLY URGENT CAUSES OF ACUTE CHEST PAIN
Acute coronary syndrome
Acute ST-elevation myocardial infarction (STEMI)
Non-ST elevation myocardial infarction (NSTEMI)
Unstable angina
Aortic dissection
Pulmonary embolus
Acute pericarditis
Esophageal rupture (Boerhaave's syndrome)

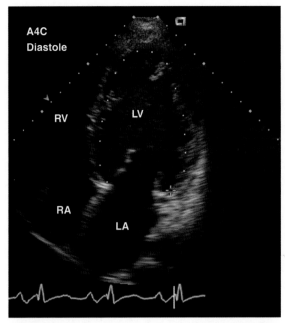

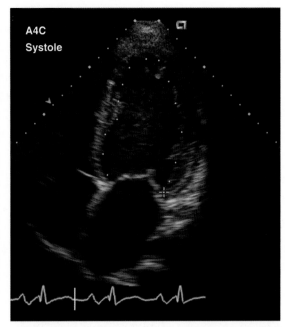

A

B

Figure 8–15 This patient with a prior non-ST elevation myocardial infarction has relatively normal wall motion when the apical four-chamber (*A4C*) diastolic (*A*) and systolic (*B*) images are compared. On the cine loops, apical hypokinesis was appreciated.

■ Often additional imaging approaches are needed for further evaluation when the clinical diagnosis remains unclear.

Key points:

❏ Evidence of aortic dilation and aortic regurgitation in a patient with acute chest pain prompts further evaluation for aortic dissection by transesophageal echocardiography (TEE) or cardiac computed tomography (CT) imaging.

❏ Although a pulmonary embolus is rarely visualized on echocardiography, findings of pulmonary hypertension and right ventricular dilation or dysfunction suggest this diagnosis be considered.

❏ A pericardial effusion is consistent with the diagnosis of pericarditis but also may be seen with acute aortic dissection (with rupture into the pericardium) and with numerous systemic diseases (see Chapter 10).

Step 4: Evaluate Cardiac Hemodynamics

■ Echocardiographic evaluation of cardiac hemodynamics is helpful in selected patients with acute chest pain.

Key points:

❏ Ischemia or infarction often is accompanied by diastolic dysfunction with evidence of

elevated left atrial (LA) pressure on the Doppler LV and LA filling curves (see Chapter 7).

❏ Pulmonary pressures may be elevated because of elevated left-sided filling pressures.

❏ Cardiac output can be measured using the LV outflow tract diameter and flow velocity integral (see Chapter 6).

Complications of Acute Myocardial Infarction

■ Echocardiography provides rapid, accurate, bedside diagnosis of mechanical complications of acute myocardial infarction (MI).

■ Mechanical complications of MI present as recurrent chest pain, a new systolic murmur, heart failure, cardiogenic shock, or a systemic embolic event.

■ Arrhythmias associated with acute MI may occur in the absence of significant structural abnormalities.

Step 1: Evaluate the Post–Myocardial Infarction Patient with Recurrent Chest Pain

■ Recurrent chest pain after myocardial infarction may be caused by recurrent ischemia, pericarditis, or noncardiac chest pain.

■ Echocardiographic evaluation focuses on evaluation of segmental wall motion and detection of a pericardial effusion.

Key points:

❏ Comparison of regional wall motion with previous studies may allow detection of recurrent ischemia in the peri-infarct region or in the distribution of a different coronary artery. However, coronary angiography often is needed for definitive diagnosis.

❏ The presence of a pericardial effusion is consistent with the diagnosis of pericarditis but also may be seen with acute aortic dissection (with rupture into the pericardium) or with LV rupture.

❏ LV rupture may present as transient chest pain. This diagnosis should be considered when a post-MI pericardial effusion is present, particularly if the episode of chest pain was accompanied by hypotension (Figs. 8–16 and 8–17).

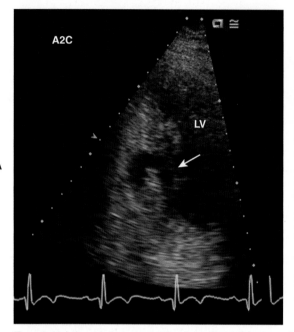
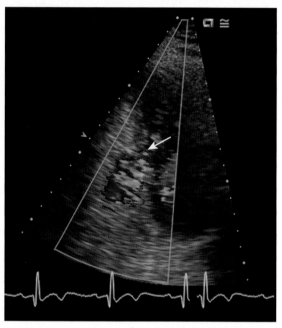

Figure 8–16 Left ventricular rupture in this patient with an inferior myocardial infarction is seen (*A*) in the apical two-chamber view (*A2C*) with an area of discontinuity in the inferior wall (*arrow*) and (*B*) with color Doppler showing flow into a narrow-necked pseudoaneurysm. The myocardial rupture is contained by pericardial adhesions, which form the wall of the pseudoaneurysm.

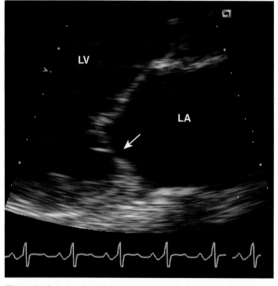
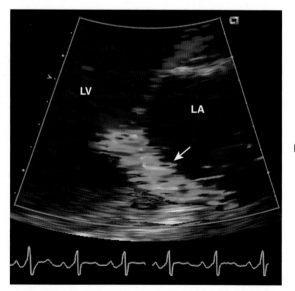

Figure 8–17 Ischemic mitral regurgitation often is characterized by tethering of the posterior leaflet caused by traction on the chords by the ischemic myocardium underlying the papillary muscle. This results in a "tented" appearance of the closed valve at end-systole (*A, arrow*) and a posterior-laterally directed jet of mitral regurgitation (*B*) as the anterior leaflet fails to coapt completely with the relatively immobile posterior leaflet.

Step 2: Evaluate the Post–Myocardial Infarction Patient with a New Systolic Murmur

- The differential diagnosis of a new post-MI murmur includes:
  - Ventricular septal defect caused by rupture of the septal myocardium
  - Acute mitral regurgitation caused by papillary muscle rupture or dysfunction
- Echocardiographic evaluation focuses on Doppler evaluation for an abnormal trans-septal or mitral regurgitant flow.

Key points:

- Mitral regurgitation after myocardial infarction most often results from ischemia or infarction of the papillary muscle or underlying inferior-lateral LV wall, resulting in "tethering" of the mitral leaflets with inadequate systolic coaptation (Fig. 8–18).
- Acute severe mitral regurgitation with pulmonary edema and cardiogenic shock occurs with partial or complete papillary muscle rupture.
- TEE often is needed to define the mechanism and evaluate severity of ischemic mitral regurgitation.
- Post-MI ventricular septal defects are detected using color Doppler showing a flow disturbance on the right ventricular side of the septum. Often the defect can be visual-

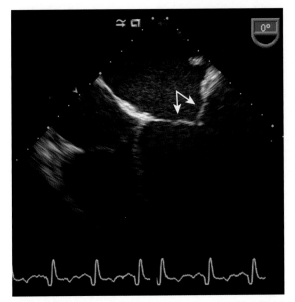

Figure 8–18 Transesophageal four-chamber view in a patient with left ventricular dilation and systolic dysfunction caused by severe three-vessel coronary disease. This mid-systolic image shows the tenting (or tethering) of the mitral leaflets caused by lateral displacement of the papillary muscles in the dilated ventricle. This restriction of leaflet motion resulted in inadequate leaflet apposition and moderate mitral regurgitation.

ized on two-dimensional (2D) imaging. Continuous wave (CW) Doppler interrogation provides information on the left-to-right ventricular systolic pressure difference (Fig. 8–19).

- With a ventricular septal defect, there is an increase in oxygen saturation from the right atrium to the right ventricle due to shunting of oxygenated blood from the left to right ventricle across the ventricular defect. If a right heart catheter is in position, measurement of oxygen saturations may be helpful when the diagnosis is unclear.

Step 3: Evaluate the Post–Myocardial Infarction Patient with Hypotension or Cardiogenic Shock

- Hypotension after MI may result from right ventricular infarction, left ventricular systolic dysfunction, or myocardial rupture with pericardial tamponade.
- Echocardiographic evaluation focuses on evaluation of global left and right ventricular systolic function and detection of a pericardial effusion.

Key points:

- Right ventricular infarction often accompanies inferior MI. The typical presentation is hypotension that responds to volume loading. Echocardiography shows a dilated hypocontractile right ventricle, despite normal pulmonary pressures (Fig. 8–20).
- With a large or recurrent MI, left ventricular systolic function may be significantly reduced, resulting in pulmonary edema and hypotension. Echocardiography allows measurement (or estimation) of ejection fraction and assessment of regional ventricular function.
- Myocardial ischemia or infarction is typically accompanied by diastolic dysfunction, often with elevated LV filling pressures. Diastolic dysfunction may lead to pulmonary congestion but rarely is the primary cause of hypotension.
- LV rupture caused by MI may result in acute cardiac tamponade and death. However, in some cases, the myocardial rupture is contained by a pericardial thrombus and adhesions.
- A contained LV rupture is called a pseudoaneurysm because its wall consists of pericardium (not myocardium) (Fig. 8–21).
- Typical characteristics of a pseudoaneurysm are a narrow neck compared with its widest diameter and an abrupt transition at an acute angle between the normal myocardium and

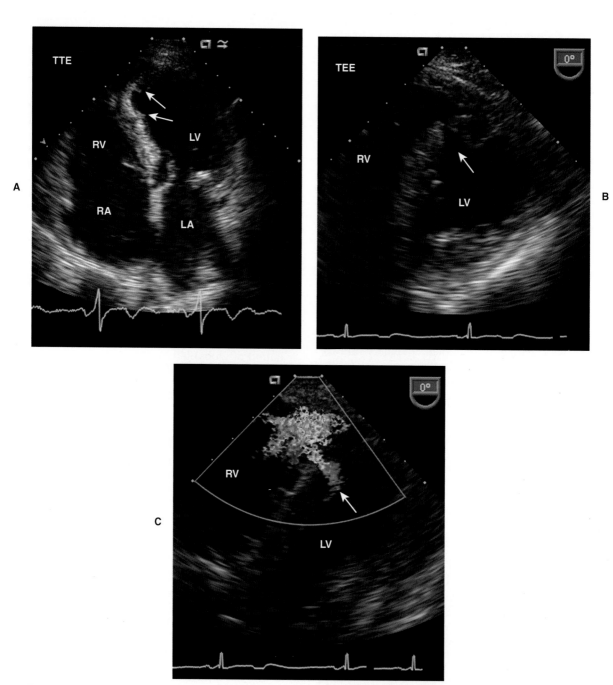

Figure 8–19 In this patient with an anterior myocardial infarction, (A) a localized area of dyskinesis (*arrows*) is seen in the apical segment of the septum in the four-chamber view on transthoracic echocardiography (*TTE*), (B) with an area of frank discontinuity in the septum (*arrow*) seen on the transgastric short axis view on transesophageal imaging (*TEE*). C, Color Doppler confirms the post-myocardial infarction ventricular septal defect with a narrow jet of flow from the left ventricle (*LV*) into the right ventricle (*RV*).

the aneurysm. Often the pseudoaneurysm is lined with thrombus.

❑ Most pseudoaneurysms require urgent surgical intervention to repair the ventricular rupture. True aneurysms typically are treated medically.

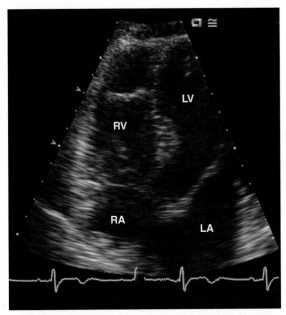

Figure 8–20 Right ventricular (*RV*) dilation and (in real time) hypokinesis in a patient with an inferior myocardial infarction is consistent with RV infarction, as seen in this apical four-chamber view.

Step 4: Evaluate for Late Complications of Myocardial Infarction

■ Late complications of MI include left ventricular aneurysm, thrombus, and systolic dysfunction.

■ Echocardiographic evaluation includes evaluation of global and regional myocardial function, calculation of ejection fraction, assessment of diastolic dysfunction, and a diligent search for apical thrombus.

Key points:

❑ Adverse ventricular remodeling after MI results in thinning and scar formation in areas of infarction, overall LV dilation, and a reduction in ejection fraction. Adverse remodeling is prevented, to some extent, by appropriate medical therapy.

❑ The myocardial thickness in diastole, wall thickening during systole, and endocardial motion are graded for each myocardial segment.

❑ An aneurysm is defined as a discrete area of the left ventricle (usually the apex) with a diastolic contour abnormality and systolic dyskinesis (Fig. 8–22).

❑ LV ejection fraction is calculated using the biplane apical approach. Single plane or M-mode evaluation of LV function may be inaccurate due to regional ventricular dysfunction.

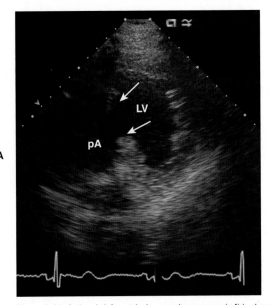

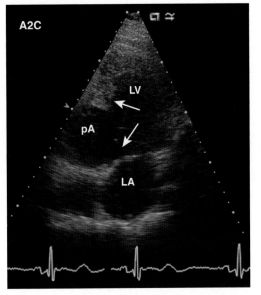

Figure 8–21 A chronic left ventricular pseudoaneurysm (*pA*) is characterized by a narrow neck (*arrows*) relative to the maximum diameter of the pseudoaneurysm, as seen in a short axis view (*A*) of the left ventricle (*LV*) and in the apical two-chamber (*A2C, B*) view. There is an abrupt transition from the normal myocardial thickness to the aneurysm, and the pseudoaneurysm has an irregular echodensity consistent with thrombus lining the cavity.

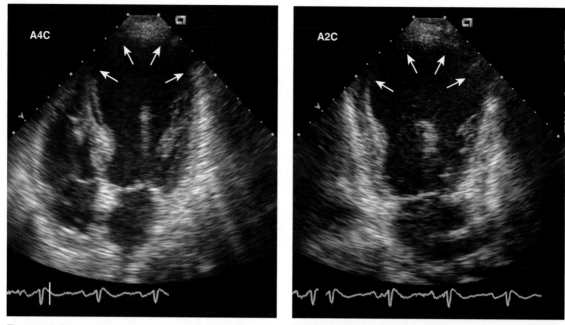

Figure 8–22 This apical true aneurysm shows a diastolic contour abnormality with a gradual, smooth transition from normal myocardial thickness to the thin scarred myocardium of the aneurysm and with systolic dyskinesis as shown by the arrows in the apical four-chamber (*A4C, A*) and two-chamber (*A2C, B*) end-systolic images.

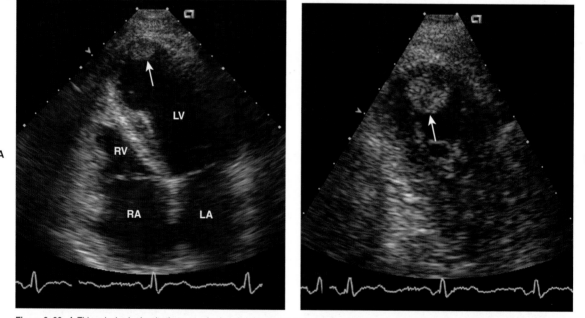

Figure 8–23 *A,* This apical echodensity that protrudes into the chamber in an area of dyskinesis is consistent with an apical thrombus. *B,* The zoomed image using a higher frequency transducer and an oblique image plane through the apex helps confirm that these echoes represent a thrombus, and not prominent trabeculation or an imaging artifact.

□ Apical thrombus is best visualized in standard and oblique apical views. Identification of thrombus is enhanced by use of a higher frequency transducer and a shallow image depth (Fig. 8–23).

□ Apical trabeculation is distinguished from thrombus by the lack of mobility, linear appearance, and attachments to the LV wall. Left-sided ultrasound contrast may be helpful when it is difficult to distinguish apical trabeculation from thrombi (Fig. 8–24).

End-Stage Ischemic Disease

■ End-stage ischemic disease, colloquially called "ischemic cardiomyopathy," has many features in common with a dilated cardiomyopathy or ventricular dysfunction caused by valvular heart disease (Table 8–3).

■ The echocardiographic features most helpful in diagnosis of end-stage ischemic disease are:
- ❏ Definite regional wall motion abnormalities with areas of thinning and akinesis (Fig. 8–25)
- ❏ Normal right ventricular size and systolic function (unless RV infarction has occurred)
- ❏ Absence of evidence for primary valvular heart disease

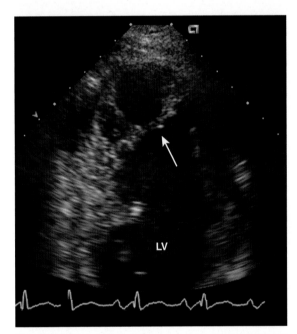

Figure 8–24 The apical trabeculation seen in this apical two-chamber view is distinguished from thrombus by similar echodensity to myocardium, a linear structure that connects to the myocardium at both ends, and the absence of an underlying wall motion abnormality.

Step 1: Evaluate Global Left Ventricular Systolic and Diastolic Function

■ Overall LV systolic function is evaluated by calculation of an apical biplane ejection fraction.

■ LV diastolic function is evaluated as described in Chapter 7.

Key points:

- ❏ Calculation of a biplane ejection fraction is performed whenever possible. If endocardial definition is suboptimal, left-sided contrast echocardiography provides better visualization of ventricular function.
- ❏ Most patients with end-stage ischemic disease have diastolic dysfunction, as well as systolic dysfunction.
- ❏ Early in the disease course, diastolic dysfunction is characterized by impaired relaxation.
- ❏ However, as systolic function deteriorates, LV filling pressures may increase, LV compliance decreases, and the increased ventricular volumes result in a rightward shift along the ventricular diastolic pressure-volume curve.

Step 2: Evaluate Regional Left Ventricular Systolic Function

■ Regional function is evaluated by grading each myocardial segment as normal, hypokinetic, akinetic, or dyskinetic.

■ Any areas of thin scarred myocardium are noted.

Key points:

- ❏ A discrete area of scarring or dyskinesis is consistent with coronary disease, rather than a primary cardiomyopathy.
- ❏ In both end-stage ischemic disease and primary cardiomyopathy, ventricular function typically is best preserved for the inferior-lateral and lateral basal segments of the left ventricle.

TABLE 8–3

DIFFERENTIATION OF LEFT VENTRICULAR SYSTOLIC DYSFUNCTION DUE TO END-STAGE ISCHEMIC DISEASE FROM DILATED CARDIOMYOPATHY OR CHRONIC VALVULAR DISEASE

FINDINGS	END-STAGE ISCHEMIC DISEASE	DILATED CARDIOMYOPATHY	CHRONIC VALVULAR DISEASE
Left ventricular ejection fraction	Moderately to severely depressed	Moderately to severely depressed	Moderately to severely depressed
Segmental wall motion abnormalities	May be present	Absent	Absent
Right ventricular systolic function	Normal	Decreased	Variable
Pulmonary artery pressures	Elevated	Elevated	Elevated
Mitral regurgitation	Moderate	Moderate	Moderate to severe
Aortic regurgitation	Not significant	Not significant	Moderate to severe

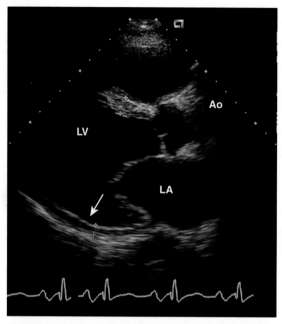
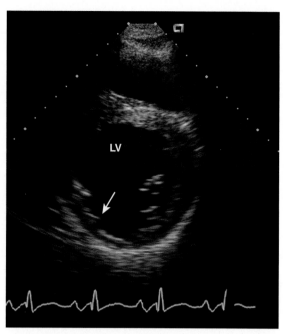

Figure 8–25 End-stage ischemic disease with a dilated left ventricular (*LV*) chamber and low ejection fraction shows thinning and more severe hypokinesis of the inferior wall (*arrows*) compared with the ventricular septum as seen in long (*A*) and short (*B*) axis views.

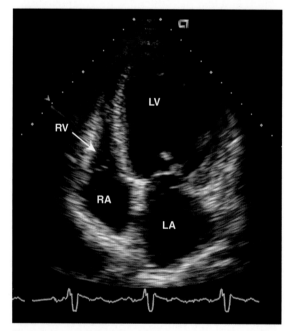

Figure 8–26 In patients with heart failure caused by end-stage ischemic disease, right ventricular size and systolic function often are normal (unless concurrent right ventricular [*RV*] infarction has occurred). Compared with the dilated and hypokinetic left ventricle (*LV*), the normal RV appears relatively small and hyperdynamic.

Step 3: Evaluate Right Ventricular Size and Systolic Function

- Right ventricular size and systolic function are qualitatively evaluated, as discussed in Chapter 6.
- Right ventricular systolic function typically is normal in patients with end-stage ischemic dis-

ease, so that the right ventricle appears small and hypercontractile compared with the dilated hypokinetic left ventricle.

Key points:

- ❏ When the right ventricular (RV) size is proportionate to the left ventricle, the degree of RV dilation is similar to the degree of LV dilation (Fig. 8–26).
- ❏ When RV systolic function appears similar to LV function, the degree of dysfunction is the same for both ventricles.
- ❏ RV function may be impaired in patients with coronary disease and a prior RV infarction.

Step 4: Estimate Cardiac Hemodynamics

- Pulmonary artery systolic pressure is estimated from the velocity of the tricuspid regurgitant jet and the appearance and respiratory variation of the inferior vena cava, as discussed in Chapter 6.
- Evidence for an elevated left atrial pressure includes a prolonged and high velocity pulmonic vein a reversal and a high ratio of transmitral flow to tissue Doppler velocity in early diastole (see Chapter 7).

Key points:

- ❏ Pulmonary pressures may be elevated because of left ventricular dysfunction, leading to chronic elevation of left atrial pressure and consequent pulmonary hypertension.

❏ Evidence for elevated filling pressures may no longer be present after optimization of medical therapy.

Step 5: Identify and Evaluate Any Associated Valve Disease

■ LV dilation and systolic dysfunction caused by chronic valve disease may be difficult to distinguish from a primary cardiomyopathy or end-stage ischemic heart disease.

■ LV systolic dysfunction of any cause commonly is accompanied by significant mitral valve regurgitation, due to displacement of the papillary muscle, leaflet tethering, and annular dilation.

Key points

❏ Primary mitral valve disease is characterized by abnormalities of the valve leaflets or chordae—for example, myxomatous or rheumatic valve disease.

❏ With secondary mitral regurgitation, the mitral valve apparatus is anatomically normal, but geometric relationships are altered by the dilated left ventricle.

❏ Mitral regurgitation caused by ischemic heart disease may improve with medical or interventional approaches for relief of ischemia.

❏ Coronary angiography may be needed to determine the contribution of coronary disease to the clinical cardiac dysfunction.

NOTES

SELF-ASSESSMENT QUESTIONS

QUESTION 1

A 67-year-old man undergoes treadmill exercise echocardiography. He exercises for 5 minutes on a Bruce protocol treadmill test, which is 30% less than predicted for age. His heart rate increases from 76 beats per minute (bpm) at rest to 110 bpm (72% maximum predicted) and blood pressures increases from 110/80 to 160/76 mm Hg. He stopped for fatigue with no chest pain or pressure. The resting ECG is normal and no ST depression occurs with exercise. Occasional premature ventricular beats are seen at peak exercise and resolve with rest. The echocardiogram shows normal wall motion at rest and after exercise (images recorded within 45 seconds of stopping exercise).

Your interpretation of this stress test is:

A. No evidence of inducible ischemia
B. Abnormal hypertensive response to exercise
C. Exercise-induced ischemia manifested as an arrhythmia
D. Limited exercise capacity due to pulmonary disease
E. Nondiagnostic test

QUESTION 2

A 74-year-old woman with a hip fracture undergoes dobutamine stress echocardiography for pre-operative evaluation. Her baseline heart rate and blood pressure are 72 bpm and 138/78 mm Hg. The resting echocardiogram is normal, so dobutamine is started at 10 mcg/kg/min and increased every 3 minutes by 10 mcg/kg/min to a maximum dose of 30 mcg/kg/min to achieve a heart rate of 125 bpm. The ECG showed 1.5 mm upsloping ST-segment depression in the inferior leads. Images recorded at maximum dose dobutamine showed hyperdynamic function with a small ventricular chamber, but her blood pressure fell to 112/72 mm Hg. She complained of feeling "jittery" but denied chest pain.

Your interpretation of this test is:

A. No evidence of inducible ischemia
B. Abnormal blood pressure response
C. A higher dobutamine dose should have been used
D. Atropine should have been given in addition to dobutamine
E. ECG changes consistent with coronary disease

QUESTION 3

A 64-year-old man reports a history of MI. His resting parasternal long axis image in mid-systole is shown in Figure 8–27.

The most likely coronary artery involved at the time of his MI was:

A. Left main
B. Left anterior descending
C. Circumflex
D. Right
E. Posterior descending

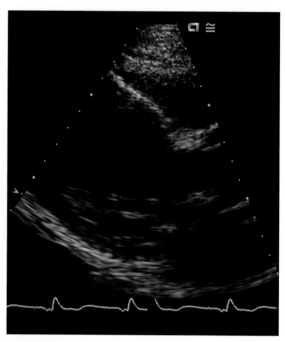

Figure 8–27

QUESTION 4

A 63-year-old man with cardiac risk factors of hypertension, smoking, and hyperlipidemia presents to the emergency department with a 12-hour history of fluctuating substernal chest pressure. The most recent episode lasted 20 minutes and was relieved by nitroglycerin in the ambulance. On arrival, the ECG showed nonspecific changes and an echocardiogram was requested. Overall LV systolic function was normal and no regional wall motion abnormalities were seen.

The likelihood that this is an acute coronary syndrome is:

A. Low
B. Intermediate
C. High

QUESTION 5

A 71-year-old woman complains of increasing shortness of breath 5 days after an acute MI. An echocardiogram is requested for a murmur on auscultation. The aortic and mitral valves show normal anatomy and motion, but the Doppler signal shown in Figure 8–28 is obtained with the transducer at the apex.

This Doppler tracing is most consistent with:

A. Acute mitral regurgitation
B. Aortic valve stenosis
C. Ventricular septal defect
D. Severe pulmonary hypertension
E. Ventricular rupture

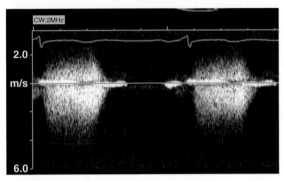

Figure 8–28

QUESTION 6

A 64-year-old man with a history of MI 1 year ago is referred for echocardiography. The apical long axis image in mid-systole shown in Figure 8–29 was recorded. Which features of the structure shown in this image most reliably distinguishes it from a ventricular pseudoaneurysm?

A. Thrombus formation
B. Narrowest diameter
C. Systolic dyskinesis
D. Diastolic contour abnormality
E. Doppler flow pattern

QUESTION 7

Echocardiography is requested on a 54-year-old man in the intensive care unit who is hypotensive. You are told he has an acute inferior MI and the medical staff are in the process of moving the patient to the cardiac catheterization laboratory. They interrupt the transfer briefly to allow echocardiographic imaging and ask you to tell them what you can in 2 to 3 minutes or less.

The first thing you should do is:

A. Parasternal long axis 2D imaging
B. Apical CW Doppler
C. Subcostal pulsed Doppler aortic flow
D. Apical four-chamber view
E. Parasternal color Doppler flow

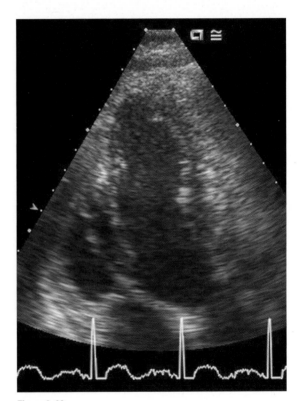

Figure 8–29

QUESTION 8

A 69-year-old man underwent emergent percutaneous coronary revascularization of a proximal
left anterior descending coronary occlusion with
a drug-eluting stent. At hospital discharge, LV
ejection fraction was 58% with the end-systolic
long axis image shown in Figure 8–30*A*. Five
days later he presented with heart failure symptoms, an ejection fraction of 40%, and the end-
systolic long axis view shown in Figure 8–30*B*.

The most likely precipitating clinical event is:

A. Excessive salt and fluid intake
B. Right coronary artery ischemia
C. Left ventricular rupture
D. Acute mitral regurgitation
E. In-stent thrombosis

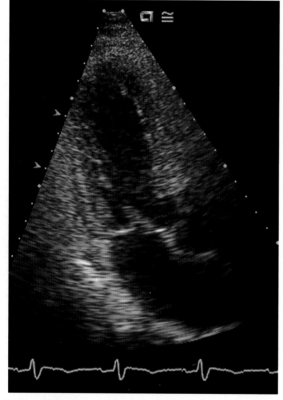
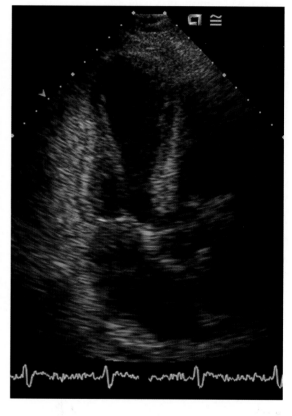

Figure 8–30

ANSWERS

ANSWER 1: E

Most clinicians consider a stress test nondiagnostic when the maximum heart rate does not exceed 85% of the maximum predicted heart rate for age. Another cause of a nondiagnostic stress echocardiogram is failure to record the post-stress images within a minute of stopping exercise at a point when heart rate is still elevated. The presence or absence of inducible ischemia cannot be deduced from this study due to the failure to achieve an appropriate heart rate. The most common cause of an inadequate heart rate response is inadequate effort. Orthopedic problems and peripheral vascular disease also may limit exercise duration without the normal rise in heart rate. Pulmonary disease is less likely as heart rate usually rises normally and respiratory symptoms are typically more prominent. A cardiopulmonary exercise test may be performed if this is of concern. Isolated unifocal premature ventricular beats with exercise are seen in normal individuals and do not indicate ischemic disease. In this patient, a pharmacologic stress test may be considered to achieve an adequate stress level.

ANSWER 2: A

This patient achieved 85% of her maximum predicted heart rate, based on the quick formula for maximum predicted heart rate of 220 minus the patient's age. Her echocardiogram appropriately shows a decreased chamber size with hyperdynamic function of all segments. Thus, this is a normal dobutamine stress echocardiogram, with no evidence for inducible ischemia. ECG changes with pharmacologic stress testing have a low sensitivity and specificity for the diagnosis of coronary disease, so the echocardiographic images provide the diagnostic data, not the ECG.

Although blood pressure often rises with dobutamine infusion, some patients have a fall in blood pressure thought to be caused by the peripheral vasodilating effects of beta-agonists. A fall in blood pressure is not predictive of coronary disease or adverse clinical outcomes. A higher dose of dobutamine or the addition of atropine would be considered only if the heart rate response was inadequate.

ANSWER 3: B

This image shows thinning and increased echogenicity of the ventricular septum, along with failure of the septum to move toward the midline of the ventricle in systole. These findings are consistent with MI caused by proximal left anterior descending coronary artery disease. The inferior-lateral wall, supplied by the posterior descending artery, is relatively normal. The posterior descending coronary artery arises from the right coronary artery in 85% of cases, with this coronary anatomy being defined as "right dominant." In the remaining 15%, the posterior descending coronary is the distal extension of the circumflex artery. The lateral wall, supplied by the circumflex coronary, is not seen in this view. Occlusion of the left main coronary artery is unlikely because the patient would probably not have survived the event.

ANSWER 4: C

These symptoms in a 63-year-old man with multiple cardiac risk factors are most consistent with an acute coronary syndrome despite the nondiagnostic ECG and the normal resting echocardiogram. The definition of acute coronary syndrome includes ST-elevation MI, non–ST-elevation MI, and unstable angina. MI usually results in a resting regional wall motion abnormality. However, with unstable angina, wall motion may be normal at rest between episodes of ischemia, as manifested by chest pain. A normal echocardiogram does not exclude the possibility of unstable angina, so careful consideration of the clinical history and other diagnostic tests is needed for clinical decision making.

ANSWER 5: C

This Doppler spectral tracing shows a systolic signal with a poorly defined peak but with a velocity of at least 4.5 m/s. Color flow imaging showed that this signal originated from a ventricular septal defect, near the apex, in the region of the previous myocardial infarction. Acute mitral regurgitation would have a similar signal in terms of timing and velocity but would be accompanied by a typical mitral inflow signal in diastole. Aortic stenosis would have a shorter ejection period (because there is no flow during isovolumic contraction and relaxation). Tricuspid regurgitation caused by severe pulmonary hypertension would be accompanied by diastolic tricuspid valve inflow. The flow signal, if any, with ventricular rupture is low velocity to-and-fro flow into and out of the pseudoaneurysm.

ANSWER 6: B

This image is most consistent with a basal ventricular aneurysm. There are many similarities between a true aneurysm and a pseudoaneurysm, including an outpouching of the ventricle or diastolic contour abnormality with systolic dyskinesis and thrombus formation in the dyskinetic region. However, unlike a true aneurysm, which is composed of scarred and thin myocardium, a pseudoaneurysm is a contained ventricular rupture with the walls of the cavity formed by pericardial adhesions. With a pseudoaneurysm, there is an abrupt transition from normal thickness myocardium to the ruptured segment and, typically, the diameter of rupture site (or "neck" of the aneurysm) is smaller than the maximum diameter of the pseudoaneurysm chamber, with a neck to cavity ratio <0.5 having a high specificity for diagnosis of a pseudoaneurysm. Although Doppler may show flow in and out of a pseudoaneurysm, the pattern of flow does not reliably differentiate a true aneurysm from pseudoaneurysm.

ANSWER 7: D

The most likely cause of hypotension after an inferior MI is right ventricular infarction. The apical four-chamber view will show overall left and right ventricular systolic function and will be most useful for immediate management. The inferior septal motion also can be seen, and the transducer can be quickly rotated to two-chamber and long axis views to assess other regional wall motion abnormalities. The apical four-chamber view also will exclude pericardial tamponade caused by a circumferential pericardial effusion, although a loculated effusion might be missed.

Parasternal imaging is less useful because only the base of the left ventricle and the right ventricular outflow tract are seen. Parasternal color Doppler might be helpful if acute mitral regurgitation caused by papillary muscle rupture or an acute ventricular septal defect are suspected. However, these might be better evaluated from the apical window with CW Doppler and color flow imaging. Subcostal pulsed Doppler aortic flow is helpful when acute aortic regurgitation is suspected, looking for holodiastolic flow reversal. However, aortic regurgitation is not a complication of MI.

ANSWER 8: E

The end-systolic image at hospital discharge is normal, suggesting recovery of function in the anterior wall and anterior septum, supplied by the revascularized left anterior descending coronary artery. The end-systolic image 5 days later shows dilation of the apex with failure of the apical half of the septum and the apex to contract in systole. In combination with the acute drop in ejection fraction, the most likely event is in-stent thrombosis of the proximal left anterior descending coronary artery with acute infarction in the same region as the original event. With excessive salt and fluid intake, heart failure would be accompanied by diffuse LV dilation, without a regional wall motion abnormality. Ischemia in the right coronary artery distribution would affect the inferior or inferior-lateral (posterior) wall. There is no evidence on this image for LV rupture (no pericardial effusion) or for acute mitral regurgitation, although a Doppler study would be needed for complete evaluation. Interestingly, on repeat catheterization there was no evidence for thrombosis or stenosis of the left anterior descending coronary artery, and the other coronary arteries showed normal flow. LV end-diastolic pressure was 40 mm Hg, and cardiac output was severely reduced. Thus the echo changes are likely caused by adverse LV remodeling after MI, despite appropriate treatment with an angiotensin-converting enzyme inhibitor.

NOTES

9

Cardiomyopathies and Hypertensive and Pulmonary Heart Disease

THE ECHO EXAM

STEP-BY-STEP APPROACH
Cardiomyopathies
  General Step-by-Step Approach
  Measure Left Ventricular Chamber Size and Systolic Function
  Evaluate for the Presence and Pattern of Ventricular Hypertrophy
  Assess Left Ventricular Diastolic Function
  Estimate Pulmonary Artery Pressures
  Evaluate Right Ventricular Size and Systolic Function
  Evaluate the Severity of Mitral and Tricuspid Regurgitation
  Evaluate Left Atrial Size

Additional Steps
  Dilated Cardiomyopathy
  Hypertrophic Cardiomyopathy
  Restrictive Cardiomyopathy
Hypertensive Heart Disease
Post-Transplant Heart Disease
Pulmonary Heart Disease
  Estimate Pulmonary Pressure
  Evaluate Right Ventricular Size and Systolic Function
  Evaluate the Severity of Tricuspid Regurgitation
  Exclude Other Causes of Pulmonary Hypertension or Right Heart Enlargement

SELF-ASSESSMENT QUESTIONS

ECHOCARDIOGRAPHIC DIFFERENTIAL DIAGNOSIS OF HEART FAILURE

Ischemic disease
Valvular disease
Hypertensive heart disease
Cardiomyopathy
  Dilated
  Hypertrophic
  Restrictive
Pericardial disease
Constriction
Tamponade
Pulmonary heart disease

CARDIOMYOPATHIES: TYPICAL FEATURES

	DILATED	HYPERTROPHIC	RESTRICTIVE
LV systolic function	Moderately to severely ↓	Normal	Normal
LV diastolic function	May be abnormal	Abnormal	Abnormal
LV hypertrophy	↑ LV mass due to LV dilation with normal wall thickness	Asymmetrical LV hypertrophy	Concentric LV hypertrophy
Chamber dilation	All four chambers	Left and right atrial dilation if MR is present	Left and right atrial dilation
Outflow tract obstruction	Absent	Dynamic LV outflow tract obstruction may be present	Absent
LV end-diastolic pressure	Elevated	Elevated	Elevated
Pulmonary artery pressures	Elevated	Elevated	Elevated

LV, *Left ventricular;* MR, *mitral regurgitation.*

DIFFERENTIATION OF CAUSE OF INCREASED WALL THICKNESS

	HYPERTENSIVE HEART DISEASE	HYPERTROPHIC CARDIOMYOPATHY	RESTRICTIVE CARDIOMYOPATHY
Left ventricular hypertrophy	+	+	+
Pattern of hypertrophy	Concentric	Asymmetrical	Concentric
Clinical history of hypertension	+	Absent	Absent
Outflow obstruction	Midventricular cavity obliteration	Dynamic subaortic obstruction	Absent
RV hypertrophy	Absent	May be present	+
Pulmonary hypertension	Mild	Mild	Moderate
LV systolic function	Normal initially but may be reduced late in disease course	Normal	Normal initially but may be reduced late in disease course
LV diastolic function	Abnormal	Abnormal	Abnormal

+, Present; LV, left ventricular; RV, right ventricular.

ECHO APPROACH TO THE CARDIOMYOPATHIES

MODALITY	ECHO VIEWS AND FLOWS	MEASUREMENTS
Imaging	LV size and systolic function	LV-EDV, LV-ESV
		Apical biplane EF
	Degree and pattern of LV hypertrophy	LV-mass
	Evidence for dynamic outflow tract obstruction	SAM of the mitral valve
		Aortic valve midsystolic closure
	RV size and systolic function	
	LA size	LA volume
Doppler Echo	Associated valvular regurgitation	Measure vena contracta, quantitate if more than mild
	LV diastolic function	Standard diastolic function evaluation with classification of severity and estimate of LV-EDP
	LV systolic function	dP/dt from MR jet
		Calculation of cardiac output
	Pulmonary pressures	TR-Jet and IVC for PA systolic pressure
		Evaluate PR jet for PA diastolic pressure
		Consider measures of pulmonary resistance
	Color, pulsed, and CW Doppler to quantitate outflow obstruction	Maximum outflow tract gradient

CW, Continuous wave; EF, ejection fraction; IVC, inferior vena cava; LV, left ventricular; LV-EDV, LV end diastolic volume; LV-ESV, LV end-systolic volume; MR, mitral regurgitation; PA, pulmonary artery; PR, pulmonary regurgitation; SAM, systolic anterior motion; TR, tricuspid regurgitation.

STEP-BY-STEP APPROACH

Cardiomyopathies

General Step-by-Step Approach

An overall approach to patients with a known or suspected cardiomyopathy is reviewed, followed by specific features of each type of cardiomyopathy.

Step 1: Measure Left Ventricular Chamber Size and Systolic Function

Left ventricular chamber size

■ Two-dimensional (2D) or 2D-guided M-mode measurement of left ventricular (LV) minor axis internal dimensions at end-diastole and end-systole (Fig. 9–1)

■ Apical biplane calculation of end-diastolic and end-systolic ventricular volumes (Fig. 9–2)

Key points:
□ LV internal dimensions are measured from the parasternal window, because the ultrasound beam is perpendicular to the blood–myocardial interface, providing high axial resolution.
□ 2D imaging in long and short axis views is used to ensure the dimension is measured in the minor axis of the ventricle (not at an oblique angle, which would overestimate size).
□ The rapid sampling rate of M-mode (compared with the slow frame rate of 2D imaging) provides more accurate identification of the endocardial borders (Fig. 9–3).
□ For sequential studies, measurements should be made at the same location.

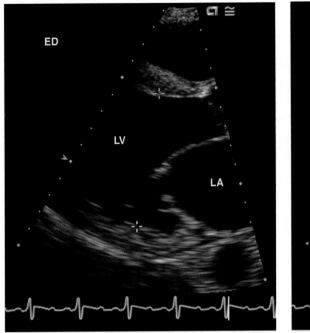
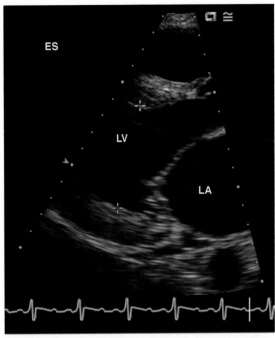

Figure 9–1 In the parasternal long axis view, left ventricular (*LV*) minor axis internal dimensions are measured at (*A*) end-diastole (*ED*, onset of the QRS) and (*B*) end-systole (*ES*, minimal LV volume just before aortic valve closure) from the septum to the posterior wall at the level of the mitral valve chords. The dimension is measured perpendicular to the long axis of the ventricle. Because the ultrasound beam is perpendicular to the myocardial–blood interface, the endocardium appears as a distinct edge, although, as in this example of a patient with a dilated ventricle, the septal endocardium typically is more clearly defined than the posterior wall endocardium, due to muscular trabeculations and overlying chords.

❏ Apical biplane ventricular volumes are indexed to body surface area.

Left ventricular systolic function

■ LV ejection fraction is calculated using the apical biplane approach.
■ LV dP/dt is calculated from the mitral regurgitation velocity curve (Fig. 9–4).
■ Forward cardiac output is measured in the LV outflow tract.
■ Regional ventricular function is evaluated qualitatively as normal, hypokinetic, akinetic, or dyskinetic for each myocardial segment (see Chapter 8).

Key points:

❏ Ejection fraction measured by the apical biplane method is compared with the visually estimated ejection fraction.
❏ The traced endocardial borders are reviewed for accuracy and retraced if the estimated and measured ejection fractions differ by more than 5 to 10 ejection fraction (EF) units.
❏ Echo-contrast is used to enhance identification of endocardial borders when image quality is suboptimal.
❏ Measured ejection fraction is reported whenever possible. The estimated ejection fraction is reported only if endocardial borders cannot be traced accurately.

❏ Ejection fraction is an imperfect measure of contractility because it is affected by loading conditions. Even so, ejection fraction is useful for clinical decision making.
❏ LV dP/dt and forward stroke volume are other useful parameters of LV systolic function (see Chapter 6).
❏ Indirect qualitative indicators of LV systolic dysfunction include M-mode findings of reduced aortic root motion and increased E-point septal separation (Fig. 9–5).

Evaluate for other cause of left ventricular dilation and systolic dysfunction

■ A cardiomyopathy is defined as a primary disease of the myocardium in the absence of coronary or valvular disease.
■ Evaluate for evidence of other causes of LV dilation and dysfunction, specifically valve disease (aortic stenosis, mitral regurgitation, or aortic regurgitation) and coronary artery disease.

Key points:

❏ LV dilation and dysfunction resulting from coronary disease with myocardial infarction or hibernation can be difficult to distinguish from a primary cardiomyopathy (see Chapter 8).

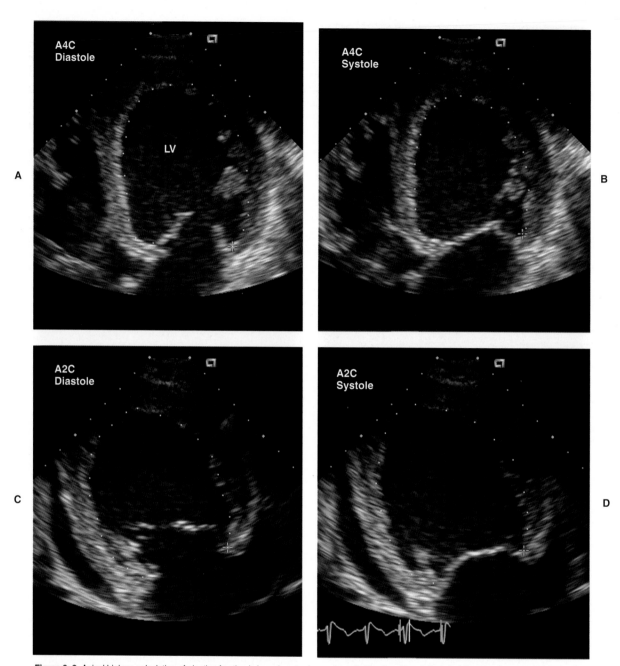

Figure 9–2 Apical biplane calculation of ejection fraction is based on tracing endocardial borders at end-diastole (*A*) and end-systole (*B*) in the four-chamber view (*A4C, A* and *B*) and in the two-chamber view (*A2C, C* and *D*). When the left ventricular (*LV*) apex appears rounded, as in this example, the view may be foreshortened, with the apparent "apex" representing an oblique view through the anterior wall. Foreshortened apical views are prevented by positioning the patient in a steep left lateral position with an apical cut-out in the stretcher to allow the transducer to be positioned on the true apex and after moving the transducer down one or more interspaces.

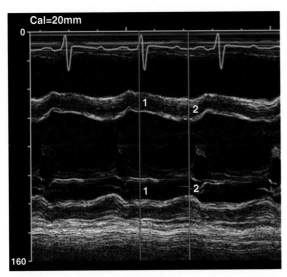

Figure 9–3 Two-dimensional (2D) echocardiography is used to ensure the M-line is perpendicular to the long axis of the left ventricle in the parasternal long axis view and in the middle of the chamber in the short axis view. The rapid sampling rate of the M-mode recording (time on the horizontal axis) provides more accurate identification and measurement of septal and posterior wall thickness and ventricular chamber dimensions at end-diastole (*1*, onset of QRS) and end-systole (*2*, maximum posterior motion of septum).

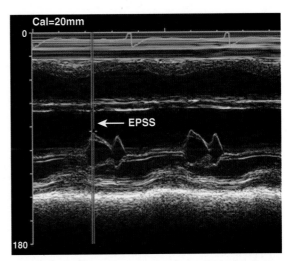

Figure 9–5 M-mode tracing at the level of the mitral valve shows a marked increase in the E-point septal separation (*EPSS*) consistent with severe left ventricular systolic dysfunction.

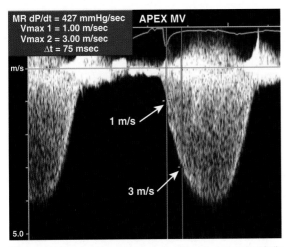

Figure 9–4 The rate of increase in velocity of the mitral regurgitant jet is markedly reduced in early systole. The calculated dP/dt of 427 mm Hg/s indicates severely reduced left ventricular contractility.

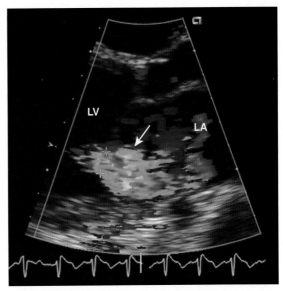

Figure 9–6 Mitral regurgitation in a patient with dilated cardiomyopathy caused by tethering of the posterior leaflet with a posteriorly directed regurgitant jet. The vena contracta width of 9 mm is consistent with severe regurgitation. Both the left ventricle (*LV*) and left atrium (*LA*) are enlarged in this view.

❐ Mitral regurgitation may be a cause or a consequence of LV dilation and dysfunction. When more than mild mitral regurgitation (vena contracta larger than 3 mm) is present, careful quantitative evaluation may be helpful (see Chapter 12; Fig. 9–6).

❐ The degree of aortic valve leaflet opening is reduced when LV dysfunction is present, making it difficult to separate severe aortic stenosis resulting in LV dysfunction from moderate aortic stenosis with coincidental LV dysfunction (see Chapter 11; Fig. 9–7).

Step 2: Evaluate for the Presence and Pattern of Ventricular Hypertrophy

Presence and severity of left ventricular hypertrophy

■ 2D-guided M-mode measurement of LV wall thickness (Fig. 9–8)

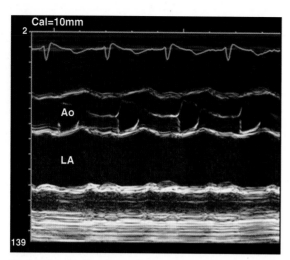

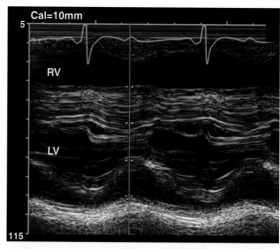

Figure 9–7 In this M-mode recording in a patient with acute viral cardiomyopathy, the aortic tracing shows reduced anterior-posterior motion of the root due to a reduced cardiac output. In addition, the aortic valve leaflets do not remain fully opened during systole due to low transaortic flow.

Figure 9–8 Two-dimensional (2D) echocardiography was used in a long axis view to ensure that the M-line was perpendicular to the long axis of the left ventricle (*LV*). The rapid sampling rate of the M-mode recording allows more accurate identification of the endocardial and epicardial LV walls.

■ Calculation of LV mass in selected cases

Key points:

❏ 2D-guided M-mode measurement of LV wall thickness at end-diastole (onset of the QRS) is adequate in most cases.

❏ Calculation of LV mass from traced 2D endocardial and epicardial borders is largely limited to research applications (see Chapter 6).

Pattern of left ventricular hypertrophy

■ Long axis, short axis, and apical views are used to evaluate the pattern of ventricular hypertrophy (Figs. 9–9 and 9–10).

Key points:

❏ 2D imaging allows evaluation of the pattern of hypertrophy in all myocardial segments.

❏ When hypertrophy is concentric, LV wall thickness measurements at one site adequately represent the degree of hypertrophy.

❏ When hypertrophy is asymmetric, measurements at key sites are reported, particularly the septal thickness in patients with hypertrophic cardiomyopathy.

❏ 2D-guided M-mode measurements are most accurate when the ultrasound beam can be aligned perpendicular to the LV wall of interest. Otherwise, 2D measurements at end-diastole are reported.

Step 3: Assess Left Ventricular Diastolic Function (See Chapter 7)

■ LV and left atrial inflow patterns (Fig. 9–11)
■ Tissue Doppler at the mitral annulus (Fig. 9–12)
■ Isovolumic relaxation time (Fig. 9–13)

Key points:

❏ Systolic LV dysfunction typically is accompanied by some degree of diastolic dysfunction.

❏ Classification of the degree of diastolic dysfunction as mild (impaired relaxation) versus severe (decreased compliance) is used in clinical decision making.

❏ LV filling pressures are estimated whenever systolic dysfunction is present.

Step 4: Estimate Pulmonary Artery Pressures (See Chapter 6)

■ Pulmonary systolic pressure is estimated from the tricuspid regurgitant jet velocity and estimated right atrial pressure (Figs. 9–14 and 9–15).

■ Other signs of pulmonary hypertension include a short time to peak velocity in the pulmonary artery velocity curve, paradoxical septal motion, and a high end-diastolic pulmonic regurgitant velocity.

Key points:

❏ Pulmonary pressures often are elevated in patients with heart failure resulting from a cardiomyopathy.

❏ Pulmonary pressures may be reduced with effective medical therapy, in conjunction with a decrease in left atrial (or LV filling) pressure.

❏ When pulmonary pressures are elevated disproportionately to the degree of left heart dysfunction, concurrent primary pulmonary disease or pulmonary thromboembolism may be present.

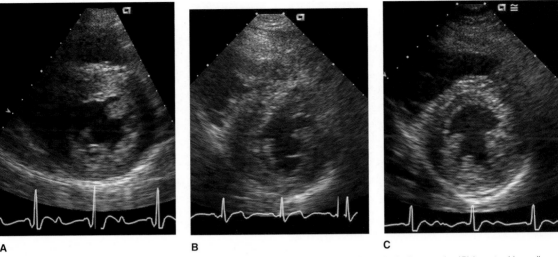

Figure 9–9 Parasternal short axis images in three different patients showing (*A*) concentric left ventricular hypertrophy, (*B*) hypertrophic cardiomyopathy involving the septum and anterior wall with sparing of the inferior-lateral and lateral walls, and (*C*) apical hypertrophic cardiomyopathy with hypertrophy of the inferior, posterior, and lateral walls but a relatively normal septum and anterior wall.

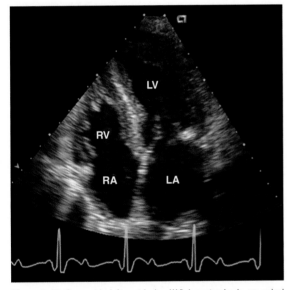

Figure 9–10 Concentric left ventricular (*LV*) hypertrophy in an apical four-chamber view shows equal thickness of the septum and lateral wall.

Step 5: Evaluate Right Ventricular Size and Systolic Function (See Chapter 6)

■ Right ventricular (RV) size and systolic function are assessed from parasternal, apical, and subcostal views (Fig. 9–16).

Key points:

❑ RV systolic dysfunction may be caused by primary myocardial disease affecting both ventricles or by the effects of pulmonary hypertension.

❑ Qualitative assessment of RV size and function takes into account the degree of LV dilation and dysfunction. If there is severe LV dilation and dysfunction and the RV appears similar in size and function, then severe RV dilation and dysfunction also is present.

❑ The apical motion of the tricuspid annulus or tricuspid annular plane systolic excursion (TASPE) is <2.0 cm when moderate or severe RV dysfunction is present.

Step 6: Evaluate the Severity of Mitral and Tricuspid Regurgitation (See Chapter 12)

■ Mitral and tricuspid regurgitation commonly are present in patients with a cardiomyopathy.

■ Regurgitant severity is evaluated using standard approaches, starting with color Doppler vena contracta and the continuous wave Doppler velocity curve.

■ The mechanism of regurgitation is evaluated using 2D imaging from multiple views.

Key points:

❑ Mitral and tricuspid regurgitation resulting from LV dilation and dysfunction are common.

❑ The mechanism of atrioventricular valve regurgitation is "tethering" of the mitral leaflets, resulting in incomplete systolic coaptation. This also has been described as an increased angle between the papillary muscles so that the leaflets are "pulled apart" relative to the mitral annulus (Fig. 9–17).

❑ The degree of annular dilation is variable, with a variable contribution to the degree of mitral regurgitation.

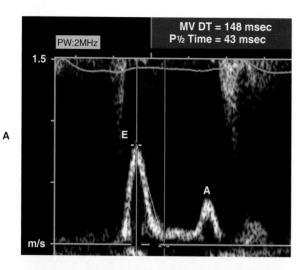

A

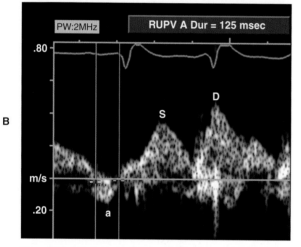

B

Figure 9–11 Left ventricular (*LV*) diastolic filling in a patient with a dilated cardiomyopathy showing an increased E/A ratio with a steep early diastolic deceleration slope, consistent with either normal diastolic function or pseudo-normalization caused by decreased LV compliance (*A*). The pulmonary vein flow pattern shows reduced systolic, compared with diastolic, inflow consistent with pseudo-normalization. *B,* The A reversal is relatively low velocity, with a short duration suggesting that left atrial pressure is not elevated on the current medical regimen.

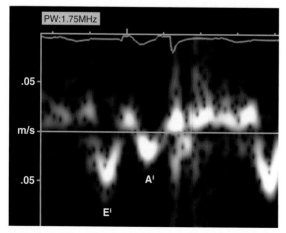

Figure 9–12 Tissue Doppler at the mitral annulus shows a relatively normal ratio of early (A') to late diastolic (E') tissue velocities in this patient with a dilated cardiomyopathy on appropriate medical therapy.

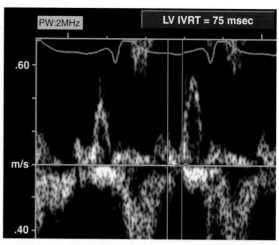

Figure 9–13 The isovolumic relaxation time (*IVRT*), measured from the end of aortic ejection flow to the onset of mitral inflow, is normal at 75 ms in this patient with dilated cardiomyopathy.

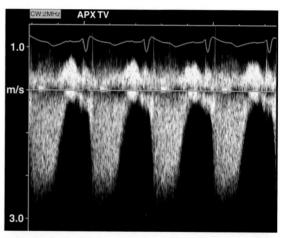

Figure 9–14 This tricuspid regurgitant jet signal has a peak somewhere around 2.5 m/s. This signal is not ideal because the peak is not well defined. This likely is due to the position of the ultrasound beam relative to the jet and the use of color coding (instead of gray scale) for the spectral display, which often obscures the peak velocity with superimposed noise. However, the peak velocity of about 2.4 m/s indicates a right ventricular to right atrial systolic pressure difference of at least 23 mm Hg.

- ❑ Mitral regurgitant severity may decrease with effective medical or resynchronization therapy for heart failure.

Step 7: Evaluate the Left Atrial Size (See Chapter 2)

- ■ Left atrial size typically is increased either because of chronic elevation of LV filling pressures or coexisting mitral regurgitation (Fig. 9–18).
- ■ Left atrial size can be evaluated qualitatively, using a simple anterior-posterior dimension, or by calculation of atrial volume from apical views.

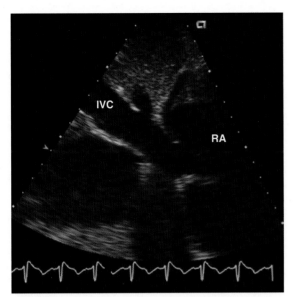

Figure 9–15 The junction of the inferior vena cava (*IVC*) and right atrium (*RA*) is visualized from the subcostal window for estimating RA pressure. In this patient, the IVC diameter is about 2.5 cm and collapses less than 50% with inspiration, consistent with a right atrial pressure of 10-15 mm Hg.

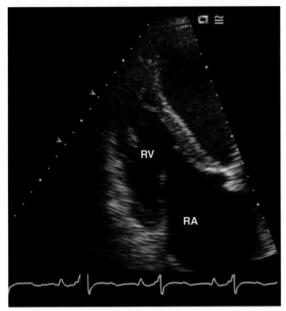

Figure 9–16 The right ventricle (*RV*) is imaged from the apical four-chamber view by tilting the transducer toward the RV and narrowing the sector.

Key points:

❒ Although atrial volumes are predictive of clinical outcome, simpler measures of atrial size suffice for clinical decision making in most cases.

❒ Left atrial anterior-posterior dimension is measured in a long axis view at end-systole (maximum left atrial dimension).

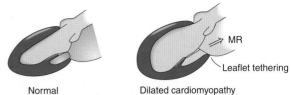

Figure 9–17 Schematic diagram showing leaflet tethering with dilated cardiomyopathy due to lateral displacement of the papillary muscles resulting in an oblique angle to the mitral annulus.

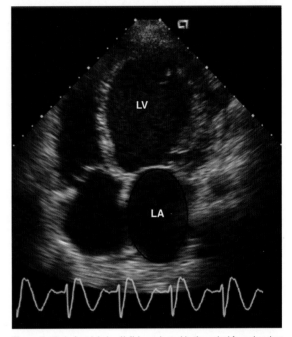

Figure 9–18 Left atrial size (*LA*) is evaluated in the apical four-chamber view by tracing the border to derive a left atrial volume. Left atrial size often is underestimated based on only the anterior-posterior diameter measured from the parasternal window.

❒ Right atrial size also may be increased and is evaluated qualitatively (as mildly, moderately, or severely dilated) in comparison with the other cardiac chambers.

Additional Steps

Dilated Cardiomyopathy

■ Evaluate for LV apical thrombus (Fig. 9–19).
■ Differentiate from end-stage coronary disease (Table 9–1).
■ Differentiate LV dysfunction caused by severe mitral regurgitation from a primary cardiomyopathy with secondary mitral regurgitation (Table 9–2).

Key points:

❒ Examination for LV apical thrombus includes oblique views of the LV apex using a high frequency transducer and shallow image depth.

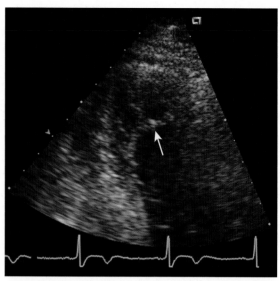

Figure 9–19 Evaluation for apical left ventricular (*LV*) thrombus using a high frequency transducer and shallow image depth from the apical four-chamber view. *A* and *B* both show normal apical trabeculation, which is distinguished from thrombus by the linear appearance with attachments to the myocardial wall.

TABLE 9–1

DIFFERENTIATION OF LEFT VENTRICULAR SYSTOLIC DYSFUNCTION DUE TO END-STAGE ISCHEMIC DISEASE FROM DILATED CARDIOMYOPATHY

FINDINGS	END-STAGE ISCHEMIC DISEASE	DILATED CARDIOMYOPATHY
Left ventricular ejection fraction	Moderately to severely depressed	Moderately to severely depressed
Segmental wall motion abnormalities	May be present	Absent
Right ventricular systolic function	Normal, except with RV infarction	Decreased
Pulmonary artery pressures	Elevated	Elevated
Other tests	Coronary disease on angiography or chest CT	No significant coronary disease

CT, *Computed tomography.*

TABLE 9–2

DIFFERENTIATION OF LEFT VENTRICULAR SYSTOLIC DYSFUNCTION DUE TO DILATED CARDIOMYOPATHY FROM PRIMAY MITRAL REGURGITATION

FINDINGS	DILATED CARDIOMYOPATHY	CHRONIC MITRAL REGURGITATION
Left ventricular ejection fraction	Moderately to severely depressed	Moderately to severely depressed
Segmental wall motion abnormalities	Absent	Absent
Right ventricular systolic function	Decreased	Variable
Pulmonary artery pressures	Elevated	Elevated
Mitral regurgitation	Moderate	Moderate to severe
Mitral valve anatomy	Dilated annulus	Primary leaflet involvement
	Abnormal papillary muscle annular angle	Rheumatic changes, leaflet prolapse
	Leaflet tethering	Flail segment

❑ Transesophageal echocardiography (TEE) is not useful to evaluate for apical thrombus because of the distance of the apex from the transducer and the likelihood that the true apex may be missed from this approach.

❑ LV systolic dysfunction resulting from coronary disease and that resulting from a primary cardiomyopathy may look similar on echocardiography. Both may show wall motion that is best preserved at the inferior-lateral base.

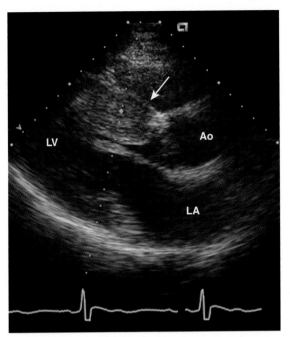

Figure 9–20 Hypertrophic cardiomyopathy in a parasternal long axis view showing marked increased thickness of the interventricular septum (*arrow*) with a normal thickness of the posterior wall.

☐ Features that suggest end-stage coronary disease include definite evidence for myocardial infarction (segmental thinning and akinesis) and normal right ventricular size and systolic function. However, direct visualization of coronary anatomy by angiography or computed tomography (CT) typically is needed.

☐ Stress echocardiography is difficult to interpret with significant resting LV systolic dysfunction with a suboptimal sensitivity and specificity for detection of ischemia.

Hypertrophic Cardiomyopathy

Step 1: Left ventricular hypertrophy

■ Describe the pattern of hypertrophy (Fig. 9–20).

■ Evaluate the wall thickness of the basal posterior wall.

■ Measure the maximal septal thickness.

Key points:

☐ The most common pattern of hypertrophy involves the ventricular septum with a normal posterior LV wall.

☐ Apical hypertrophy may be missed unless echo-contrast is used to opacify the ventricle because the endocardial border in the mid-left ventricle may be difficult to visualize (Fig. 9–21).

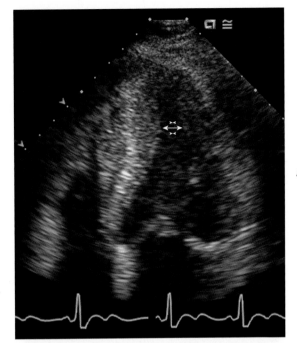

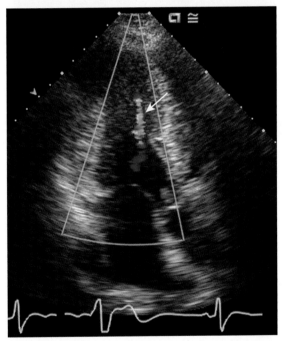

Figure 9–21 Apical four-chamber view (*A*) in a young woman with hypertrophic cardiomyopathy showing the small chamber (*double arrow*) and thick walls at the apex on a diastolic frame. In systole, the long axis view (*B*) shows flow acceleration at the midventricular level (*arrow*), instead of the subaortic obstruction seen with the more typical basal septal hypertrophy in patients with hypertrophic cardiomyopathy.

☐ Even with atypical patterns of hypertrophy, the basal posterior wall thickness typically is normal.

☐ The maximal septal thickness is a predictor of sudden death risk. Septal thickness is mea-

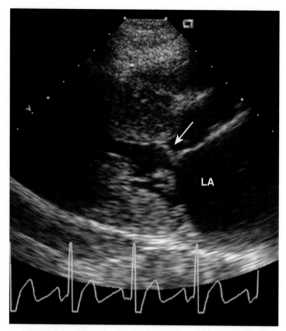

Figure 9–22 Hypertrophic cardiomyopathy in a parasternal long axis view showing systolic anterior motion of the mitral leaflet (*arrow*) causing dynamic subaortic obstruction.

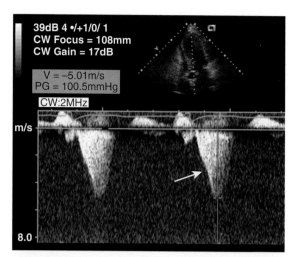

Figure 9–23 Continuous wave Doppler recording from an apical approach of outflow velocity in a patient with obstructive hypertrophic cardiomyopathy. This waveform is consistent with dynamic obstruction with a late-peaking high velocity systolic signal. The level of obstruction is not defined using continuous wave Doppler because the signal includes velocities from the entire length of the ultrasound beam.

sured at end-diastole, taking care to exclude RV trabeculations from the measurement.

◻ Screening of first-degree relatives is recommended when hypertrophic cardiomyopathy is diagnosed, because early detection and treatment can prevent sudden death.

Step 2: Dynamic subaortic outflow obstruction

■ Evaluate dynamic subaortic outflow obstruction.
■ Evaluate the mechanism and severity of mitral regurgitation.

Key points:

◻ Subaortic obstruction is caused by systolic anterior motion (SAM) of the mitral leaflet and a hypertrophied septum (Fig. 9–22).
◻ The Doppler velocity curve peaks in late systole, instead of in mid-systole as seen with valvular obstruction (Fig. 9–23).
◻ The level of obstruction is established with pulsed or high pulse repetition frequency (HPRF) Doppler, with continuous wave Doppler used to measure the maximum velocity.
◻ The severity of obstruction varies with loading conditions, increasing when afterload is decreased or when ventricular volume is reduced—exercise testing may be used to evaluate the change in outflow obstruction with exertion.
◻ Mitral regurgitation may be caused by SAM of the mitral leaflet, resulting in inadequate

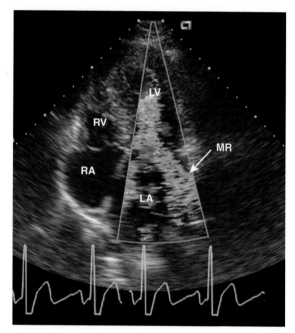

Figure 9–24 Mitral regurgitation in a patient with obstructive hypertrophic cardiomyopathy with the posterior-lateral jet direction demonstrated in this apical four-chamber view.

coaptation with a typical posteriorly directed regurgitant jet (Fig. 9–24).

Step 3: Distinguish from hypertensive heart disease

■ Hypertensive heart disease may be mistaken for hypertrophic cardiomyopathy.
■ Left ventricular hypertrophy in a patient with a clinical history of hypertension is nearly always caused by hypertensive heart disease.

Key points:

❐ Hypertension results in concentric LV hypertrophy; even the basal posterior wall is thickened.

❐ Dynamic outflow obstruction may occur with hypertensive heart disease, but the location of obstruction is mid-ventricular and SAM occurs in the mitral chordal region, instead of at the leaflet level.

Restrictive Cardiomyopathy

■ Perform a more detailed evaluation of LV diastolic function (Fig. 9–25).

■ Differentiate restrictive cardiomyopathy from constrictive pericarditis (see Chapter 10).

Key points:

❐ Restrictive cardiomyopathy is a primary disease of the myocardium, often related to an infiltrative or inflammatory process.

❐ Restrictive cardiomyopathy is characterized by predominant diastolic, rather than systolic, dysfunction, so detailed evaluation of diastolic function is helpful.

❐ Restrictive cardiomyopathy and constrictive pericarditis result in similar changes in ventricular filling but can be differentiated based on several features (see Table 10–2).

❐ LV systolic dysfunction may also be present, especially late in the disease course.

❐ Pulmonary systolic pressure usually is moderately to severely elevated.

Hypertensive Heart Disease

■ Evaluation of the patient with hypertensive heart disease follows the general approach outlined for a patient with a cardiomyopathy (Fig. 9–26).

■ Blood pressure should be recorded at the time of every echocardiographic examination. In some patients, a diagnosis of hypertension may be made only after echocardiographic examination.

Key points:

❐ Hypertension results in LV hypertrophy with impaired diastolic relaxation.

❐ Prolonged poorly controlled hypertension may eventually result in more severe diastolic dysfunction and systolic dysfunction.

❐ Effective treatment of hypertension results in regression of LV hypertrophy.

❐ LV hypertrophy may be accompanied by dynamic mid-cavity obstruction due to a small, thick-walled, hyperdynamic ventricle (Fig. 9–27).

❐ Obstruction may only be present or may increase with hypovolemia or hyperdynamic states (such as anemia, fever, sepsis, etc.).

❐ Aortic valve sclerosis and mitral annular calcification are typically seen in patients with hypertensive heart disease (Fig. 9–28).

❐ Hypertension is associated with dilation and increased tortuosity of the ascending aorta resulting in a more acute angle between the ventricular septum and the aortic root, some-

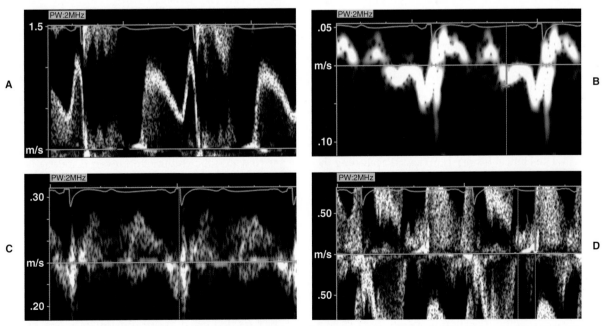

Figure 9–25 Evaluation of diastolic function in a patient with a restrictive cardiomyopathy includes (*A*) transmitral flow, (*B*) tissue Doppler velocity at the mitral annulus, (*C*) pulmonary vein flow, and (*D*) the isovolumic relaxation time. These tracings show impaired diastolic relaxation (transmitral and tissue Doppler E that is less than A, prolonged deceleration time, and prolonged isovolumic relaxation time). Left atrial pressure also may be elevated with an E/E' ratio >30, even though the pulmonary venous A wave is low velocity and short in duration.

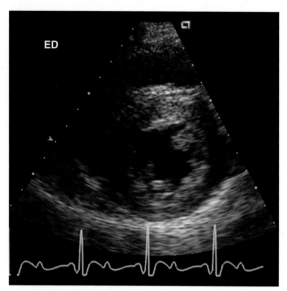

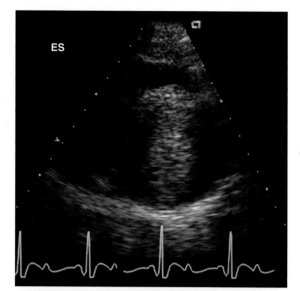

Figure 9–26 Parasternal short axis view in a patient with hypertensive heart disease showing a small ventricular cavity and concentric hypertrophy and end-diastole (*ED*).

times mistaken for focal basal septal thickening (Fig. 9–29).

Post-Transplant Heart Disease

■ Evaluation of the patient after heart transplantation follows the general approach outlined for a patient with a cardiomyopathy.

■ Early after heart transplantation, the major issues are surgical (e.g., pericardial effusion) and myocardial preservation (e.g., right and left ventricular systolic function).

■ Echocardiographic signs of transplant rejection include diastolic and systolic LV dysfunction.

■ Long-term, post-transplant patients are followed with dobutamine stress echocardiography for detection of graft coronary artery disease.

Key points:

❏ The clinical history is reviewed regarding the type of surgical anastomoses (bicaval versus atrial level suture lines; Fig. 9–30).

❏ Biatrial enlargement is typical after heart transplantation, sometimes with massive atrial enlargement with the older approach of biatrial anastomoses.

❏ Complications of percutaneous myocardial biopsy include cardiac perforation with pericardial effusion and tamponade and tricuspid valve damage resulting in regurgitation.

❏ Detection of rejection based on diastolic dysfunction is challenging, and this approach is used only by experienced transplant centers.

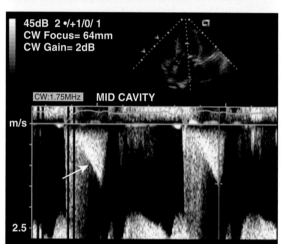

Figure 9–27 In the same patient as in Figure 9–26, (*A*) the end-systolic parasternal short axis view shows complete obliteration of the chamber at end-systole (*ES*) and (*B*) continuous wave Doppler from the apex shows a late-peaking systolic velocity of 1.4 m/s consistent with mid-cavity obstruction caused by a small, thick-walled chamber with normal systolic function.

❏ New systolic dysfunction, even if mild, may indicate acute rejection and requires prompt evaluation by the transplant team.

❏ When dobutamine stress echocardiography is performed after heart transplantation, atropine is unlikely to increase heart rate due to cardiac denervation.

Pulmonary Heart Disease

■ Pulmonary hypertension in the absence of significant left-sided heart disease indicates primary pulmonary or pulmonary vascular disease.

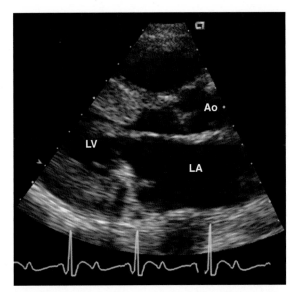

Figure 9–28 Parasternal long axis view in a patient with hypertension showing mild ventricular hypertrophy and aortic valve sclerosis.

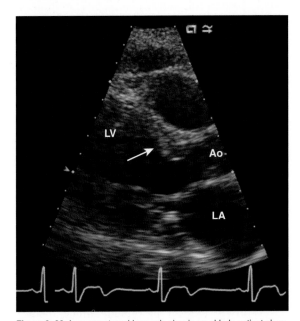

Figure 9–29 Low parasternal long axis view in an elderly patient showing prominence of the base of the septum (sometimes called a "septal knuckle," *arrow*) caused by an increased angle between the long axes of the aorta (*Ao*) and left ventricle (*LV*). Mild mitral annular calcification is present, but there is no evidence of left ventricular hypertrophy.

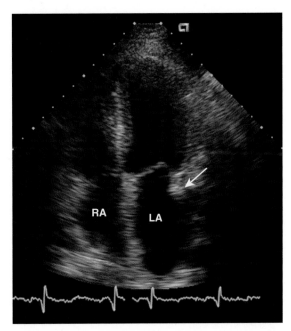

Figure 9–30 In this patient with biatrial anastomoses at heart transplantation, the enlarged left and right atria (caused by suturing of the native and donor atrium; *arrow* shows suture line) are seen in the apical four-chamber view.

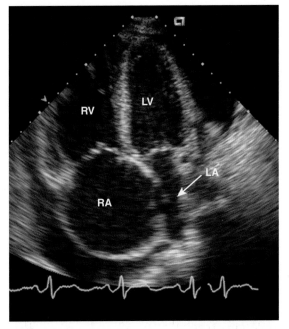

Figure 9–31 Cor pulmonale in a patient with severe pulmonary hypertension resulting in severe right ventricular hypertrophy and dilation and severely reduced right ventricular (*RV*) systolic function. The right atrium (*RA*) is severely enlarged with bulging of the atrial septum from right to left suggesting that right atrial pressure is higher than left atrial (*LA*) pressure. A moderate pericardial effusion (*PE*) also is seen.

■ The effects of pulmonary hypertension on the right heart result in pulmonary heart disease (or cor pulmonale; Fig. 9–31).

Step 1: Estimate Pulmonary Pressure

■ Pulmonary systolic pressure is determined based on the velocity in the tricuspid regurgitant jet and the estimated right atrial pressure (see Chapter 6; Fig. 9–32).

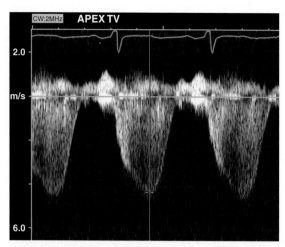

Figure 9–32 Tricuspid regurgitant jet recorded with continuous wave Doppler from an apical window. This recording shows a well-defined peak velocity with a dark band of velocities along the outer edge of the velocity curve, consistent with a good quality signal. A nonparallel intercept angle cannot be excluded, but this velocity indicates a right ventricular to right atrial systolic pressure difference of 76 mm Hg consistent with severe pulmonary hypertension.

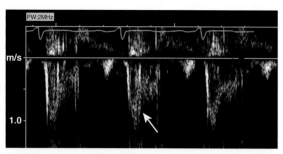

Figure 9–33 Pulsed Doppler recording of antegrade flow in the pulmonary artery from the parasternal right ventricular outflow view, in the same patient as Figure 9–32, shows a short time to peak velocity and a mid-systolic notch (*arrow*) in the velocity curve, which are specific for severe pulmonary hypertension.

- Additional signs of pulmonary hypertension also are evaluated.

Key points:

❑ When 2D echo findings show right heart dysfunction, a diligent search for the highest velocity tricuspid regurgitant jet is especially important.

❑ Other findings that suggest pulmonary hypertension include a short time to peak velocity, mid-systolic deceleration of the pulmonary artery velocity curve, and paradoxical septal motion (Fig. 9–33).

❑ The velocity of the tricuspid regurgitant jet reflects the systolic pressure difference between the right ventricle and atrium, not the volume of regurgitation. Thus severe pulmonary hypertension may be present with only mild tricuspid regurgitation.

❑ Overestimation of pulmonary pressures is prevented by using a gray-scale velocity display, increasing the high-pass (or wall) filter, and adjusting the gain level appropriately. The low intensity linear signals outside the edge of the velocity envelope are not included in the velocity measurement.

Step 2: Evaluate Right Ventricular Size and Systolic Function

- The right ventricle responds to chronic pressure overload by hypertrophy of the wall and dilation of the chamber, often accompanied by systolic dysfunction.

- RV size is compared with LV size and graded as mildly, moderately, or severely enlarged (Fig. 9–34).
- RV systolic function is qualitatively evaluated as mildly, moderately, or severely reduced.
- The pattern of ventricular septal motion is evaluated in a parasternal short axis view.

Key points:

❑ If the left ventricle is normal in size, the right ventricle is severely dilated if the 2D area in a four-chamber view is larger than the left ventricle, moderately dilated if equal to the left ventricle, and mildly dilated if greater than normal but not equal to the left ventricle.

❑ If the left ventricle is dilated or hypovolemic, estimates of RV size are adjusted accordingly.

❑ RV size and systolic function are evaluated based on parasternal, apical, and subcostal views.

❑ The tricuspid annular plane systolic excursion also is a helpful marker of RV function.

❑ RV size and function often are best evaluated from the subcostal window, because the right ventricle is seen in oblique image planes from the parasternal view and the RV free wall may be difficult to visualize on apical views.

❑ Elevated RV pressure results in flattening of the ventricular septum during both systole and diastole, whereas right heart volume overload results in flattening mostly during diastole.

Step 3: Evaluate the Severity of Tricuspid Regurgitation

- Pulmonary hypertension often results in dilation of the tricuspid annulus with inadequate leaflet coaptation and tricuspid regurgitation.

■ Tricuspid regurgitant severity is evaluated based on the vena contracta width of the regurgitant jet, the density of the continuous wave Doppler velocity curve, and the pattern of flow in the hepatic veins.

Key points:
❐ Vena contracta width is best measured in the parasternal RV inflow view; a width >7 mm indicates severe regurgitation.
❐ The density of the continuous wave Doppler signal is compared with antegrade flow; equal density indicates severe regurgitation.
❐ The normal hepatic vein pattern of systolic flow into the right atrium is reversed when tricuspid regurgitation is severe. However, systolic flow reversal may be seen when the patient is not in sinus rhythm, even when regurgitation is not severe.

Step 4: Exclude Other Causes of Pulmonary Hypertension or Right Heart Enlargement

■ Pulmonary hypertension and right heart enlargement also may be caused by left-sided heart disease or congenital heart disease.
■ Right heart enlargement without severe pulmonary hypertension is seen with volume overload caused by valve regurgitation or a left-to-right shunt.

Key points:
❐ Left-sided and congenital heart disease results in secondary pulmonary hypertension, which is easily distinguished from primary pulmonary disease.
❐ Right-sided volume overload in the absence of an obvious atrial septal defect or severe right-sided valve regurgitation prompts TEE to exclude a sinus venosus atrial septal defect or partial anomalous pulmonary venous return.

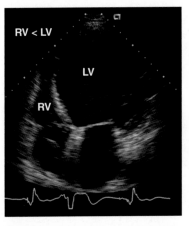 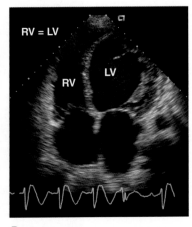 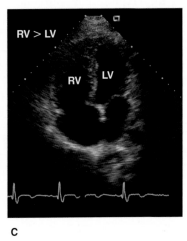

A   **B**   **C**

Figure 9–34 Examples of estimating right ventricular size compared with the left ventricle (*LV*) in the apical four-chamber view. *A,* The LV is severely dilated, so the normal-size right ventricle (*RV*) appears very small. *B,* Although the right ventricular area is not as large as the LV, the LV is moderately dilated. In addition, the right ventricular apex extends beyond the left ventricular apex (instead of being about two thirds of the left ventricular basal–apical distance). These findings are consistent with moderate right ventricular enlargement. *C,* This patient has a normal-size LV with an RV that is larger in area than the LV, and a right ventricular apex at the same level as the LV, consistent with severe right ventricular enlargement. In addition, right ventricular free wall thickness is increased, indicating right ventricular pressure overload and hypertrophy.

NOTES

SELF-ASSESMENT QUESTIONS

QUESTION 1

Echocardiography is requested in an 82-year-old woman for dyspnea on exertion. The following measurements are recorded:

LV dimension, end-diastole:	34 mm
End-systole:	20 mm
Wall thickness, septum:	10 mm
Posterior wall:	9 mm
Ejection fraction:	68%
Left atrial dimension:	4.8 cm
Tricuspid regurgitant jet:	3 m/s
Estimated right atrial pressure:	5 mm Hg

Her LV inflow, tissue Doppler, and LA inflow velocities are shown in Figure 9–35.

These findings are most consistent with:

A. Dilated cardiomyopathy
B. Hypertrophic cardiomyopathy
C. Restrictive cardiomyopathy
D. Hypertensive heart disease
E. Pulmonary heart disease
F. Normal heart

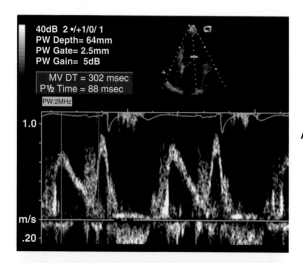

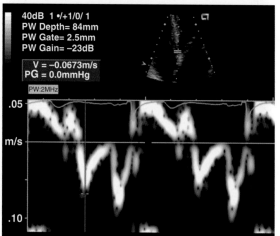

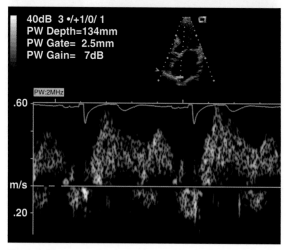

Figure 9–35

QUESTION 2

A 58-year-old man is referred for echocardiography for evaluation of a murmur during a hospital admission for gastrointestinal bleeding. His past medical history is remarkable for smoking, diabetes, hypertension, and hyperlipidemia. He has a positive family history for heart disease, with an uncle who died at age 56 years and his father, who died at age 62 years. The Doppler signal shown in Figure 9–36 is recorded.

The most likely diagnosis is:

A. Dilated cardiomyopathy
B. Hypertrophic cardiomyopathy
C. Restrictive cardiomyopathy
D. Hypertensive heart disease
E. Pulmonary heart disease
F. Normal heart

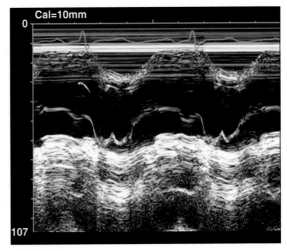

Figure 9–37

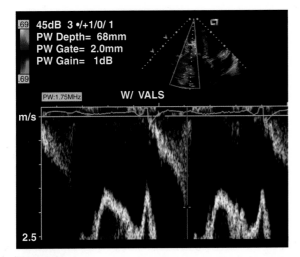

Figure 9–36

QUESTION 3

A 37-year-old woman is referred for echocardiography for dyspnea. She denies a previous cardiac history. Evaluation of cardiac risk factors reveals she does not smoke, has a normal blood pressure, has no family history of heart disease, and has not had her cholesterol or glucose checked. Early in the examination, the pulmonic valve M-mode shown in Figure 9–37 is recorded. At this point, the most likely diagnosis is:

A. Dilated cardiomyopathy
B. Hypertrophic cardiomyopathy
C. Restrictive cardiomyopathy
D. Hypertensive heart disease
E. Pulmonary heart disease
F. Normal heart

QUESTION 4

A colleague asks you to look at the parasternal long axis view shown in Figure 9–38.

The most likely clinical diagnosis is:

A. Dilated cardiomyopathy
B. Hypertrophic cardiomyopathy
C. Restrictive cardiomyopathy
D. Hypertensive heart disease
E. Pulmonary heart disease
F. Normal heart

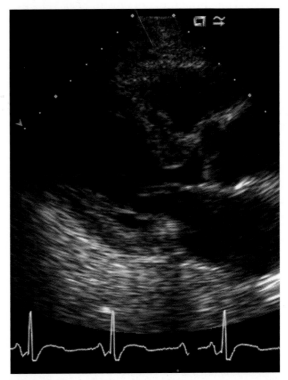

Figure 9–38

QUESTION 5

A 38-year-old woman with hypertrophic cardio-myopathy presents with decreased exercise toler-ance over the past year. Her echocardiogram shows septal hypertrophy with a maximum thick-ness of 2.6 cm, a normal ejection fraction, and impaired early diastolic relaxation but an outflow tract velocity of only 1.8 m/s. Pulmonary systolic pressure is estimated at 42 mm Hg.

The most useful next step in evaluation of her symptoms is:

A. Pulmonary function tests
B. Transesophageal echocardiogram
C. Coronary angiography
D. Saline contrast echo study
E. Exercise echocardiography

QUESTION 6

A 26-year-old man with hypertrophic cardiomy-opathy has both subaortic outflow obstruction and moderate mitral regurgitation. From an api-cal view, the two Doppler signals shown in Figure 9–39 are recorded.

Which specific feature convinces you that the velocity curve B is due to outflow obstruction?

A. Peak velocity
B. Duration of flow
C. Time from onset of flow to peak velocity
D. Density of signal
E. Diastolic flow signal

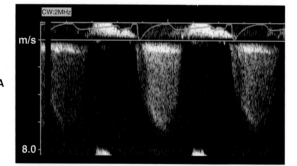

A

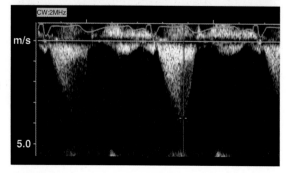

B

Figure 9–39

QUESTION 7

A 28-year-old woman with a diagnosis of primary pulmonary hypertension is referred to re-evaluate pulmonary pressures after 6 months of medical therapy with bosentan. You obtain a pulmonary pressure of 36 mm Hg, based on a tricuspid regur-gitant jet velocity of 2.8 m/s and an estimated right atrial pressure of 5 mm Hg. Her previous study was done at another laboratory with the tricuspid regurgitant jet shown in Figure 9–40.

Comparing your results to the previous study and assuming no change in right atrial pressure, you conclude that pulmonary systolic pressure has:

A. Decreased
B. Increased
C. Not changed

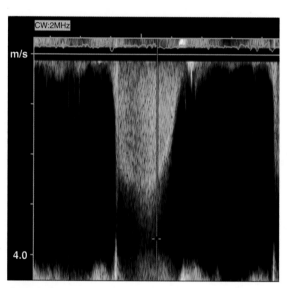

Figure 9–40

QUESTION 8

A 64-year-old man is referred for a new diagnosis of heart failure. Echocardiography shows an ejection fraction of 28%. The feature most helpful in distinguishing whether this is a primary dilated cardiomyopathy or results from coronary artery disease is:

A. Pulmonary systolic pressure
B. Severity of mitral regurgitation
C. Right ventricular systolic function
D. Regional wall motion abnormalities
E. Left atrial size

NOTES

ANSWERS

ANSWER 1: F

This elderly woman has a normal (to small) ventricular chamber with wall thickness at the upper limits of normal. Systolic function is normal based on ejection fraction. The Doppler tracings show a reduced transmitral and tissue Doppler E velocity, consistent with impaired relaxation (mild diastolic dysfunction), and the left atrium is moderately enlarged. However, all these findings are typical for the patient's age with no convincing evidence of ventricular dilation, hypertrophy, systolic dysfunction, or significant diastolic dysfunction to suggest a cardiomyopathy. Based on the tricuspid regurgitant jet velocity and estimated right atrial pressure, there is mild pulmonary hypertension with a systolic pressure of 41 mm Hg–again, a finding typical for age.

ANSWER 2: D

The figure shows an anteriorly angulated apical four-chamber view, with a pulsed Doppler sample volume positioned in the LV outflow tract at the mid-ventricular level. The baseline has been shifted to the top of the scale to measure the peak systolic velocity, so the mitral inflow toward the transducer is effectively aliased and is shown at the bottom of the display. This late peaking outflow velocity signal with a maximum velocity of 1.8 m/s is atypical for hypertrophic cardiomyopathy based on location (mid-ventricular instead of subaortic) and the abrupt brief late systolic peak, suggesting cavity obliteration, rather than the smooth concave upward velocity curve seen with dynamic obstruction related to systolic motion of the anterior mitral leaflet. This patient has a history of hypertension, so mid-LV obstruction most likely is caused by the combination of concentric hypertrophy, normal systolic function, and a small chamber related to hypovolemia with gastrointestinal bleeding.

ANSWER 3: E

Using the electrocardiogram for timing, note that in mid-systole, the opened pulmonic valve leaflet briefly partially closes; this mid-systolic closure, sometimes called a "flying w," suggests significant pulmonary hypertension. This M-mode finding is equivalent to the mid-systolic notch seen on the pulmonary artery antegrade flow spectral Doppler tracing. This M-mode tracing suggests a pos-

sible diagnosis of pulmonary hypertension, mandating a careful search for the highest tricuspid regurgitant jet velocity. Pulmonary hypertension may be secondary to left sided heart disease, such as a cardiomyopathy, with a chronically elevated left atrial pressure. However, given the absence of risk factors for heart disease in this patient, it is more likely that primary pulmonary hypertension is present.

ANSWER 4: D

This parasternal long axis view at end-diastole shows a normal-size LV chamber with mildly increased thickness (about 12 mm) of the septum and posterior wall. There is prominence of the basal septum due to the increased angle between the aorta and long axis of the left ventricle. All these features are typical for hypertensive heart disease. In addition, there is mild mitral annular calcification and mild aortic leaflet thickening, also typical features of hypertensive heart disease.

This is not a dilated cardiomyopathy, because the LV is not dilated and the lack of asymmetric hypertrophy argues against hypertrophic cardiomyopathy. There are no findings to suggest pulmonary heart disease with a normal diastolic shape of the septum and a normal-size RV outflow tract. It is more difficult to exclude restrictive cardiomyopathy, but the increase in wall thickness is only mild and hypertensive heart disease is far more common than a restrictive cardiomyopathy.

ANSWER 5: E

Exercise echocardiography to evaluate the severity of outflow obstruction after exertion would be the most helpful next step. Many patients with hypertrophic cardiomyopathy who have only mild outflow obstruction at rest will develop more severe obstruction with exercise that may account for symptoms. Pulmonary function tests should be considered when cardiac studies are unrevealing or when history or physical examination findings suggest concurrent pulmonary disease. Transesophageal echocardiography may provide improved images of septal thickness but is less useful for hemodynamics because the Doppler beam usually cannot be aligned parallel to LV outflow. Coronary angiography is not helpful for evaluation of small vessel disease related to hypertrophic cardiomyopathy and is reserved for patients with risk factors for epicardial coronary disease. A patent foramen ovale would not explain the patient's symptoms, so a saline contrast study is not indicated.

ANSWER 6: B

The most reliable distinguishing factor between these two Doppler curves is the systolic ejection period. Mitral regurgitation (curve A) includes isovolumic contraction and relaxation periods, as well as the systolic ejection period, and thus is longer in duration than LV outflow obstruction (curve B). Both LV outflow obstruction and mitral regurgitation have a high peak velocity in systole. Although curve A has a higher velocity (6.5 m/s) than curve B (3.5 m/s), underestimation may be due to a nonparallel intercept angle between the ultrasound beam and direction of flow. The time from onset of flow to peak velocity can be difficult to measure reliably, especially with mitral regurgitation, which typically has a rounded peak. The density of mitral regurgitation, relative to antegrade flow, is a reflection of regurgitant severity. However, outflow obstruction often is accompanied by significant mitral regurgitation (as the anterior motion of the mitral leaflet results in inadequate coaptation), so both signals may be similar in intensity. The diastolic flow signal may not be helpful because the wide beam width of continuous wave Doppler results in LV inflow being recorded with both systolic signals.

ANSWER 7: C

This Doppler recording from the previous study is difficult to measure. The Doppler gain is too high and the color (instead of gray scale) displays noise with hue and intensity similar to the Doppler signal. The Doppler velocity can be discerned as the dense smooth rounded curve within the combined noise and signal displayed in color. Doppler flow curves reflect physiologic pressure differences, with smooth increases and decreases in velocity. The Doppler curve should show a smooth dense outer edge, often called "envelope of flow," indicating the modal Doppler velocity. The Doppler curve and correct peak velocity

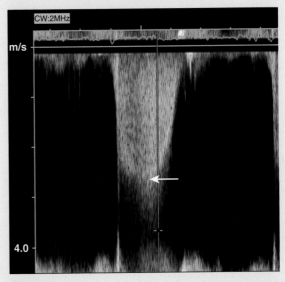

Figure 9–41

(*arrow*) is shown in Figure 9–41. Based on a maximum tricuspid regurgitant jet velocity of 2.8 m/s, pulmonary systolic pressure is unchanged compared with the previous study.

ANSWER 8: D

It is difficult to distinguish a primary dilated cardiomyopathy from systolic dysfunction caused by coronary disease based on echocardiography alone; many of these patients require evaluation of coronary anatomy. However, the finding of clear regional wall motion abnormalities is consistent with coronary artery disease. This finding is most reliable if some segments are thin, bright, and akinetic (scarred from previous infarction) and some segments are normal. Mitral regurgitation, left atrial enlargement, and pulmonary hypertension typically are seen with LV systolic dysfunction of any cause. Normal RV size and systolic function with a dilated, hypokinetic left ventricle suggests coronary disease is likely. However, RV size and function may be abnormal with coronary disease if there has been an RV infarction. Conversely, some cardiomyopathies affect the myocardium asymmetrically, so LV dysfunction may be more severe than RV involvement.

NOTES

10 Pericardial Disease

THE ECHO EXAM: PERICARDIAL DISEASE

PERICARDIAL EFFUSION

Views

Parasternal

Apical

Subcostal

Distinguish From Pleural Fluid

Size

Small (< 0.5 cm)

Moderate (0.5-2.0 cm)

Large (> 2.0 cm)

Diffuse Versus Loculated

Evaluate for Tamponade Physiology if Moderate or Large

CONSTRICTIVE PERICARDITIS

M-Mode/2D

Pericardial thickening

Normal LV size and systolic function

LA enlargement

Flattened diastolic wall motion

Abrupt posterior motion of the ventricular septum in early diastole

Dilated inferior vena cava and hepatic veins

Doppler

Prominent *y* descent on hepatic vein or superior vena cava flow pattern

LV inflow shows prominent E velocity with a rapid early diastolic deceleration slope and a small or absent A velocity

Increase in LV-IVRT by > 20% on first beat after inspiration

Respiratory variations in RV/LV diastolic filling (difference > 25%) with ↑ RV and ↓ LV filling with inspiration

Pulmonary venous flow shows prominent A wave and blunting of systolic phase

PERICARDIAL TAMPONADE

Clinical Findings

Low cardiac output

Elevated venous pressures

Pulsus paradoxus

Hypotension

2D-Echo

Moderate to large pericardial effusion

RA systolic collapse (duration >⅓ of systole)

RV diastolic collapse

Reciprocal respiratory changes in RV and LV volumes

Inferior vena cava plethora

Doppler

Respiratory variation in RV and LV diastolic filling

Increased RV filling on first beat after inspiration

Decreased LV filling on first beat after inspiration

LV PSEUDOANEURYSM

Abrupt transition from normal myocardium to aneurysm

Acute angle between myocardium and aneurysm

Narrow neck

Ratio of neck diameter to aneurysm diameter < 0.5

May be lined with thrombus

↑, *Increased;* ↓, *decreased;* 2D, *two-dimensional;* LA, *left atrial;* LV, *left ventricular;* LV-IVRT, *left ventricular isovolumic relaxation time;* RA, *right atrial;* RV, *right ventricular.*

STEP-BY-STEP APPROACH

Pericardial Effusion

■ There are numerous causes for accumulation of fluid in the pericardial space (Table 10–1).

■ A pericardial effusion may be asymptomatic or may be associated with pericarditis or with tamponade physiology.

■ Pericarditis is a clinical diagnosis based on the triad of typical pericardial pain, a pericardial rub, and diffuse ST elevation on the electrocardiograph (ECG; Fig. 10–1).

■ Tamponade physiology is present when systemic blood pressure or cardiac output are reduced because of compression of the cardiac chambers by the pericardial fluid.

Key points:

❏ In patients with pericarditis, the effusion ranges from absent to large in size.

❏ The presence of a pericardial rub does not correlate with the size of the effusion.

❏ In a patient with a large pericardial effusion and hypotension or a low cardiac output, tamponade physiology likely is present, even if other echocardiographic signs are not present.

Step 1: Record the Patient's Blood Pressure and Heart Rate

■ The first step in echocardiographic evaluation of a patient with suspected pericardial disease is to measure and record blood pressure and heart rate (as for any echocardiographic examination).

■ Pulsus paradoxus is a decline in the systolic blood pressure by more than 20 mm Hg with inspiration (Fig. 10–2).

Key points:

❏ Hypotension and tachycardia are nonspecific but are seen in patients with tamponade physiology.

❏ To measure pulsus paradoxus, the blood pressure cuff is deflated until the first Korotkoff sound is intermittently heard during expiration. The cuff is then slowly deflated until the Korotkoff sound is heard on every beat. The difference between these two pressures is the paradoxical pulse.

❏ A physician should be present for the echocardiographic study when the patient is hemodynamically compromised (hypotension or significant tachycardia).

TABLE 10–1

DIFFERENTIAL DIAGNOSIS OF PERICARDIAL EFFUSION/PERICARDITIS

I. Infections
  A. Postviral pericarditis
  B. Bacterial
  C. Tuberculosis
II. Malignant
  A. Metastatic disease (e.g., lymphoma, melanoma)
  B. Direct extension (lung carcinoma, breast carcinoma)
  C. Primary cardiac malignancy
III. "Inflammatory"
  A. Post-myocardial infarction (Dressler's syndrome)
  B. Uremia
  C. Collagen-vascular disease
  D. Post-cardiac surgery
IV. Intracardiac–pericardial communications
  A. Blunt or penetrating chest trauma
  B. Post-catheter procedures (electrophysiology studies, percutaneous coronary intervention, valvuloplasty)
  C. Left ventricular rupture post-myocardial infarction

From Otto CM: Textbook of Clinical Echocardiography, 3rd ed. Philadelphia: Elsevier, 2004.

Step 2: Evaluate for the Presence of Pericardial Fluid

■ An echo-free space adjacent to the heart is consistent with a pericardial effusion (Figs. 10–3*A* and *B*).

■ The pericardial sac extends completely around both the left and right ventricles, from the apex to the base, and extends around the right atrium to the bases of the superior and inferior vena cava.

■ The pericardial sac extends posterior to the left atrium, between the pulmonary vein orifices (the oblique sinus of the pericardium), and there is a small cuff of pericardial space around the base of the great vessels (the transverse sinus; Fig. 10–4).

Key points:

❏ An isolated anterior relatively echo-free space usually is caused by the normal epicardial fat pad. With an effusion, the echo-free space usually is seen both anteriorly and posteriorly (Fig. 10–5).

❏ A pericardial effusion is seen anterior to the descending thoracic aorta, whereas a pleural effusion extends posteriorly to the descending aorta (Figs. 10–6*A* and *B*).

❏ Fluid adjacent to the right atrium in the apical four-chamber view may be caused by pericardial or pleural fluid. The specific diagnosis is based on evidence of pericardial or pleural fluid in other views (Fig. 10–7).

❏ If the pericardial fluid contains thrombus or fibrinous debris, the effusion may be echogenic, rather than echolucent (Fig. 10–8).

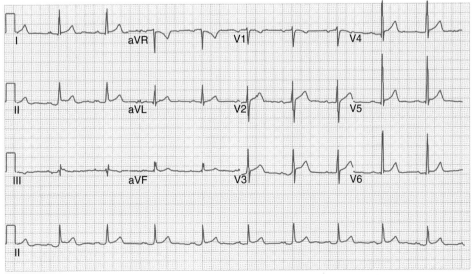

Figure 10–1 This 12-lead electrocardiograph shows diffuse upsloping ST elevation and PR segment depression, consistent with pericarditis, in this 42-year-old man with a 2-week history of persistent dull chest pain and a pericardial rub on physical examination.

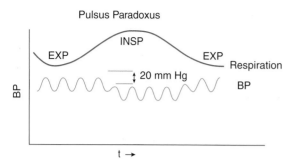

Figure 10–2 This schematic shows that with inspiration (*INSP*), systolic blood pressure (*BP*) falls by at least 20 mm Hg when pulsus paradoxus is present.

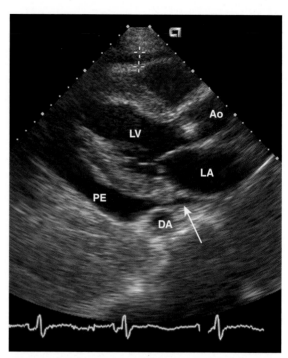

Figure 10–4 Pericardial fluid is seen posterior to the left atrium (*LA, arrow*) in the oblique sinus of the pericardium in this parasternal long axis view. This is clearly a pericardial effusion (*PE*), not pleural fluid, as it tracks anteriorly to the descending aorta (*DA*).

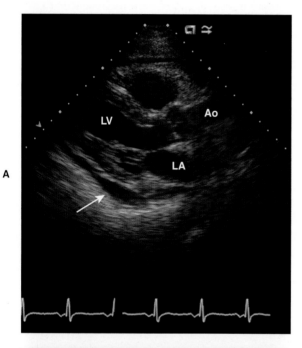

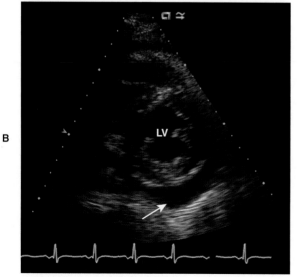

Figure 10–3 A small pericardial effusion is seen posterior to the left ventricle (*LV*) in both the parasternal long axis view (*A*) and the short axis view at the mid-ventricular level (*B*).

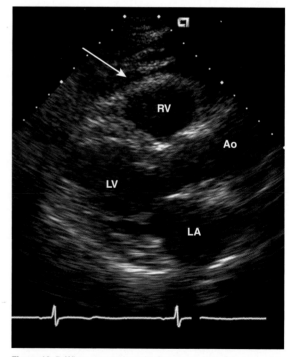

Figure 10–5 When an anterior echo free space (*arrow*) is seen, as in this parasternal long axis view, without evidence for posterior effusion, the most likely diagnosis is normal epicardial adipose tissue, or a "fat pad."

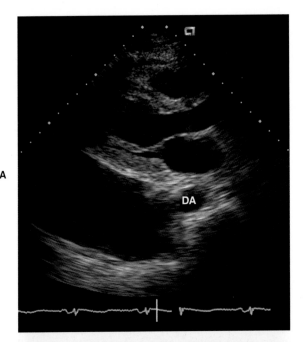

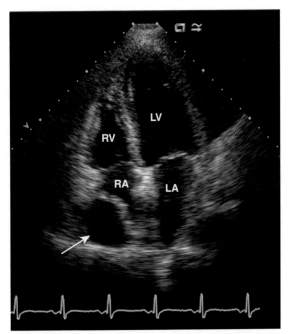

Figure 10–7 Fluid (*arrow*) adjacent to the right atrium (*RA*) seen in the apical four-chamber view most likely is pericardial, although pleural effusion also may extend adjacent to the RA in this view.

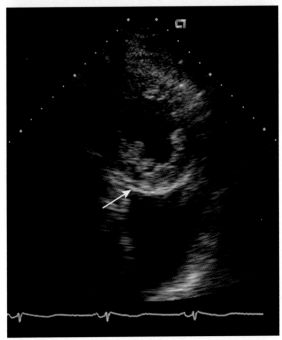

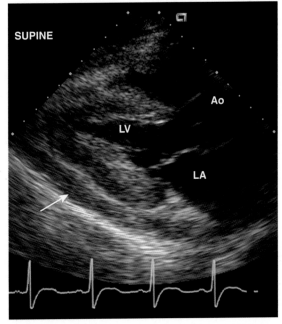

Figure 10–6 A large left pleural effusion is seen in this parasternal long axis (*A*) and short axis (*B*) view. The pleural effusion extends posterior to the descending thoracic aorta (*DA*). In the short axis view, the slight normal separation of the pericardial layers is seen (*arrow*).

Figure 10–8 In this parasternal long axis view, the pericardial space (*arrow*) is filled with echodense material, consistent with hematoma, tumor, or fibrinous debris.

Step 3: Evaluate the Distribution of Pericardial Fluid

■ Effusions may be circumferential or loculated, so evaluation in multiple views from parasternal, apical, and subcostal windows is essential (Fig. 10–9).

■ Loculation of fluid caused by adhesions often is seen after cardiac surgery or trauma or with malignant effusions.

Key points:

❑ Loculated fluid may be missed unless multiple views are examined; sometimes transesophageal echocardiography (TEE) is needed to identify loculated fluid posterior to the left atrium.

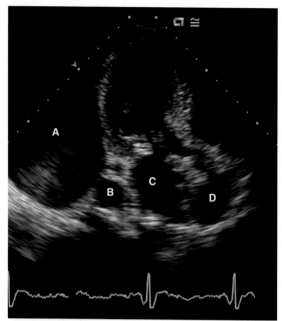

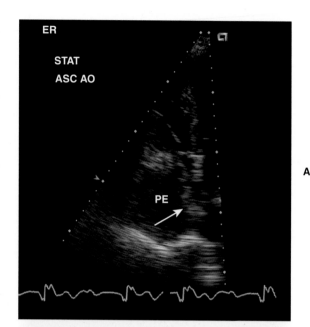

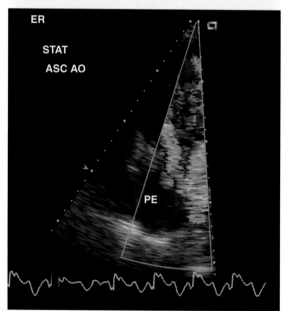

Figure 10–9 This apical long axis view was obtained in a 58-year-old woman after renal transplantation with an enlarged heart on chest X-ray. The large left pleural effusion (*A*) is identified based on its relationship to the descending thoracic aorta (*B*). There is a space that most likely is the left atrium (*C*) and another space that may be the ascending aorta (*D*). However, the space labeled *D* seems unusual in size and shape for the aorta and raises the concern of a loculated effusion. In addition, a loculated effusion can fill the space normally occupied by the left atrium. The location of the mitral annular calcification and the shape of the basal posterior wall are worrisome for a compressed left atrium. Color flow imaging would be helpful for confirming whether the left atrium is compressed. The structure labeled *D* should be imaged from another view and interrogated with color and pulsed Doppler.

❏ Loculated fluid occasionally may be mistaken for a normal cardiac chamber–for example, when loculated fluid compresses the left or right atrium (Figs. 10–10*A* and *B*).

Step 4: Estimate the Size of the Pericardial Effusion

■ A small, normal amount of pericardial fluid appears as a trivial or absent effusion on echocardiography.
■ The volume of an abnormal pericardial effusion ranges from 50 ml to more than 1 liter.
■ The size of the effusion is qualitatively graded as small, moderate, or large.

Key points:

❏ A small effusion on two-dimensional (2D) imaging can be confirmed by the M-mode finding of flat motion of the parietal pericardium with systolic separation of the epicardium (Figs. 10–11*A* and *B*).
❏ There is no precise approach to estimate pericardial fluid volume by echocardiography.

Figure 10–10 In an apical four-chamber orientation, the sector has been narrowed to focus on the right heart. The right ventricle is small, with a catheter seen in the chamber. *A,* The area normally occupied by the right atrium consists primarily of loculated pericardial fluid, with the right atrial free wall (*arrow*) compressed so that it almost touches the interatrial septum. *B,* Color Doppler confirms the severe compression of the right atrium with a very narrow flow stream into the right ventricle.

❏ One useful approach is to consider the effusion small if the distance between the epicardium and pericardium is less than 0.5 cm, moderate if it is 0.5 to 2 cm, and large if it is greater than 2 cm (Fig. 10–12).
❏ With loculated effusions, size is described in a similar fashion, along with the location of the fluid.

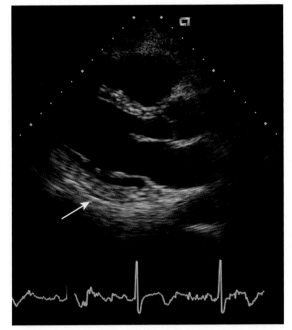

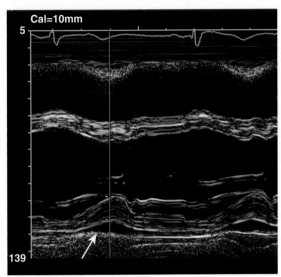

Figure 10–11 A very small pericardial effusion is seen (*A*) on two-dimensional imaging posterior to the left ventricle. *B*, The M-mode tracing demonstrates the small effusion more clearly with flat motion of the parietal pericardium, so there is a more prominent posterior echo free space in systole than diastole.

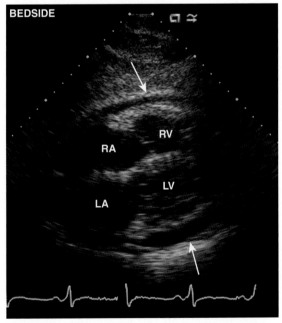

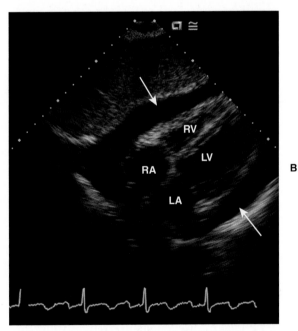

Figure 10–12 The size of a pericardial effusion is graded qualitatively, but measurement of the distance between the epicardium and pericardium is helpful. On a subcostal view, both these patients have a circumferential pericardial effusion, with a moderate effusion (*A*) showing between 0.5 and 2 cm maximal pericardial separation, compared with more than 2 cm with a large effusion (*B*).

❏ Evaluation from the subcostal view is especially important, because this approach often is used for pericardiocentesis (Fig. 10–13).

Tamponade Physiology

■ Pericardial pressure depends on both the volume and rate of accumulation of pericardial fluid.

■ Tamponade physiology occurs when pericardial pressure exceeds intracardiac pressure.

■ With tamponade physiology, cardiac output and blood pressure are reduced because of impaired cardiac filling caused by compression of the cardiac chambers.

■ Pulsus paradoxus is an excessive fall (more than 20 mm Hg) in systolic blood pressure with

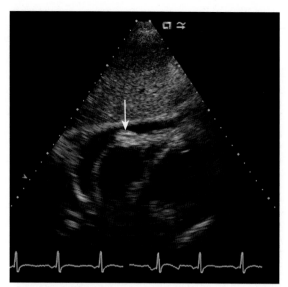

Figure 10–13 The subcostal window is key in evaluation of pericardial effusions, because this approach often is used for drainage of pericardial fluid. In this patient, the effusion between the liver and right heart is seen. The normal adipose tissue at the right atrioventricular groove (*arrow*) often is highly visible when a pericardial effusion is present. If pericardiocentesis is planned, a transducer position where the effusion is closer to the site of needle entry, with less intervening hepatic tissue, is preferred. This effusion is only small to moderate in size, so many clinicians would defer pericardiocentesis.

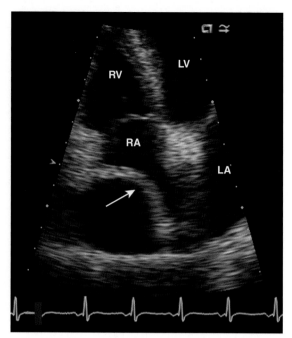

Figure 10–14 The right atrial (*RA*) free wall is examined frame by frame in the apical four-chamber plane using zoom mode and a narrow sector. This end-systolic frame shows persistent systolic compression (or collapse) of the right atrial free wall consistent with tamponade physiology.

inspiration, resulting from the fall in cardiac output with inspiration.

Key points:

❏ Tamponade physiology may occur with a rapidly accumulating moderate-size effusion (for example, with aortic dissection or trauma) but may not occur even with very large effusions if the rate of increase in size was gradual.

❏ Thin-walled low pressure cardiac chambers (e.g., the right atrium) are compressed at lower pericardial pressures than thicker-walled chambers (e.g., the right ventricle).

❏ Cardiac compression is most evident during the phase of the cardiac cycle when the chamber pressure is low (e.g., systole for the atrial chambers, diastole for the right ventricle).

❏ With inspiration, intrathoracic pressure falls, resulting in increased filling of the right heart. If total cardiac volume is fixed (as with tamponade physiology), the increased filling of the right heart limits filling of the left heart, resulting in a lower forward stroke volume and blood pressure.

❏ If the patient has a low cardiac output or hypotension and a large pericardial effusion is present, further echocardiographic evaluation is not needed–prompt therapy is more appropriate.

Step 1: Look for Right Atrial Systolic Collapse

■ When intrapericardial pressure exceeds right atrial pressure, the right atrial free wall collapses in systole (Fig. 10–14).

■ Right atrial free wall inversion for more than one third of systole is sensitive and specific for the diagnosis of tamponade physiology.

Key points:

❏ Brief systolic inversion of the right atrial free wall may be seen without tamponade physiology.

❏ The right atrial free wall is best evaluated in the apical and subcostal four-chamber views.

❏ Zoom mode provides optimal image resolution; a narrow 2D sector improves frame rate.

❏ Frame-by-frame analysis, to determine the number of frames with free wall inversion compared with the total frames in systole, improves the accuracy of this approach.

Step 2: Evaluate Right Ventricular Diastolic Collapse

■ When intrapericardial pressure exceeds right ventricular diastolic pressure, the right ventricular (RV) free wall collapses in diastole (Fig. 10–15).

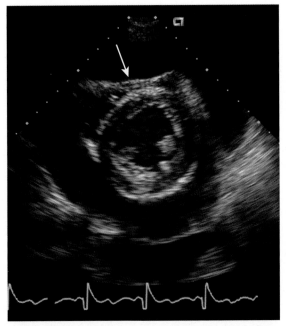
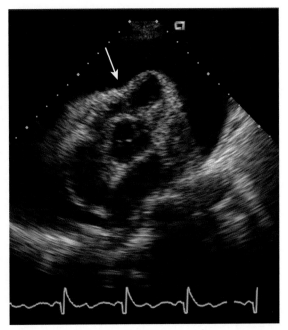

A

B

Figure 10–15 Parasternal short axis views in mid-diastole in a patient with a large pericardial effusion show right ventricular (RV) diastolic collapse at the mid-ventricular (*A*) and RV outflow tract (*B*) levels. The RV chamber is very small, with concave indentation of the RV free wall by the pericardial effusion.

Key points:

- Frame-by-frame analysis or use of an M-mode cursor through the RV free wall may be helpful for evaluation of the timing of RV free wall motion.
- RV diastolic collapse may be appreciated in parasternal long- and short-axis and in apical and subcostal four-chamber views.
- RV diastolic collapse is less sensitive, but more specific, than brief right atrial (RA) systolic collapse for the diagnosis of pericardial tamponade.
- If the RV free wall is thickened because of hypertrophy or an infiltrative process, diastolic collapse may not occur even with elevated pericardial pressures.

Step 3: Examine for Reciprocal Respiratory Changes in Right Ventricular and Left Ventricular Volumes

- An effusion with tamponade physiology results in a fixed total cardiac volume.
- With a fixed total volume, the increase in right-sided filling with inspiration is matched by a reciprocal decrease in left-sided volumes.
- Conversely, with expiration, there is a relative increase in left, compared with right, heart filling.

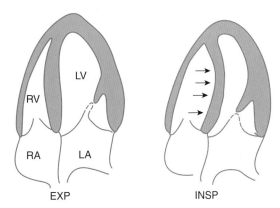

Figure 10–16 Schematic diagram showing an apical four-chamber view at end-expiration (*EXP*) and during inspiration (*INSP*) with pericardial constriction. The increase in right ventricular filling with inspiration results in a compensatory decrease in left ventricular size, as the total cardiac volume is constrained by the thickened and adherent pericardium. This results in "septal shift" with inspiration.

Key points:

- The reciprocal changes in right- and left-sided filling with respiration are best seen on 2D imaging in a four-chamber view (Fig. 10–16).
- With inspiration, the ventricular septum shifts to the left, followed by a shift toward the right with expiration.
- An M-mode tracing of the septum from the parasternal window also may be helpful.

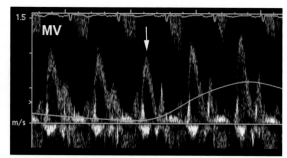

Figure 10–17 In this patient with a larger pericardial effusion, ventricular inflow velocities across the tricuspid valve (*TV, A*) and mitral valve (*MV, B*) were recorded at a slow sweep speed simultaneously with a respirometer tracing. The cyan-colored respirometer tracing indicates inspiration as an upward deflection and expiration as a downward deflection. The TV tracing shows a peak velocity of only 0.4 m/s in expiration with an increase during inspiration (*arrow* in A) to 0.8 m/s (an increase of 100%). There are reciprocal changes in transmitral flow with the peak velocity decreasing from 1.2 m/s during expiration to 0.8 m/s on the first beat after inspiration (*arrow* in B).

Step 4: Evaluate for Reciprocal Respiratory Changes in Right Ventricular and Left Ventricular Filling Velocities

■ Analogous to the changes in right and left ventricular volumes with respiration, the volume of inflow across the atrioventricular valves varies with respiration.
■ With inspiration, there is an increase (more than 25%) in RV diastolic filling; with expiration, LV diastolic filling increases by more than 25% (Figs. 10–17*A* and *B*).

Key points:

❑ The phase of respiration is recorded (using a respirometer) simultaneously with the ECG and Doppler velocity data.
❑ A slow sweep speed is used to include more than one respiratory cycle on the recording.
❑ The Doppler sample volume is positioned and a 2D image is recorded for several beats to ensure the intercept angle between the Doppler beam and direction of inflow does not vary significantly with respiration. If there is a significant variation in intercept angle, observed differences in velocity with respiration may be an artifact caused by assuming a constant angle in the Doppler equation.
❑ With tamponade physiology, RV diastolic filling increases and left ventricular (LV) diastolic filling decreases on the first beat after inspiration.
❑ Evaluation of filling dynamics is challenging, so an apparent lack of respiratory variation does not exclude the possibility of tamponade physiology.

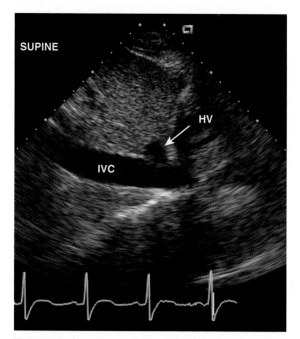

Figure 10–18 Subcostal view showing a dilated inferior vena cava (*IVC*) and hepatic vein (*HV*) in a patient with pericardial tamponade. With inspiration, there was no change in IVC diameter.

Step 5: Determine Whether Right Atrial Filling Pressures Are Elevated

■ Elevated RA filling pressures are a sensitive, but not specific, sign of cardiac tamponade.
■ Echocardiographic evaluation of RA filling pressure is based on the size and respiratory variation of the inferior vena cava–a dilated inferior vena cava (IVC) without respiratory variation and with dilated hepatic veins is termed "plethora of the IVC" (Fig. 10–18).

Key points:

❏ Images of the IVC are obtained from the subcostal view in spontaneously breathing patients.

❏ This method is not applicable in patients on mechanical ventilation.

❏ There are many other causes for elevated RA pressures, other than tamponade physiology, so this finding is interpreted in the context of the other imaging findings.

❏ Tamponade may be present without plethora of the IVC if the patient is hypovolemic.

Step 6: Perform Echo-Guided Pericardiocentesis, If Clinically Indicated

■ Echocardiography may be used to guide the percutaneous pericardiocentesis procedure either to define the best approach to percutaneous drainage or to confirm the needle position in the pericardial space (Fig. 10–19).

■ Echocardiography is used after pericardiocentesis to assess the amount of residual fluid (Fig. 10–20).

Key points:

❏ Evaluation from apical and subcostal approaches demonstrates the depth and amount of pericardial fluid from the position of the transducer. Usually a subcostal approach is used, but an apical approach may be preferable in some cases.

❏ Visualization of the tip of the needle is problematic, because any segment of the needle passing through the image plane may be mistaken for the tip.

❏ The position of the needle is confirmed by injection of a small amount of agitated saline to produce a contrast effect.

Pericardial constriction

■ Pericardial constriction is the result of pericardial thickening and fibrosis with fusion of the parietal and visceral pericardium.

■ The thickened and rigid pericardium constricts the cardiac chambers, resulting in a limited total cardiac volume and a reduced cardiac output.

Key points:

❏ Common causes of pericardial constriction include prior cardiac surgery or trauma, radiation therapy, and recurrent pericarditis.

❏ Like tamponade physiology, the fixed total cardiac volume with pericardial constriction results in reciprocal changes in right- and left-sided heart filling.

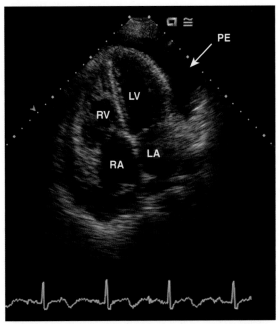

Figure 10–19 Apical four-chamber view showing a large circumferential pericardial effusion (*PE*), with relatively more fluid posterior and lateral to the left ventricle (*LV*), as is typical on echocardiography. Fluid is seen adjacent to the right atrium (*RA*), and a small amount of fluid is seen superior to the left atrium (*LA*), in the oblique sinus of the pericardium that extends between the right and left pulmonary veins.

❏ Typically, there is no significant pericardial effusion when constrictive pericarditis is present, although there are rare cases of "effusive-constrictive" physiology.

❏ Clinically, the differentiation of constrictive pericarditis (which is treated by pericardiotomy) and restrictive cardiomyopathy (which is treated medically) is problematic.

Step 1: Look for Evidence of Pericardial Thickening

■ Pericardial thickening may be evident on 2D echocardiography as areas of increased echogenicity in the pericardial region (Fig. 10–21).

■ On M-mode tracings, pericardial thickening is evident as multiple dense parallel lines posterior to the LV endocardium that persist even with low gain settings (Fig. 10–22).

Key points:

❏ Echocardiography is not sensitive for detection of pericardial thickening; cardiac computed tomography (CT) or magnetic resonance (MR) imaging are preferred when measurement of pericardial thickness is needed.

❏ Pericardial thickening may be asymmetric, so a complete evaluation includes evaluation from parasternal, apical, and subcostal windows.

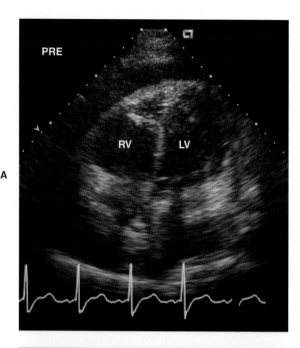

A

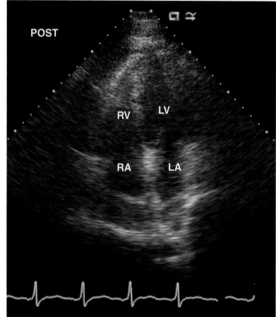

B

Figure 10–20 Echocardiographic monitoring of pericardiocentesis in the cardiac catheterization lab. At baseline (*A, PRE*), a foreshortened apical view shows a large pericardial effusion. *B,* After drainage of 1 L of fluid, repeat imaging (*POST*) shows a much smaller effusion at the apex, although some fluid persists adjacent to the right ventricle (*RV*) and right atrium (*RA*). Image quality is suboptimal, because the patient is supine and removal of the fluid resulted in poorer acoustic access.

Step 2: Evaluate for Anatomic Evidence of Constriction

■ Typical findings in patients with pericardial constriction are enlarged atria (due to chroni-

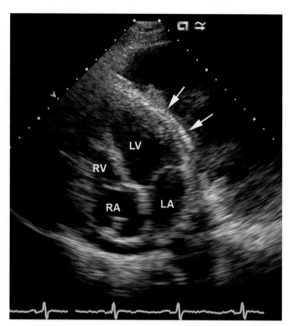

Figure 10–21 This apical view shows marked thickening and calcification of the pericardium (*arrows*) in a 30-year-old man with constrictive pericarditis and recurrent pleural effusion 10 years after radiation therapy for Hodgkin's disease.

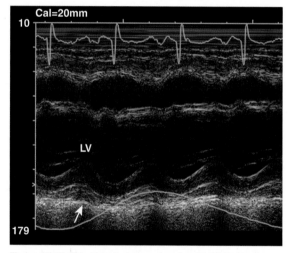

Figure 10–22 This M-mode image of pericardial thickening demonstrates a thick posterior pericardium that moves with the epicardium during the cardiac cycle. Septal motion also is typical for constrictive pericarditis.

cally elevated filling pressures) and small ventricles with normal systolic function.

■ M-mode findings in constrictive pericarditis include reduced posterior motion of the LV posterior wall endocardium in diastole (less than 2 mm) and a brief rapid posterior motion of the ventricular septum in early diastole.

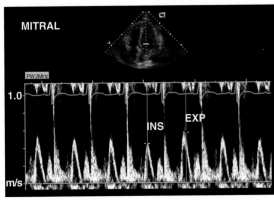
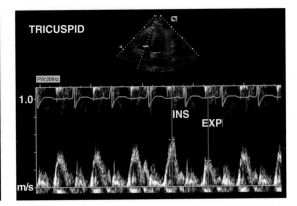

Figure 10–23 Ventricular inflow patterns in this patient with constrictive pericarditis show a marked (more than 25%) increase in right ventricular filling during inspiration (*INS*) with a reciprocal respiratory decrease of more than 25% in left ventricular diastolic filling. *EXP,* Expiration.

Key points:

❑ There are no specific 2D-imaging findings in patients with constrictive pericarditis.

❑ The diagnosis of constrictive pericarditis should be considered in the appropriate clinical setting (cardiac symptoms in a patient at risk of constrictive disease) if the echocardiogram does not show other causes for the patient's symptoms; that is, constrictive pericarditis most often is diagnosed in patients with unremarkable echocardiographic images.

Step 3: Perform Doppler Studies to Diagnose Constriction

■ Reciprocal respiratory changes in right and left ventricular diastolic filling, in the absence of a pericardial effusion, suggest the diagnosis of constrictive pericarditis (Fig. 10–23).

■ Typically, pulmonary pressures are normal in patients with constrictive pericarditis but elevated (greater than 60 mm Hg) in those with restrictive cardiomyopathy.

Key points:

❑ With pericardial constriction, the normal myocardium allows rapid early diastolic filling of the chamber with normal relaxation and compliance. Once the chamber has reached the limit of total cardiac volume imposed by the rigid pericardium, ventricular filling abruptly halts.

❑ The ventricular inflow pattern shows a prominent early (E) filling velocity, a normal deceleration slope, and a very small atrial contribution to filling (due to elevated end-diastolic LV pressures).

❑ The RA inflow (hepatic vein) pattern shows a prominent atrial reversal, with prominent diastolic (and blunted systolic) ventricular filling.

❑ Pulmonary pressures are estimated based on the velocity in the tricuspid regurgitant jet and an estimate of RA pressure.

Step 4: Distinguish Constrictive Pericarditis from Restrictive Cardiomyopathy

■ Echocardiography alone often is inadequate to distinguish constrictive pericarditis from restrictive cardiomyopathy (Table 10–2).

■ However, the possibility of these diagnoses often is first suggested by the echocardiographic findings.

Key points:

❑ Right and left atrial filling pressures are increased in both conditions.

❑ Right and left ventricular diastolic pressures are equal, even after volume loading, when constrictive pericarditis is present.

❑ Pulmonary systolic pressure typically is severely elevated with restrictive cardiomyopathy.

❑ Early diastolic filling is rapid with constrictive pericarditis and is reduced with restrictive cardiomyopathy early in the disease course.

❑ However, with advanced restrictive physiology, ventricular compliance is reduced, so early diastolic filling may appear similar to the pattern seen with constrictive pericarditis.

❑ The LV myocardium is normal with constrictive pericarditis. With restrictive cardiomyopathy, LV wall thickness often is increased.

❑ Additional helpful studies are CT and/or MR direct imaging of pericardial thickness, cardiac catheterization for simultaneous measurement of LV and RV diastolic pressures, and endomyocardial biopsy.

TABLE 10–2

COMPARISON OF PERICARDIAL TAMPONADE, CONSTRICTION, AND RESTRICTIVE CARDIOMYOPATHY

	PERICARDIAL TAMPONADE	CONSTRICTIVE PERICARDITIS	RESTRICTIVE CARDIOMYOPATHY
HEMODYNAMICS			
Right atrial pressure	↑	↑	↑
RV/LV filling pressures	↑, RV = LV	↑, RV = LV	↑, LV > RV
Pulmonary artery pressures	Normal	Mild elevation (35-40 mm Hg systolic)	Moderate to severe elevation (≥60 mm Hg systolic)
RV diastolic pressure plateau		> ⅓ peak RV pressure	> ⅓ peak RV pressure
Radionuclide diastolic filling		Rapid early filling, impaired late filling	Impaired early filling
2D ECHO	Moderate to large PE	Pericardial thickening without effusion	Left ventricular hypertrophy Normal systolic function
DOPPLER ECHO	Reciprocal respiratory changes in RV and LV filling Inferior vena cava plethora	E > A on LV inflow Prominent *y* descent in hepatic vein Pulmonary venous flow = prominent *a* wave, reduced systolic phase Respiratory variation in IVRT and in *E* velocity	(1) Early in disease E < A on LV inflow (2) Late in disease E > A (3) Constant IVRT (4) Absence of significant respiratory variation
OTHER DIAGNOSTIC TESTS	Therapeutic/diagnostic pericardiocentesis	CT or MRI for pericardial thickening	Endomyocardial biopsy

↑, *Increased;* 2D, *two-dimensional;* CT, *computed tomography;* IVRT, *isovolumic relaxation time;* LV, *left ventricular;* MRI, *magnetic resonance imaging;* PE, *pericardial effusion;* RV, *right ventricular.*
From Otto CM: *Textbook of Clinical Echocardiography, 3rd ed. Philadelphia: Elsevier, 2004.*

NOTES

SELF-ASSESSMENT QUESTIONS

QUESTION 1

In the parasternal long axis view shown in Figure 10–24, identify the structures labeled A through E.

A. _____

B. _____

C. _____

D. _____

E. _____

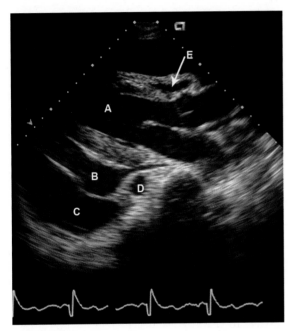

Figure 10–24

QUESTION 2

A 34-year-old man with lymphoma presents with a 3-week history of decreased exercise tolerance. Physical examination shows a diaphoretic man with a blood pressure of 90/60 mm Hg, pulse of 120 beats per minute (bpm), and respiratory rate of 24 per minute. His lungs are clear, and heart sounds are distant. A handheld bedside echocardiogram shows a large circumferential pericardial effusion.

The most appropriate next step is:

A. Evaluate for RA systolic and RV diastolic collapse.
B. Record Doppler left and right ventricular filling velocities with a respiration tracing.
C. Insert a Swan-Ganz (right heart) catheter.
D. Perform pericardiocentesis.
E. Call cardiac surgery.

QUESTION 3

In a 56-year-old woman with breast cancer and a moderate-sized pericardial effusion, inflow velocities across the tricuspid (Fig. 10–25A) and mitral (Fig. 10–25B) valves were recorded along with a respirometer showing inspiration as an upward deflection of the tracing. These tracings show:

A. Normal respiratory variation in inflows
B. Reduced RV filling with inspiration
C. Tamponade physiology
D. Electrical alternans
E. Pulsus paradoxus

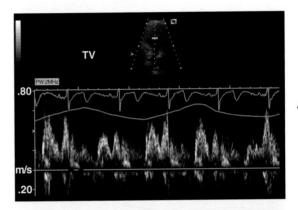

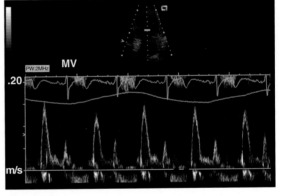

Figure 10–25

QUESTION 4

Echocardiography is requested in a 52-year-old man with dyspnea and a long history of asthma. There is a small pericardial effusion, and the LV and RV inflow patterns are recorded with a respirometer. The tracings for this patient, shown in Figures 10–26A and B, are most consistent with:

A. Normal respiratory variation in inflows
B. Reduced RV filling with inspiration
C. Tamponade physiology
D. Respiratory distress
E. Restrictive cardiomyopathy

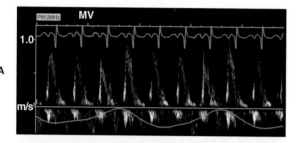

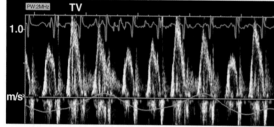

Figure 10–26

QUESTION 5

The M-mode tracing in Figure 10–27 shows:

A. Pericardial constriction
B. Cardiac tamponade
C. Aortic regurgitation
D. Pericardial effusion
E. Hypertrophic cardiomyopathy

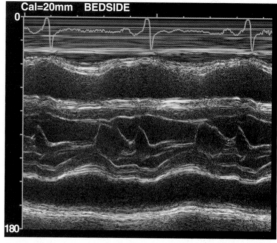

Figure 10–27

QUESTION 6

A 34-year-old woman presents with decreased exercise tolerance and increased abdominal girth over the last year. Her past medical history is remarkable for radiation therapy for Hodgkin's disease 16 years ago. Physical examination shows a blood pressure of 124/74 mm Hg, with a decline in systolic blood pressure to 110 mm Hg with inspiration. Heart rate is 92 bpm, respiratory rate is 20 per minute, and her jugular venous pressure is more than 20 cm H_2O. There is a grade 2/6 holosystolic murmur at the apex, but no gallops are appreciated. Her lungs are clear, but her abdomen is distended with a fluid wave and there is 3+ ankle edema. Echocardiography shows a small left ventricle with normal systolic function, but image quality is poor. The left ventricular inflow pattern shows an E velocity of 1.4 m/s and an A velocity of 0.6 m/s. Tissue Doppler signals are poor quality, and pulmonary vein flow cannot be recorded. There is about a 16% decline in LV inflow velocities with respiration.
The most useful next step is:

A. Coronary angiography
B. TEE
C. Endomyocardial biopsy
D. Right heart catheterization
E. Chest CT

QUESTION 7

In the apical view shown in Figure 10–28, an echo lucent space (*arrow*) is seen lateral to the left ventricle. Which of the following views would be most helpful in determining whether this is a pleural or pericardial effusion?

A. Parasternal long axis
B. Subcostal four-chamber
C. Apical two-chamber
D. Left sub-scapular
E. Suprasternal

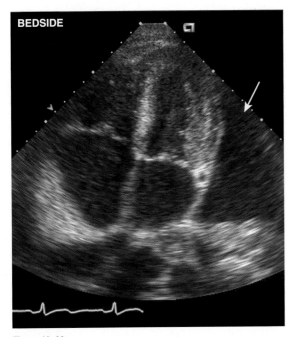

Figure 10–28

QUESTION 8

A 68-year-old woman presents with a 2-month history of increasing dyspnea on exertion and decreased exercise tolerance. Her past medical history is remarkable for rheumatoid arthritis, hypertension treated with a diuretic, and coronary bypass grafting surgery 10 years ago. Physical examination shows equal blood pressures in both arms at 138/86 mm Hg, with systolic blood pressure falling to 116 mm Hg during inspiration. Heart rate is 88 bpm, respiratory rate is 14 per minute, jugular venous pressure is 18 cm H_2O, and lungs are clear. There are no murmurs, gallops, or rubs.

Echocardiography shows an LV dimension of 50 mm at end-diastole and 32 mm at end-systole with a diastolic wall thickness of 10 mm and an ejection fraction of 56%. There is no significant pericardial effusion. Estimated pulmonary systolic pressure is 32 mm Hg. The transmitral E velocity is 1.2 m/s with a deceleration time of 100 ms and an A velocity of 0.4 m/s. Tissue Doppler at the medial mitral annulus shows E_M is greater than A_M, and pulmonary venous flow shows a predominance of diastolic inflow. The transmitral E velocity falls from 1.2 m/s to 0.9 m/s with inspiration, and the transtricuspid E velocity increases from 0.8 to 1.2 m/s with inspiration.

The most likely diagnosis is:

A. Pericardial tamponade
B. Constrictive pericarditis
C. Restrictive cardiomyopathy
D. Dilated cardiomyopathy
E. Hypertensive heart disease

ANSWERS

ANSWER 1

A. Left ventricle
B. Pericardial effusion
C. Pleural effusion
D. Descending thoracic aorta
E. Right ventricle (compressed consistent with tamponade physiology)

ANSWER 2: D

This patient has a large pericardial effusion and is hypotensive, so the most appropriate next step is pericardiocentesis to relieve tamponade physiology. The effusion is not loculated, so percutaneous drainage is reasonable; cardiac surgery would be called only if the effusion was loculated or if recurrent effusions suggested the need for a pericardial window. Further echocardiographic evaluation for signs of tamponade physiology is not needed because the diagnosis is evident on physical examination—the finding of a large effusion is enough to proceed with therapy. Further diagnostic evaluation would unnecessarily prolong the time to treatment. A right heart catheter is helpful for monitoring right and left heart filling pressures and to measure cardiac output but would not add useful information in this case.

ANSWER 3: A

The tricuspid valve tracing is noisy. However, the lowest E velocity (second beat) is about 0.35 m/s and increases with inspiration (note the third and fourth beats) to about 0.45 m/s. Although this increase in flow velocity is greater than 20%, right-sided filling normally increases with inspiration. The transmitral velocity shows an E velocity of about 1.4 m/s with inspiration (second and fifth beats) with an apparent slight increase in velocity to 1.5 m/s at end expiration. If tamponade were present, the expected finding is a decrease in transmitral velocity by at least 20% with inspiration. Normally, there is little change in mitral inflow velocity with respiration; the apparent slight variation on this tracing might reflect slight changes in the intercept angle between the Doppler beam and inflow velocity as the heart position moves in the chest with respiration and the sonographer maintains a steady transducer position.

Electrical alternans may be seen with very large pericardial effusions where the heart "swings" from side to side on alternate beats, resulting in a decrease in the amplitude of the QRS on the ECG on every other beat. Pulsus paradoxus refers to the physical examination findings of an inspiratory fall in systolic blood pressure of at least 20 mm Hg, appreciated on auscultation of the blood pressure or palpation of a peripheral pulse.

ANSWER 4: D

The patient is tachycardic, with a heart rate of about 130 bpm resulting in fusion of the E and A velocities on both tracings. The RV inflow shows a marked increase in velocity, from 0.6 to 1.1 m/s with inspiration, suggesting a marked increase in RV diastolic filling with the negative intrathoracic pressure of inspiration. There are several possible underlying causes for this observation. With cardiac tamponade, the negative intrathoracic pressure of inspiration allows rapid right heart filling, but the fixed total cardiac volume results in a reciprocal decrease in LV diastolic filling with inspiration. In the LV inflow tracing, flow decreases with inspiration but only from about 0.7 to 0.6 cm/s (less than 20%). In addition, tamponade is very unlikely with a small effusion. Thus these tracings are most consistent with exaggerated variation in right-sided filling due to respiratory distress with a greater negative intrathoracic pressure compared with normal quiet respiration. Respiratory variation in patients with restrictive cardiomyopathy tends to be similar to normal.

ANSWER 5: D

This M-mode tracing at the mitral valve level shows a pericardial effusion both anterior to the right ventricle and, more prominently, posterior to the left ventricle. The flat motion of the posterior pericardium with the normal motion of the posterior wall epicardium are diagnostic. With constriction, multiple parallel echodense signals would be seen in the pericardial region. There are no signs of tamponade physiology; the inward motion of the RV free wall in systole is caused by normal RV contraction. Aortic regurgitation would result in high frequency fluttering of the anterior mitral valve leaflet, and hypertrophic cardiomyopathy would be associated with increased diastolic thickness of the ventricular septum.

ANSWER 6: E

The clinical history (prior radiation therapy), physical examination (ascites, elevated right-sided filling pressures), and the echocardiographic findings suggest constrictive pericarditis. The most useful test at this point is a chest CT to evaluate the thickness of the pericardium. If pericardial thickening and constriction are present, surgical pericardiectomy is beneficial. Patients with prior radiation are at risk for accelerated coronary disease; however, her symptoms do not suggest this diagnosis, so coronary angiography should not be the first diagnostic step. TEE would provide better visualization of chamber anatomy and function and would allow recording of pulmonary vein inflow. However, TEE is not accurate for assessment of pericardial thickening. Endomyocardial biopsy may show myocardial fibrosis in patients with prior mediastinal radiation but has a low yield when the differential diagnosis is pericardial constriction versus restrictive cardiomyopathy. Right heart catheterization alone would confirm elevated right-sided filling pressures, but a combined right and left heart catheterization is needed when constriction is suspected to demonstrate the equalization of intracardiac diastolic pressures.

ANSWER 7: A

The parasternal long axis view is most likely to be helpful, because it will show whether the fluid tracks anteriorly (pericardial) or posteriorly (pleural) to the descending thoracic aorta. Identification of a small amount of pericardial fluid with parallel lines indicating the parietal and visceral pericardium also may be seen. The subcostal view might show pericardial fluid anterior to the right ventricle but would not help with identification of the fluid lateral to the left ventricle. The pericardial and pleural spaces are not easily seen in the apical two-chamber view. Obtaining views from the posterior left chest, using the left pleural effusion as an acoustic window, may be used for cardiac visualization when other views are inadequate but is only feasible with large pleural fluid collections. The pericardial space is not easily seen from the suprasternal notch.

ANSWER 8: B

The diastolic filling parameters in this patient are consistent with any of these five possible diagnoses. However, the echocardiographic findings are most suggestive of constrictive pericarditis because there is a greater than 20% inspiratory increase in RV filling concurrent with a reciprocal respiratory decrease in LV filling. The more than 20 mm Hg fall in systolic blood pressure with inspiration (pulsus paradoxus) and the elevated jugular venous pressure also are consistent with this diagnosis. In this patient with rheumatoid arthritis and previous coronary surgery, constrictive pericarditis may be the end-stage result of repeated episodes of inflammatory pericarditis, or it may be due to her previous surgical procedure.

Similar clinical and Doppler findings are seen with pericardial tamponade, but there was no significant pericardial effusion in this case. Restrictive cardiomyopathy also might show a similar pattern of diastolic dysfunction but would also be characterized by increased LV wall thickness, elevated pulmonary pressures, and lack of respiratory variation in right and left ventricular filling. With a dilated cardiomyopathy, the ventricular dimensions would be larger and the ejection fraction would be lower. Hypertensive heart disease is defined as concentric ventricular hypertrophy caused by hypertension, often with early diastolic and late systolic dysfunction. The normal wall thickness in this patient and the respiratory variation in filling patterns argue against this diagnosis.

NOTES

Valvular Stenosis

11

AORTIC STENOSIS	MITRAL STENOSIS
THE ECHO EXAM	**THE ECHO EXAM**

AORTIC STENOSIS

THE ECHO EXAM
　Step-by-Step Evaluation
　　Determine the Etiology of Stenosis
　　Evaluate Severity of Stenosis Based on Jet Velocity, Mean Gradient, and Valve Area
　　Evaluate Aortic Regurgitation and Ascending Aorta
　　Evaluate the Consequences of Chronic Pressure Overload
　　Consider Additional Evaluation of Aortic Stenosis Severity in Select Cases

MITRAL STENOSIS

THE ECHO EXAM
　Step-by-Step Evaluation
　　Evaluate Mitral Valve Morphology
　　Evaluate the Severity of Mitral Stenosis
　　Evaluate Mitral Regurgitation
　　Examine Aortic and Tricuspid Valves for Rheumatic Involvement
　　Evaluate the Consequences of Mitral Valve Obstruction

PULMONIC STENOSIS

SELF-ASSESSMENT QUESTIONS

AORTIC STENOSIS

THE ECHO EXAM: AORTIC VALVE STENOSIS

VALVE ANATOMY
Calcific
Bicuspid (two leaflets in systole)
Rheumatic

STENOSIS SEVERITY
Jet velocity (V_{max})
Mean pressure gradient (ΔP_{mean})
LVOT/AS velocity ratio
Aortic valve area (AVA)

CO-EXISTING AR
Qualitative evaluation of severity

LV RESPONSE
LV hypertrophy
LV dimensions or volumes
LV ejection fraction

Other findings
Pulmonary pressures
Mitral regurgitation

EXAMPLE
An 82-year-old woman presents with dyspnea on exertion and is noted to have a 3/6 systolic murmur at the base, radiating to the carotids with a single S2 and diminished carotid upstrokes. Echocardiography shows a calcified aortic valve with:

Aortic jet velocity (V_{max})	4.2 m/s
Velocity time integral (VTI_{AS})	68 cm
Mean gradient	45 mm Hg
LV outflow tract diameter ($LVOT_D$)	2.1 cm
LVOT velocity (V_{LVOT})	0.9 m/s
Velocity time integral (VTI_{LVOT})	14 cm

The *maximum jet velocity* of 4.2 m/s indicates severe stenosis, which is confirmed by calculation of maximum and mean pressure gradients.

Maximum pressure gradient is calculated from maximum aortic jet velocity (V_{max}) as:

$$\Delta P_{max} = 4\,(V_{max})^2 = 4\,(4.2)^2 = 71 \text{ mm Hg}$$

Mean pressure gradient is calculated by tracing the outer edge of the CW Doppler velocity curve, with the echo instrument calculating and then averaging instantaneous pressure gradients over the systolic ejection period. The simplified method for estimation of mean gradient is:

$$\Delta P = 2.4\,(V_{max})^2 = 2.4\,(4.2)^2 = 42 \text{ mm Hg}$$

In order to correct for transvalvular volume flow rate, the velocity ratio and valve area are calculated:

Velocity ratio is:

$$V_{LVOT}/V_{max} = 0.9/4.2 = 0.21 \text{ (dimensionless index)}$$

Aortic valve area is:

$$AVA = (CSA_{LVOT} \times VTI_{LVOT})/\,VTI_{AS\text{-}Jet}$$

Where cross-sectional area (CSA) of the LVOT is:

$$CSA_{LVOT} = \pi(\,LVOT_D\,/2)^2 = 3.14(2.1/2)^2 = 3.46 \text{ cm}^2$$

Thus:

$$AVA = (3.46 \text{ cm}^2 \times 14 \text{ cm})/68 \text{ cm} = 0.71 \text{ cm}^2$$

Simplified formula for valve area is:

$$AVA = (CSA_{LVOT} \times V_{LVOT})/V_{max}$$

Thus:

$$AVA = (3.46 \text{ cm}^2 \times 0.9 \text{ cm/s})/4.2 \text{ cm/s} = 0.74 \text{ cm}^2$$

This mean gradient (> 40 mm Hg), velocity ratio (< 0.25), and valve area (< 1.0 cm^2) are all consistent with severe stenosis.

CLASSIFICATION OF AORTIC STENOSIS SEVERITY

	MILD	SEVERE
Jet velocity (m/s)	< 3.0	> 4.0
Mean gradient (mm Hg)	< 20	> 40
Velocity ratio	> 0.50	< 0.25
Valve area (cm²)	> 1.5	< 1.0

AR, *Aortic regurgitation;* AS, *aortic stenosis;* CSA, *cross-sectional area;* CW, *continuous wave;* LV, *left ventricle;* LVOT, *left ventricular outflow tract.*

QUANTITATION OF AORTIC STENOSIS SEVERITY

COMPONENTS	MODALITY	VIEW	RECORDING	MEASUREMENTS
LVOT diameter ($LVOT_D$)	2D	Parasternal long axis	Adjust depth, optimize endocardial definition, zoom mode	Inner edge to inner edge of LVOT, parallel and adjacent to aortic valve, mid-systole
LVOT flow V_{LVOT} VTI_{LVOT}	Pulsed Doppler	Apical 4-chamber (anteriorly angulated)	Sample volume 2-3 mm, envelope of flow with defined peak, start with sample volume at valve and move apically	Trace modal velocity of spectral velocity curve
AS- Jet V_{max} $VTI_{AS\text{-}Jet}$	CW Doppler	Apical, SSN, other	Examination from multiple windows, careful positioning, and transducer angulation to obtain highest velocity signal	Measure maximum velocities at edge of intense velocity signal

2D, *Two-dimensional*; AS, *aortic stenosis*; CW, *continuous wave*; LVOT, *left ventricular outflow tract*; SSN, *suprasternal notch*; VTI, *velocity time integral*.

A
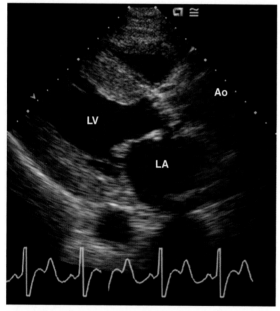

B
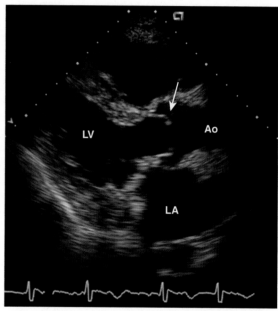

Figure 11–1 The etiology of aortic valve stenosis is evident on imaging the valve in these long axis views. With calcific valve disease (*A*), there is increased echogenicity of the leaflets, caused by calcification and thickening, with reduced systolic opening of the leaflets. Short axis views may show a trileaflet or bicuspid valve, but the number of leaflets may be difficult to determine when significant calcification is present. In a patient with a congenitally bicuspid, noncalcified valve (*B*), the long axis view shows thin leaflets with reduced systolic opening caused by "doming" of the leaflets in systole (*arrow*), as seen by the curve at the tips of the leaflets.

Step-by-Step Evaluation

Step 1: Determine the Etiology of Stenosis

- Parasternal two-dimensional (2D) images of the valve in long and short axis views (Fig. 11–1)
- Number of leaflets, mobility, thickness, and calcification
- Level of obstruction: valvular, subvalvular, or supravalvular

Key points:

- ❏ Calcific changes usually start in the central part of the leaflets, resulting in a three-pointed star-shaped orifice.
- ❏ Rheumatic aortic valve disease affects the commissures and leaflet edges, with a triangular-shaped systolic orifice, and is accompanied by rheumatic mitral valve changes.
- ❏ A bicuspid valve may appear trileaflet in diastole because of a raphe in one leaflet; the number of leaflets must be visualized when the valve is open in systole.

□ Subvalvular or supravalvular stenosis is distinguished from valvular stenosis based on the site of the increase in velocity and on the anatomy of the entire outflow tract.

Step 2: Evaluate Severity of Stenosis Based on Jet Velocity, Mean Gradient, and Valve Area

Aortic jet velocity (Fig. 11–2)

■ Continuous wave Doppler (CWD) gray-scale spectral recording of aortic jet velocity

Key points:

□ Use multiple acoustic windows (apical, supra-sternal, right parasternal) with careful patient positioning and transducer angulation to avoid underestimation of velocity.

□ A dedicated small CWD transducer provides the optimal signal-to-noise ratio and allows optimal angulation of the transducer.

□ Decrease the gain, increase the wall filter, and adjust the baseline and scale to optimize identification of the maximum velocity.

□ Use the gray-scale spectral displays, because with some color displays the edge of the spectral envelope may be blurred, leading to overestimation of velocity.

□ A smooth velocity curve with a dense outer edge and clear maximum velocity should be recorded; fine linear echoes at the peak of the curve are due to the transit time effect and are not included in measurements.

□ Color Doppler is usually not helpful for jet direction, because the jet is short with post-stenotic turbulence and because the elevational plane is not visualized.

Mean gradient

■ Transaortic pressure gradient (ΔP) is calculated from velocity (v) using the Bernoulli equation as $\Delta P = 4v^2$ (Fig. 11–3).

Key points:

□ Maximum gradient is calculated from maximum velocity: $\Delta P_{max} = 4v_{max}^2$.

□ When proximal velocity is faster than 1.0 m/s, it should be included in the Bernoulli equation so that $\Delta P = 4(v_{max}^2 - v_{proximal}^2)$.

□ Mean gradient is calculated by tracing the velocity curve so that the instantaneous gradients are averaged over the systolic ejection period (Fig. 11–4).

□ Any underestimation of aortic velocity results in an even greater underestimation in gradients.

Continuity equation valve area (Fig. 11–5)

■ Aortic valve area (AVA) is calculated as: AVA = $(CSA_{LVOT} \times VTI_{LVOT})/ VTI_{AS\text{-}Jet}$, where CSA is the cross-sectional area, LVOT is left ventricular outflow tract, and VTI is velocity time integral.

■ The simplified continuity equation, which uses maximum velocities instead of velocity time integrals (VTI), also can be used: AVA = $(CSA_{LVOT} \times V_{LVOT})/ V_{max}$

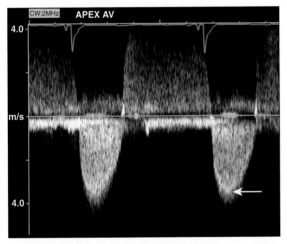

Figure 11–2 Aortic jet velocity is recorded using continuous wave Doppler. An optimal signal-to-noise ratio is obtained using a small dedicated transducer; the small footprint of this transducer also allows optimal positioning and angulation to align the ultrasound beam parallel to the direction of the stenotic jet. In this example, the scale has been adjusted to show both aortic stenosis and regurgitation. The aortic jet should show a denser signal around the edge and a smooth velocity curve. The difficulty in identifying the maximum velocity is seen in this example, with fuzzy linear signals at peak velocity that are due to the transit time effect. Maximum velocity is measured at the edge of the denser signal, as shown by the arrow.

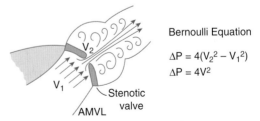

Bernoulli Equation

$\Delta P = 4(V_2^2 - V_1^2)$

$\Delta P = 4V^2$

Figure 11–3 This schematic diagram of the Bernoulli equation demonstrates aortic stenosis with laminar low velocity flow on the ventricular side of the valve, a small area of acceleration into the narrow orifice, and the high velocity jet of flow through the narrowed valve. The distal flow disturbance is shown by the curved arrows. The instantaneous pressure gradient (ΔP) across the valve is related to the proximal velocity (V1) and jet velocity (V2) as shown. Because the proximal velocity is much less than the jet velocity, and usually is less than 1 m/s, the simplified Bernoulli equation uses only jet velocity.

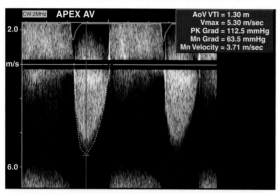

Figure 11–4 In a different patient with aortic stenosis, the highest velocity aortic jet was obtained from an apical window. The baseline is moved and the scale is adjusted so that the stenotic signal fills the vertical range of the display. The horizontal axis or "sweep speed" is adjusted to 100 mm/s to allow accurate measurement. The Doppler curve is traced along the outer edge of the dark signal to obtain the velocity time integral (VTI). The instantaneous pressure gradients over the systolic ejection period are averaged by the analysis package to provide the mean systolic gradient. Note that the mean gradient is *not* calculated by using the mean velocity in the Bernoulli equation.

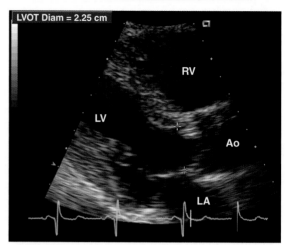

Figure 11–6 Left ventricular (*LV*) outflow tract diameter is measured in a parasternal long axis view in mid-systole from the inner edge of the septum to the inner edge of the anterior mitral leaflet, immediately adjacent to the aortic valve leaflets (*caliper marks*). A magnified image allows more accurate measurement, and typically several beats are measured to ensure a reproducible value. In this patient, the standard parasternal view was suboptimal, so a lower parasternal window was used (this is evident by the angle of the septum relative to the transducer position). However, the LV outflow tract diameter still can be measured accurately. A typical outflow tract diameter is 2.2 to 2.6 cm in adult men and 2.0 to 2.4 cm in adult women. Outflow tract diameter in adults with aortic stenosis rarely changes over time, so the same value should be used when comparing sequential studies.

CONTINUITY EQUATION

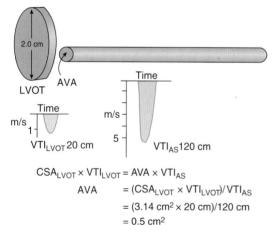

$$CSA_{LVOT} \times VTI_{LVOT} = AVA \times VTI_{AS}$$
$$AVA = (CSA_{LVOT} \times VTI_{LVOT})/VTI_{AS}$$
$$= (3.14 \text{ cm}^2 \times 20 \text{ cm})/120 \text{ cm}$$
$$= 0.5 \text{ cm}^2$$

Figure 11–5 The continuity equation is based on the principle that the volume of flow proximal to and in the narrowed valve must be equal. Flow for one cardiac cycle in the left ventricular outflow tract (*LVOT*) is shown as a cylinder with a diameter equal to LVOT diameter and length equal to the velocity time integral (*VTI*) of LVOT flow (because the integral of velocity over time is distance; e.g., like traveling in a car). The flow through the orifice is shown as a cylinder, with the cross section equal to aortic valve area (*AVA*) and length equal to the VTI of the aortic stenosis (*AS*) jet. Because the volume of both cylinders is the same, the equation is solved for AVA as shown.

Key points:
- ❏ Outflow tract diameter is measured in the parasternal long axis view in mid-systole using zoom mode and by adjusting gain settings to optimize the blood–tissue interface (Fig. 11–6).
- ❏ Diameter (D) is measured immediately adjacent to the aortic leaflets from inner edge to

inner edge. Calculate the circular cross-sectional area: $(CSA_{LVOT}) = 3.14(D/2)^2$
- ❏ Outflow tract velocity is recorded with pulsed Doppler from the apical window with the sample volume positioned just apically from the flow acceleration into the valve. An aortic closing click on the spectral tracing indicates correct sample volume positioning.
- ❏ Move the baseline, adjust the velocity scale, and use an expanded time scale for accurate measurements (Fig. 11–7).
- ❏ Trace the modal systolic velocity (VTI_{LVOT}) and measure peak velocity (V_{LVOT}).
- ❏ If outflow tract diameter cannot be accurately measured, calculate the ratio of outflow tract to aortic jet velocity: Ratio = V_{LVOT}/V_{max} (a ratio of less than 0.25 indicates severe stenosis).

Step 3: Evaluate Aortic Regurgitation and Ascending Aorta (Fig. 11–8)

- ■ If regurgitation is significant (vena contracta >3 mm), evaluate as detailed in Chapter 12.
- ■ Dilation of the ascending aorta may accompany aortic stenosis, particularly with a bicuspid valve.

Key points:
- ❏ Most patients with aortic stenosis have some degree (usually mild) of aortic regurgitation.

□ With combined moderate stenosis and regurgitation, quantitation of both lesions is needed.

□ The diameter of the aorta is measured at the sinuses, sinotubular junction, and mid-ascending aorta when aortic valve disease is present.

Step 4: Evaluate the Consequences of Chronic Pressure Overload (Fig. 11–9)

■ Measure left ventricular (LV) size and wall thickness and calculate the ejection fraction as detailed in Chapter 6.

■ Evaluate ventricular diastolic function as detailed in Chapter 7.

■ Evaluate coexisting mitral regurgitation (if vena contracta is >3 mm) as detailed in Chapter 12.

■ Estimate pulmonary pressures as detailed in Chapter 6.

Key points:

□ Aortic stenosis typically results in concentric LV hypertrophy.

□ Systolic function and ejection fraction remain normal in most patients, but occasionally systolic dysfunction is identified in an asymptomatic patient.

□ Diastolic dysfunction, usually impaired relaxation, is common.

□ Pulmonary pressures may be elevated with longstanding severe aortic stenosis.

Step 5: Consider Additional Evaluation of Aortic Stenosis Severity in Select Cases

Key points:

□ The degree of valve calcification (mild, moderate, severe) is a simple, important parameter that is predictive of clinical outcome.

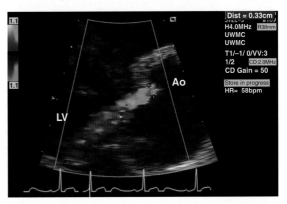

Figure 11–8 Aortic regurgitation is common in adults with aortic stenosis. Often evaluation based on vena contracta width, as shown here, and the continuous wave Doppler signal is adequate. If further evaluation is needed, the approaches detailed in Chapter 12 are used.

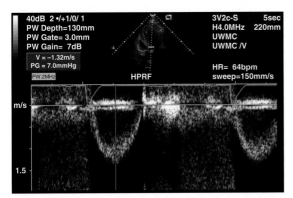

Figure 11–7 Although left ventricular (*LV*) outflow tract diameter is measured from the parasternal window, to provide axial resolution of the tissue–blood interfaces, with ultrasound imaging, LV outflow tract velocity is recorded from the apical window to allow parallel alignment between the ultrasound beam and flow direction. Pulsed (or high pulse repetition frequency [*HPRF*]) Doppler is used to measure the velocity signal on the ventricular side of the aortic valve, in an anteriorly angulated four-chamber view (as shown here) or in a long axis view. The sample volume length or gate is adjusted to 2 to 3 mm, and the sample volume is positioned as close to the valve as possible (often the closing click is seen), avoiding the small area of flow acceleration immediately adjacent to the stenotic orifice. The sample volume position should correspond to the site where LV outflow tract diameter was measured. The velocity range and baseline are adjusted so the signal fits but fills the scale, using a fast (100 to 150 mm/s) horizontal axis scale. A smooth curve with a dense band of velocities ("envelope of flow") with a well-defined peak velocity should be seen. If there is spectral broadening at the peak, the sample volume position is moved slightly apically until a clear signal is obtained.

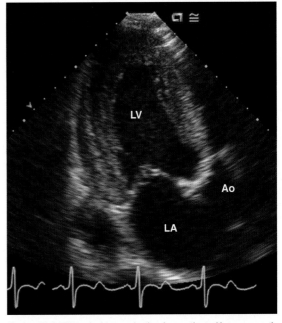

Figure 11–9 This apical long axis view in a patient with severe aortic stenosis (note calcified valve) demonstrates a normal-sized chamber with concentric hypertrophy, as expected with chronic pressure overload of the ventricle.

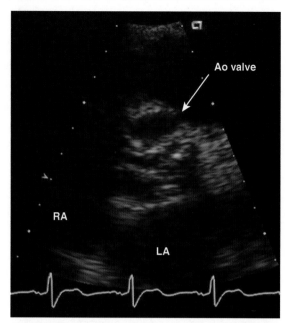

Figure 11–10 In the short axis view of the aortic valve (*Ao valve*), on transthoracic echocardiography or transesophageal echocardiography imaging, the apparent opening of the leaflets often can be visualized. In selected cases, planimetry of this apparent orifice may be helpful. Caution is needed to ensure the image plane is at the level of the orifice (particularly with bicuspid valves), and that shadowing and reverberations from calcification do not obscure the leaflet edges.

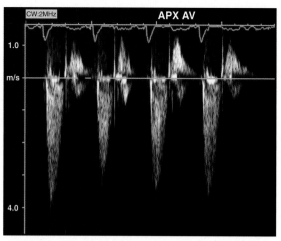

Figure 11–11 When the cardiac rhythm is irregular, the velocity (and pressure gradient) across a stenotic valve varies with the length of the R-R interval because of an increased stroke volume with a longer diastolic filling period. This example shows the variation in aortic jet velocity (at a slow sweep speed to include multiple beats) in a patient in atrial fibrillation. Ideally, heart rate should be controlled before evaluation of stenosis severity is performed. Several beats are then averaged for each measurement. Signal quality in this example is suboptimal, so additional efforts to improve patient or transducer positioning are needed.

- ❐ The dimensionless ratio of outflow tract–to–aortic jet velocity provides a simple index of stenosis severity (normal, 1.0; mild stenosis, 0.5; severe stenosis, 0.25).
- ❐ Planimetry of valve area can be helpful in select cases with excellent images but should be used cautiously because of reverberations and shadowing from leaflet calcification (Fig. 11–10).
- ❐ Blood pressure should be recorded at the time of the velocity data acquisition; stenosis severity may be underestimated in hypertensive patients.
- ❐ With atrial fibrillation, several beats should be averaged for each measurement (Fig. 11–11).
- ❐ With low output aortic stenosis and a low LV ejection fraction, evaluation of hemodynamics at two different flow rates (e.g., at rest and with dobutamine) may be helpful.

NOTES

MITRAL STENOSIS

THE ECHO EXAM: MITRAL STENOSIS

Valve anatomy	Valve thickness and mobility
	Calcification
	Commissural fusion
	Subvalvular involvement
Stenosis severity	2D valve area
	Mean pressure gradient
	Pressure half-time valve area
Left atrium	Size
	TEE for thrombus pre-valvuloplasty
Co-existing MR	Qualitative evaluation of severity
Pulmonary vasculature	Pulmonary systolic pressure
	Right ventricular size and function
Other findings	Aortic valve involvement
	Left ventricular size and systolic function

EXAMPLE

A 26-year-old pregnant woman presents with dyspnea and is noted to have a diastolic murmur at the apex. Echocardiography shows rheumatic mitral stenosis with:

MVA$_{2D}$	0.8 cm^2
Mean ΔP	5 mm Hg
T$_{1/2}$	260 ms
Mitral valve morphology score	
Leaflet thickness	2
Mobility	1
Calcification	1
Subvalvular	2
TOTAL	6

Tricuspid regurgitant jet velocity	3.1 m/s
Estimated RA pressure	10 mm Hg
Mitral regurgitation	Mild

Mean pressure gradient is calculated by tracing the outer edge of the CW Doppler velocity curve, with the echo instrument calculating and then averaging instantaneous pressure gradients over the systolic ejection period.

*Doppler mitral valve area (*MVA$_{Doppler}$*)* is calculated as:

$$MVA_{Doppler} = 220/T\{1/2\} = 220/260 = 0.85\ cm^2$$

The 2D mitral valve area and the pressure half time valve area show reasonable agreement, and both are consistent with severe mitral stenosis.

Pulmonary artery pressure (PAP) is:

$$PAP = 4(V_{TR})^2 + RAP = 4(3.1)^2 + 10\ mm\ Hg = 48\ mm\ Hg$$

Pulmonary pressure is moderately elevated, consistent with a secondary response to severe mitral stenosis.

The mitral morphology score is low, and only mild mitral regurgitation is present, indicating a high likelihood of immediate and long-term success with balloon mitral valvuloplasty. A transesophageal echo is needed just before mitral valvuloplasty to evaluate for left atrial thrombus.

CLASSIFICATION OF MITRAL STENOSIS SEVERITY

	MILD	SEVERE
Mean gradient (mm Hg)	< 5	> 15
Pulmonary pressure (mm Hg)	< 30	> 60
Valve area (cm^2)	> 1.5	< 1.0

2D, *Two-dimensional;* CW, *continuous wave;* RA, *right atrial.*

QUANTITATION OF MITRAL STENOSIS SEVERITY

PARAMETER	MODALITY	VIEW	RECORDING	MEASUREMENTS
2D valve area (MVA$_{2D}$)	2D	Parasternal short axis	Scan from apex to base to identify minimal valve area.	Planimetry of inner edge of dark–light interface
Mean gradient (Mean ΔP)	PW or HPRF Doppler	Apical four-chamber or long axis	Align Doppler beam parallel to MS jet. Adjust angle to obtain smooth envelope, clear peak, and linear deceleration slope.	Trace maximum velocity of spectral velocity curve
Pressure half-time (T$_{1/2}$)	PW or HPRF Doppler	Apical four-chamber or long axis	Same as mean gradient. Adjust scale so velocity curve fills the screen. HPRF Doppler often has less noise than CW Doppler signal.	Place line from maximum velocity along mid-diastolic linear slope

2D, *Two-dimensional;* CW, *continuous wave;* HPRF, *high pulse repetition frequency;* MS, *mitral stenosis;* MVA, *mitral valve area;* PW, *pulsed wave.*

Step-by-step evaluation

Step 1: Evaluate Mitral Valve Morphology *(Fig. 11–12)*

■ Use long and short axis views of the mitral valve to demonstrate the typical findings of rheumatic valve disease (commissural fusion resulting in diastolic doming, chordal shortening, and fusion).

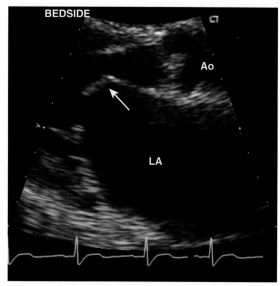

Figure 11–12 In this parasternal long axis view, the typical changes of rheumatic mitral stenosis are seen. There is diastolic doming (*arrow*) of the anterior mitral leaflet due to commissural fusion. The left atrium (*LA*) is enlarged, but left ventricular size is normal, as expected with mitral stenosis.

■ Evaluate mitral valve leaflet mobility, thickening, calcification, and subvalvular disease using the morphology score (Table 11–1) or French classification (Table 11–2).

Key points:

❑ Rheumatic valve disease is the most common cause of mitral stenosis.

❑ Rarely, severe mitral annular calcification encroaches on the mitral orifice, but calcific stenosis is rarely severe.

❑ In addition to a numerical score, a description of valve anatomy is helpful for deciding on the optimal intervention.

❑ The extent of commissural calcification and asymmetry of leaflet calcification should be noted.

❑ The subvalvular apparatus may be best seen on apical views (and may be poorly visualized on transesophageal echocardiography [TEE]).

Step 2: Evaluate the Severity of Mitral Stenosis

Two-dimensional planimetry of valve area *(Fig. 11–13)*

■ Valve area is measured directly by tracing the orifice in a short axis view at the leaflet tips.

Key points:

❑ In a parasternal short axis orientation, the image plane is slowly moved from the apex toward the base to identify the orifice of the funnel-shaped stenotic valve.

❑ The zoom mode is used to focus on the valve orifice, with the gain reduced to clearly show the tissue–blood interface.

TABLE 11–1

MITRAL VALVE MORPHOLOGY* BY TWO-DIMENSIONAL ECHOCARDIOGRAPHY

GRADE	MOBILITY	SUBVALVULAR THICKENING	THICKENING	CALCIFICATION
1	Highly mobile valve with only leaflet tips restricted	Minimal thickening just below the mitral leaflets	Leaflets near normal in thickness (4-5 mm)	A single area of increased echo brightness
2	Leaflet mid- and base portions have normal mobility	Thickening of chordal structures extending up to one third of the chordal length	Mid-leaflets normal, considerable thickening of margins (5-8 mm)	Scattered areas of brightness confined to leaflet margins
3	Valve continues to move forward in diastole, mainly from the base	Thickening extending to the distal third of the chords	Thickening extending through the entire leaflet (5-8 mm)	Brightness extending into the mid-portion of the leaflets
4	No or minimal forward movement of the leaflets in diastole	Extensive thickening and shortening of all chordal structures extending down to the papillary muscles	Considerable thickening of all leaflet tissue (> 8-10 mm)	Extensive brightness throughout much of the leaflet tissue

*The total echocardiographic score is derived from an analysis of mitral leaflet mobility, valvar and subvalvar thickening, and calcification. These elements are graded from 0 to 4 according to the above criteria. This gives a total score of 0 to 16.
From Wilkins GT, Weyman AE, Abascal VM, et al: Br Heart J 60:299-308, 1988.

TABLE 11–2

THE FRENCH THREE-GROUP GRADING OF MITRAL VALVE ANATOMY

ECHOCARDIOGRAPHIC GROUP	MITRAL VALVE ANATOMY
Group 1	Pliable noncalcified anterior mitral leaflet and mild subvalvular disease (i.e., thin chordae ≥10 mm long)
Group 2	Pliable noncalcified anterior mitral leaflet and severe subvalvular disease (i.e., thickened chordae < 10 mm long)
Group 3	Calcification of mitral valve of any extent, as assessed by fluoroscopy, whatever the state of the subvalvular apparatus

From Lung B, Cormier B, Discimetiere P, et al: J Am Coll Cardiol 27:407-414, 1996.

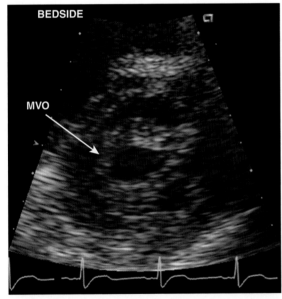

Figure 11–13 The rheumatic mitral valve orifice (*MVO*) is imaged in short axis, with care taken to scan from the apex toward the base to identify the smallest area of the funnel-shaped stenotic orifice. The inner edge of the white–dark interface is traced to obtain valve area. The distance between the left ventricular wall and the edge of the orifice reflects the degree of commissural fusion. These leaflets are uniformly echogenic, consistent with symmetric fibrosis and little calcification.

- ❏ The inner border of the black–white interface is traced to obtain valve area.
- ❏ The orifice typically is a smooth elliptical shape in patients with no prior procedures.
- ❏ After percutaneous or surgical valvotomy, the orifice is more irregular due to splitting of the fused commissures.

Mean gradient *(Fig. 11–14)*

- ■ The Doppler velocity curve across the narrowed mitral orifice is recorded from the apical window.

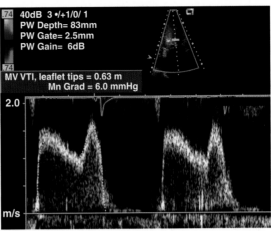

Figure 11–14 Measurement of the mean transmitral pressure gradient in a patient with mitral stenosis. The transmitral velocity is recorded with pulsed Doppler (including HPRF) or continuous wave Doppler if needed to prevent signal aliasing, from an apical window with the baseline shifted and the velocity scale adjusted so that the Doppler velocity fits the vertical axis of the tracing. The time scale is set at 100 to 150 mm/s, with the electrocardiograph included for timing. After a smooth Doppler curve with a narrow band along the outer edge and a clearly defined peak is obtained, the outer edge of the signal is traced. The analysis package averages the instantaneous gradients over the diastolic filling period. This patient is in sinus rhythm, which does not affect the accuracy of Doppler evaluation of stenosis severity, as long as the early diastolic deceleration slope is clearly defined.

- ■ Mean gradient is determined using the Bernoulli equation to average the instantaneous pressure gradients over the diastolic filling period.

Key points:

- ❏ The mitral stenosis jet is directed toward the apex, so only minor adjustment of transducer position and angulation is needed to obtain a parallel angle between the Doppler beam and mitral jet; color flow can help with alignment.
- ❏ Transducer position and gain are adjusted to demonstrate a clear outer boundary of the velocity curve with a well-defined peak and a linear deceleration slope.
- ❏ The baseline is moved toward the edge of the display, the scale adjusted so the Doppler curve fits but fills the space, and gain and wall filters adjusted to decrease signal noise.
- ❏ Pulsed or high pulse-repetition frequency Doppler may provide a more clearly defined velocity curve than CW Doppler.
- ❏ Movement of the heart with respiration may result in variation in the Doppler curve resulting from a variation in the intercept angle; if this occurs, have the patient suspend respiration briefly during data recording.

Pressure half time valve area *(Fig. 11–15)*

- ■ The pressure half time is calculated from the Doppler curve at the time interval between peak velocity and the peak velocity, divided by 1.4.

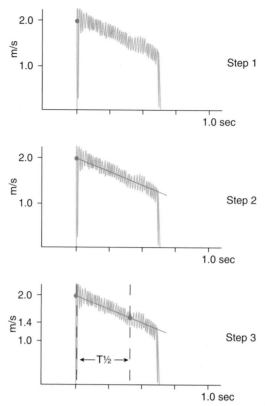

Figure 11–15 The mitral pressure half time is calculated as shown. In this example, the pressure half time is 320 milliseconds. The mitral valve area then is 220/320 = 0.69 cm², consistent with severe stenosis.

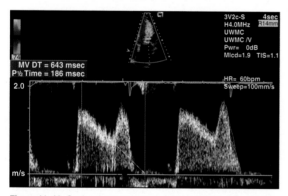

Figure 11–16 On the ultrasound system, the pressure half time is measured by identifying the peak early diastolic velocity and then placing a line along the mid-diastolic deceleration slope. The quantitation software then calculates the time interval between the peak gradient and one half the peak gradient. The empiric constant 220 is divided by the pressure half time to obtain valve area.

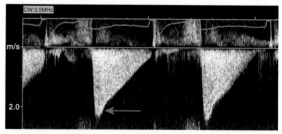

Figure 11–17 This transesophageal imaging in a 64-year-old woman with rheumatic mitral valve disease shows continuous Doppler antegrade flow (away from the transducer) across the stenotic mitral valve. The initial diastolic slope (*arrow*) is steeper than the mid-diastolic slope. When there is an initial steep decline in velocity (often called a "ski-slope" pattern) with a flatter mid-diastolic slope, the pressure half time is measured along the mid-diastolic portion of the curve, as shown on the second beat, extrapolating back to the onset of flow.

■ The empiric constant 220 is divided by the pressure half time (T½ in milliseconds) to estimate mitral valve area (MVA in cm²): MVA = 220/T½.

Key points:

❑ The peak velocity occurs at the onset of diastole, with flow deceleration in mid-diastole.

❑ A clearly defined peak velocity is needed for an accurate pressure half time measurement (Fig. 11–16).

❑ The diastolic slope should be linear with a clearly defined edge; if a nonlinear slope is obtained, the mid-diastolic segment of the curve should be used for the pressure half time calculation (Fig. 11–17).

❑ The pressure half time may be inaccurate if left atrial (LA) or LV compliance is abnormal.

□ If an atrial contraction is present, only the early diastolic portion of the curve is included in the pressure half time calculation.

Continuity equation valve area

■ If further evaluation of mitral stenosis severity is needed, a continuity equation valve area can be calculated.

■ Transmitral stroke volume (SV) is divided by the velocity time integral of the mitral stenosis jet

(VTI_{MS}) to obtain mitral valve area: MVA = SV/VTI_{MS}

Key points:

□ Transmitral stroke volume is determined in the LV outflow tract or across the pulmonic valve.

□ This approach is only accurate when there is no mitral regurgitation.

Step 3: Evaluate Mitral Regurgitation (Fig. 11–18)

■ If regurgitation is significant (vena contracta >3 mm), evaluate as detailed in Chapter 12.

Key points:

□ Most patients with rheumatic mitral stenosis have some degree of mitral regurgitation.

□ With combined moderate stenosis and regurgitation, quantitation of both lesions is needed.

□ The degree of mitral regurgitation may need to be evaluated by TEE, because moderate or greater regurgitation is a contraindication to percutaneous valvotomy.

Step 4: Examine Aortic and Tricuspid Valves for Rheumatic Involvement

■ When rheumatic mitral stenosis is present, careful evaluation of aortic and tricuspid valves is needed to detect rheumatic involvement (Fig. 11–19).

A
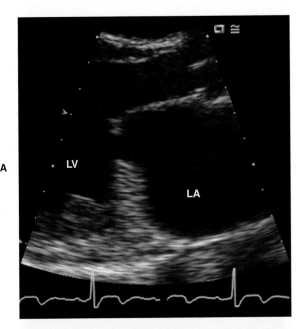

B
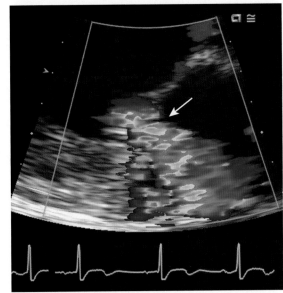

Figure 11–18 In this patient with mitral stenosis, the parasternal long axis view shows typical diastolic doming caused by commissural fusion (*A*). In systole, there is moderate to severe mitral regurgitation with a vena contracta (*arrow*) width of 1.0 cm (*B*).

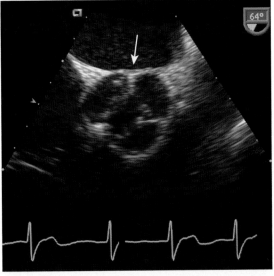

Figure 11–19 In the same patient as Figure 11–17, there is rheumatic involvement of the aortic valve with fusion (*arrow*) at all three commissures of the aortic valve and restricted leaflet opening. On transthoracic echo, her aortic jet velocity was 4.2 m/s, with a functional valve area of 0.8 cm². She was scheduled for aortic valve replacement for severe symptomatic aortic stenosis; the purpose of the transesophageal echocardiograph was to determine whether concurrent mitral valve replacement or repair was needed.

Key points:

- ❑ Rheumatic disease typically affects the mitral valve first, causing stenosis or regurgitation.
- ❑ The aortic valve is affected in about 35% of patients and the tricuspid valve in about 6% of patients with rheumatic mitral valve disease.
- ❑ The appearance of rheumatic disease affecting the aortic and tricuspid valves is similar to the mitral valve disease, with commissural fusion being the most consistent feature.
- ❑ Evaluation of rheumatic tricuspid stenosis is similar to evaluation of mitral stenosis, although pressure gradients may be lower for the tricuspid compared with the mitral valve (Fig. 11–20).

Step 5: Evaluate the Consequences of Mitral Valve Obstruction

- ■ Measure LA size (Fig. 11–21).
- ■ Estimate pulmonary pressures as detailed in Chapter 6.
- ■ Evaluate right ventricular (RV) size and systolic function.

Key points:

- ❑ LA enlargement is usually present in patients with mitral stenosis and is related to the severity and chronicity of mitral valve obstruction.
- ❑ Pulmonary pressures are elevated passively because of the increased LA pressure. In addition, reactive pulmonary hypertension is seen with changes in the pulmonary vasculature that may persist after relief of mitral stenosis.
- ❑ RV enlargement and systolic dysfunction in patients with mitral stenosis may be due to pulmonary hypertension (pressure overload)

or to rheumatic tricuspid regurgitation (volume overload).

PULMONIC STENOSIS

- ■ The velocity across the pulmonic valve is recorded using pulsed Doppler or CWD from a parasternal approach (Fig. 11–22).

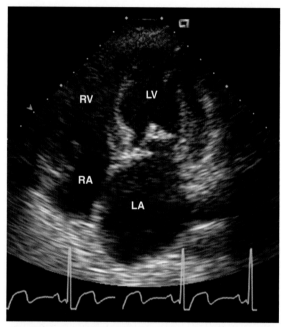

Figure 11–21 The marked degree of left atrial (*LA*) enlargement in this patient with rheumatic mitral stenosis is seen in an apical four-chamber view. The LA area appears larger than the left ventricular (*LV*) area in this diastolic frame.

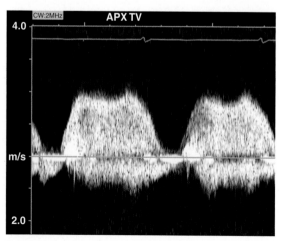

Figure 11–20 Antegrade flow across a stenotic tricuspid valve recorded with continuous wave Doppler from an apical view. The velocity is markedly increased, with a mean gradient of 12 mm Hg, and the diastolic slope is very flat, with a pressure half time of 400 ms and a valve area of 0.6 cm².

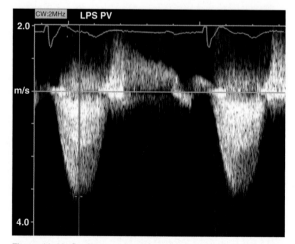

Figure 11–22 Continuous wave Doppler recording of pulmonary valve flow showing an antegrade velocity of 3.2 m/s consistent with a maximum gradient of 41 mm Hg, or moderate pulmonic stenosis. Pulmonic regurgitation is seen above the baseline and appears to be moderate based on the relative density of retrograde versus antegrade flow. Pulmonary pressures are low, based on the low end-diastolic velocity of the regurgitant signal.

- Maximum gradient is calculated using the Bernoulli equation.
- Coexisting pulmonic regurgitation is evaluated by color Doppler and CWD.

Key points:

❐ Pulmonic stenosis usually is due to congenital heart disease and may be an isolated defect or a component of more complex congenital disease, such as tetralogy of Fallot.

❐ Visualization of the pulmonic valve is challenging both on transthoracic and transesophageal imaging in adults; often Doppler data are used to infer valve pathology.

❐ Grading of stenosis severity is based on the maximum transvalvular pressure gradient (mild, less than 25 mm Hg; moderate, 25 to 50 mm Hg; and severe, greater than 50 mm Hg).

❐ Pulmonic stenosis often is accompanied by significant pulmonic regurgitation, particularly if there has been a prior surgical or percutaneous procedure.

❐ Branch pulmonary artery stenosis may also be present and is difficult to evaluate by echocardiography, although evaluation of the proximal right and left pulmonary arteries may be possible from a high parasternal short axis view.

NOTES

SELF-ASSESSMENT QUESTIONS

QUESTION 1

An 82-year-old man presented with symptoms of exertional dyspnea. The aortic valve was severely calcified, with an outflow tract diameter of 2.4 cm and a velocity time integral of 12 cm (Fig. 11–23). Aortic jet velocity and VTI were 3.9 m/s and 86 cm from the apical window and 3.96 m/s and 94 cm from the suprasternal notch approach (Fig. 11–24). VTIs were calculated as the area under the Doppler curve by tracing the outer edge of the curve.

Based on these data, perform the following calculations:

Transaortic stroke volume: _____
Cardiac output: _____
Continuity equation aortic valve area: _____
_____
Velocity ratio: _____
Overall, the degree of aortic stenosis is: _____
_____

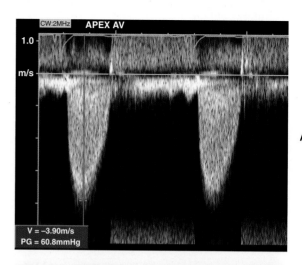

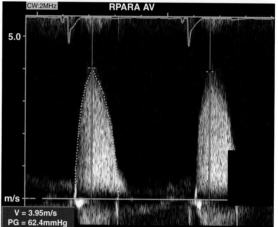

A

B

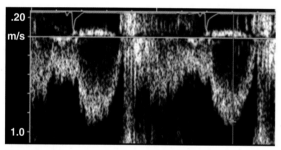

Figure 11–23

Figure 11–24

QUESTION 2

A 42-year-old woman being evaluated for liver transplantation has a CWD LV outflow velocity of 3.8 m/s. The aortic valve M-mode is shown in Figure 11–25.

The most likely diagnosis is:

A. Bicuspid aortic valve
B. Hypertrophic cardiomyopathy
C. Subaortic membrane
D. Mitral regurgitation jet mistaken for LV outflow

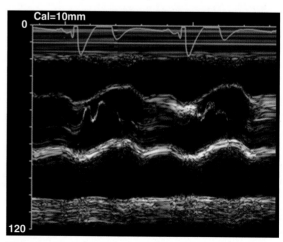

Figure 11–25

QUESTION 3

2D images of the aortic valve in a 56-year-old man referred for evaluation of a murmur are shown in Figures 11–26A and B.

The most likely diagnosis is:

A. Rheumatic valve disease
B. Calcific valve disease
C. Bicuspid valve
D. Subaortic membrane
E. Normal valve

QUESTION 4

During evaluation of a 76-year-old man with calcific aortic stenosis, you are having difficulty obtaining a left ventricular outflow tract (LVOT) diameter measurement from the parasternal window. You have already adjusted the depth and used zoom mode to maximize the frame rate and readjusted the gain setting to optimize the blood–tissue interface. You also tried repositioning the patient and had him hold his breath at end exhalation. At this point, the next best step is to:

A. Use a default value of 2.0 cm for outflow tract diameter
B. Calculate the LVOT–to–aortic jet velocity ratio instead of valve area
C. Recommend transesophageal echocardiography
D. Refer for cardiac catheterization
E. Measure LVOT diameter in the apical long axis view

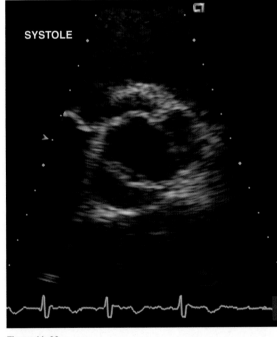

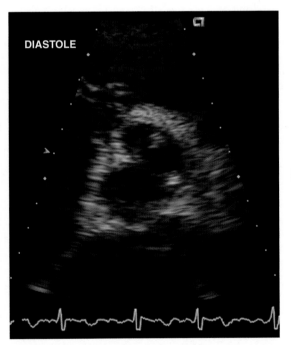

A   B

Figure 11–26

QUESTION 5

An 84-year-old man presented with heart failure symptoms. Coronary angiography was normal, but echocardiography showed an LV ejection fraction of 24%. In addition, the aortic valve was moderately calcified, with a maximum jet velocity of 2.4 m/s, an LV outflow tract diameter of 2.4 cm, an LV outflow tract velocity of 0.6 m/s, and a continuity equation valve area of 1.0 cm^2. A dobutamine stress echocardiogram was requested and the Doppler flows shown in Figure 11–27 were obtained:

These findings are most consistent with:

   A. Severe aortic stenosis
   B. Primary myocardial dysfunction
   C. Lack of contractile reserve
   D. Inadequate test

QUESTION 6

A 23-year-old man was referred to echocardiography for evaluation of hypertension. Parasternal short axis views showed a bicuspid aortic valve. The long axis view is shown in Figure 11–28.

Which of the following Doppler data is essential in this patient?

   A. Doppler tissue imaging at the mitral annulus
   B. Pulmonary vein Doppler velocities
   C. Doppler descending aortic velocities
   D. Mitral regurgitant jet dP/dt measurement
   E. Tricuspid regurgitant jet

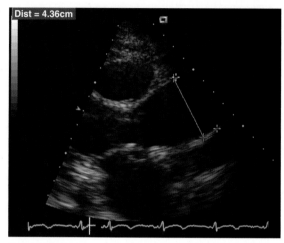

Figure 11–28

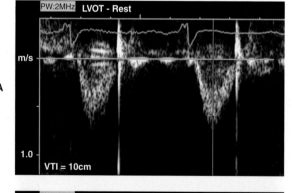
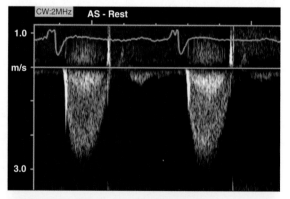
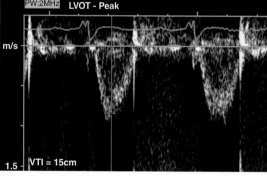
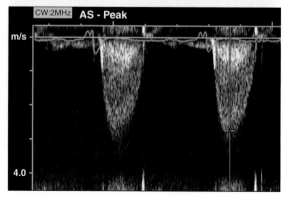

Figure 11–27

QUESTION 7

A 23-year-old woman is referred for possible balloon mitral valvuloplasty for rheumatic mitral stenosis. Parasternal long and short axis views in diastole are shown in Figure 11–29.

Calculate the mitral valve morphology score:

_____

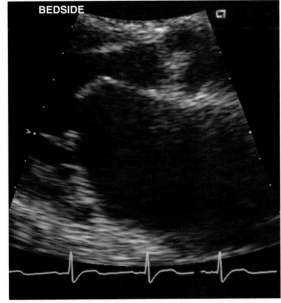

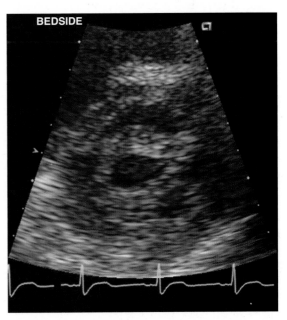

Figure 11–29

QUESTION 8

The Doppler velocity curve across the mitral valve in the same patient as shown in Question 7 is shown in Figure 11–30.

Measure the pressure half time:_____
Calculate valve area: _____

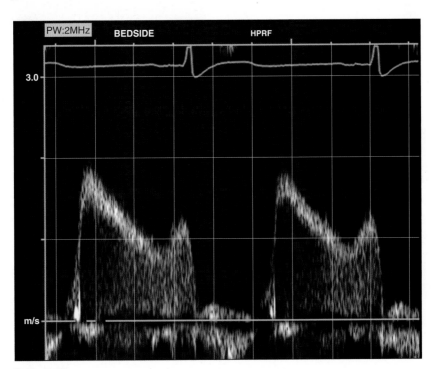

Figure 11–30

QUESTION 9

An apical Doppler signal across the mitral valve in a patient with mitral stenosis is recorded (Fig. 11–31). The patient is in a steep left lateral decubitus position on a stretcher with an apical cutout.

The best approach to measuring the pressure half time in this patient is to:

A. Use the CWD recording instead.
B. Place a line from the peak velocity to the end-diastolic velocity.
C. Place the line along the mid-diastolic section of the velocity curve.
D. Use a higher transducer frequency for the Doppler recording.
E. Use a lower transducer frequency for the Doppler recording.

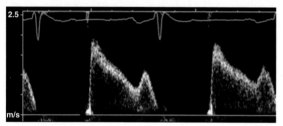

Figure 11–31

QUESTION 10

The Doppler recording in Figure 11–32 shows:

A. Severe mitral stenosis
B. Severe mitral regurgitation
C. Severe aortic stenosis
D. Severe aortic regurgitation

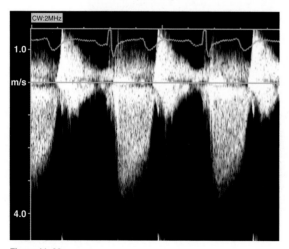

Figure 11–32

QUESTION 11

A patient with rheumatic mitral stenosis underwent treadmill stress testing, with the Doppler recordings at baseline (*A*) and immediately post-exercise (*B*) shown in Figure 11–33.

This data is most consistent with:

A. Normal exercise response
B. Exercise-induced mitral regurgitation
C. Dynamic outflow obstruction
D. Primary pulmonary hypertension
E. Severe mitral stenosis

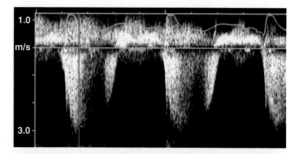

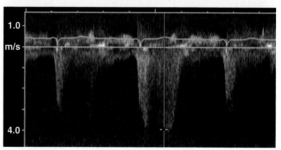

Figure 11–33

QUESTION 12

A 26-year-old man with a history of repaired tetralogy of Fallot is referred for echocardiography. The request form notes that a systolic murmur is present. The CWD recordings obtained in this patient are shown in Figure 11–34. What is the most likely diagnosis?

A. Residual ventricular septal defect
B. Severe pulmonic regurgitation
C. Severe pulmonic stenosis
D. Severe pulmonary hypertension
E. Severe tricuspid regurgitation

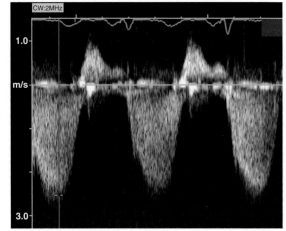
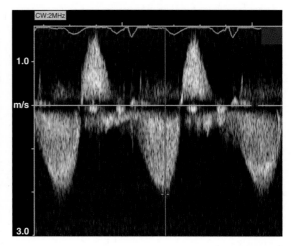

Figure 11–34

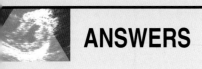

ANSWERS

ANSWER 1

The first step is to calculate the outflow tract cross-sectional area:

$$CSA_{LVOT} = \pi(\,LVOT_D\,/2)^2 = 3.14(2.4/2)^2 = 4.5\ cm^2$$

$$Transaortic\ stroke\ volume\ (SV) = CSA_{LVOT} \times VTI_{LVOT} = 4.5\ cm^2 \times 12\ cm = 54\ cm^3 = 54\ ml$$

Heart rate is calculated as 60 seconds/minute divided by the R-R interval in seconds. In this case, the R-R interval is 0.9 second (see the ECG and time markers at the standard 0.2 second intervals), so heart rate is 67 beats per minute.

Cardiac output is SV × heart rate (66 beats per minute [bpm]) = 3564 ml = 3.56 L/min

The aortic jet is examined from both apical and high right parasternal windows, with the highest jet velocity representing the most parallel intercept angle between the jet and ultrasound beam. The highest velocity signal is used to measure the VTI.

Continuity equation aortic valve area is

$$AVA = SV/VTI_{AS\text{-}Jet} = 54\ cm^3/94\ cm = 0.6\ cm^2$$

The velocity ratio is

$$V_{LVOT}/V_{max} = 0.9/4.0 = 0.23$$

These findings are all consistent with severe aortic stenosis.

ANSWER 2: C

This M-mode recording shows early systolic closure of the aortic valve, but the leaflets then open fully in late systole, as is typical with a fixed subaortic obstruction, such as a subaortic membrane. With a bicuspid valve, leaflet closure is eccentric and opening is normal unless there is superimposed calcification. With dynamic subaortic obstruction caused by hypertrophic cardiomyopathy, the leaflets close in mid (not early) systole, followed by coarse fluttering of the leaflets in late systole. If a high velocity jet is found with a normal aortic valve, the possibility of having mistaken the mitral regurgitant jet for the aortic stenosis jet should be considered. The mitral regurgitant jet is longer in duration than LV outflow and has a velocity of faster than 5 m/s if blood pressure is greater than 100 mm Hg.

ANSWER 3: C

These images show a bicuspid aortic valve. In diastole, there appear to be three leaflets, because there is a raphe in the anterior leaflet (the fused right and left coronary cusps). The systolic image is diagnostic, showing only two leaflets with only two points of attachment to the aorta (commissures). Often, frame-by-frame analysis of a zoomed short axis view of the valve is needed to make this diagnosis. In a short axis view, with rheumatic aortic disease there is commissural fusion. With calcific disease of either a bicuspid or trileaflet valve, there is calcification in the base of the leaflets. With a subaortic membrane, the aortic valve may appear normal or may be mildly sclerotic due to the impact of the high velocity jet. With a normal trileaflet valve, all three leaflets can be seen in systole.

ANSWER 4: B

LVOT diameter can be accurately measured in more than 95% of patients if care is taken in optimizing patient position and instrument settings. LVOT diameter varies widely and is not accurately predicted by body size in adults, although it tends to be smaller in women, so using a "default" value is not appropriate. The ratio of outflow tract to aortic jet velocity does not require an LVOT diameter measurement and is a useful measure of stenosis severity. Transesophageal imaging might provide better images of the valve itself and might be considered if the velocity ratio and other data do not provide sufficient information of clinical decision making. Transesophageal images allow better evaluation of valve anatomy and may allow direct planimetry of valve area in some cases but rarely provide accurate velocity data because of the intercept angle from this approach. Cardiac catheterization is reserved for cases when the aortic jet velocity also is nondiagnostic or if clinical data are discrepant with the echocardiographic findings. LVOT diameter measurements from an apical view are likely to be imprecise because of the lateral beam width at this depth from this approach.

ANSWER 5: B

From the data shown, the maximum aortic velocities can be directly measured. Mean gradient was estimated using the formula Mean gradient

$= 2.4v^2$. Stroke volume was calculated as LV outflow tract CSA times the VTI of flow. Valve area was calculated with the continuity equation. This study shows:

	Rest	Dobutamine
Stroke volume	45 ml	68 ml
Aortic velocity	2.4 m/s	2.7 m/s
Mean gradient	14 mm Hg	17 mm Hg
Aortic valve area	1.0 cm^2	1.4 cm^2

This is an adequate test because there was an increase in aortic jet velocity. There is a normal contractile response to dobutamine with an increase in stroke volume. There also was an improvement in the biplane ejection fraction from 24% to 30%. The increase in valve area with dobutamine indicates the valve leaflets are flexible and that severe stenosis is not present. Thus this patient has a primary cardiomyopathy with the incidental finding of moderate aortic valve stenosis. The stenosis appears more severe at rest because the valve leaflets only open to an area of 1.0 cm^2 because of the combination of moderately calcified leaflets and inadequate force to open the leaflets in systole.

ANSWER 6: C

A bicuspid aortic valve is associated with an aortic coarctation in 10% of cases, so it is essential to evaluate descending aortic flow signals in this patient, especially given the history of hypertension. Conversely, more than 50% of patients with an aortic coarctation have a bicuspid valve. The finding of a dilated ascending aorta is also associated with a bicuspid aortic valve and is not related to the severity of valve dysfunction. These patients are at increased risk of aortic dissection. Doppler tissue imaging and pulmonary venous inflow patterns would be helpful for evaluation of ventricular diastolic dysfunction but are not essential in this patient. The mitral regurgitant jet dP/dt would be helpful if ventricular systolic dysfunction was present. The tricuspid regurgitant jet would allow estimation of pulmonary pressures but is likely to be normal in this patient.

ANSWER 7

A score of 1 (mild) to 4 (severe) is assigned to each of four characteristics of the valve: reduction in leaflet mobility, leaflet thickening, calcification, and subvalvular (chordal) involvement. In this patient, classical rheumatic changes are present, with commissural fusion resulting in diastolic doming of the leaflets with little separation of the leaflet tips. However, the base and mid-portion of the leaflet move relatively normally, consistent with a score of 1 for leaflet mobility. Thickening is very mild and restricted to the leaflet tips (score 1), and there is minimal valve calcification (score 1). The chordae do not appear to be thickened (score 1) but might be better evaluated in an apical view. The total Wilkins morphology score thus is 4, indicating a favorable morphology for a valvotomy and a low likelihood of procedural complications. Using the French classification, this is a group I valve, thin pliable leaflets with normal chordal length.

ANSWER 8

The pressure half time is the time interval between the peak pressure gradient and $\frac{1}{2}$ the peak gradient. The peak velocity in early diastole (1.8 m/s) corresponds to the peak pressure gradient. A line is drawn from the peak velocity along the diastolic deceleration slope of the flow signal. The velocity corresponding to $\frac{1}{2}$ the peak gradient is calculated ($V_{T\frac{1}{2}}$) using the simplified Bernoulli equation for the pressure gradient at each velocity. Thus:

$$4\,(V_{T\frac{1}{2}})^2 = 4(V_{max})^2/2$$

and solving for $V_{T\frac{1}{2}}$:

$$V_{T\frac{1}{2}} = V_{max}/\sqrt{2} = V_{max}/1.4$$

With an ultrasound system or a computer analysis system, the pressure half time is displayed from the line placed on the diastolic deceleration slope. By hand, a vertical line is drawn at the peak velocity, and the point on this line corresponding to $\frac{1}{2}$ the peak gradient (1.3 m/s) and the time interval between these two lines is measured in milliseconds (175 msec). Valve area is calculated by dividing the empiric constant 220 by the pressure half time, so valve area in this case is 1.3 cm^2.

ANSWER 9: C

This Doppler recording shows a deceleration slope that is not linear, with a steep slope in early and mid-diastole, followed by a flatter slope in late diastole, possibly related to pulmonary venous inflow contributing to the transmitral flow curve. If efforts to obtain a more parallel intercept angle do not improve the signal, the best approach is to draw the line along the mid-diastolic slope, ignoring the end-diastolic signal, and using the intersection of this line with the onset of flow as the peak velocity. The CWD signal will have the same slope as the pulsed Doppler signal and is measured the same way. Changing the transducer frequency will not affect the slope of the diastolic velocity deceleration.

ANSWER 10: B

This CWD velocity signal recorded from an apical window shows a diastolic signal of LV inflow. Although the antegrade mitral velocity is high, the deceleration slope is steep, consistent with a high antegrade volume flow rate, without significant stenosis. In systole, the mitral regurgitant signal is as dense as antegrade flow, consistent with severe mitral regurgitation. The relatively low velocity suggests a low systolic blood pressure and high left atrial pressure. With aortic stenosis, the systolic ejection period is shorter than for mitral regurgitation, and there is a gap between the end of forward mitral flow and the onset of aortic flow (isovolumic contraction) and between the end of aortic flow and the onset of mitral flow (isovolumic relaxation). With aortic regurgitation, the diastolic velocity reflects the aortic–to–left ventricular diastolic pressure difference, which is typically greater than 50 mm Hg, or a velocity of faster than 3.5 m/s, which is much higher than transmitral velocities, even when mitral stenosis is present. The aortic regurgitant flow is longer in duration than antegrade mitral flow as aortic regurgitation continues from aortic valve closure to valve opening.

ANSWER 11: E

These Doppler recordings show tricuspid regurgitation at rest and post-exercise. The resting tricuspid regurgitant (TR) jet of 2.8 m/s indicates an RV to RA systolic pressure gradient of 31 mm Hg. Assuming an RA pressure of 5 mm Hg, estimated resting pulmonary artery (PA) pressure is 36 mm Hg. The post-exercise TR jet of 3.6 m/s is consistent with a pressure difference of 52 mm

Hg and a PA systolic pressure of 57 mm Hg (moderate pulmonary hypertension). The primary goal in exercise testing with mitral stenosis is to evaluate the rise in PA pressure with exercise. A small increase is normal, but an exercise PA systolic pressure of more than 50 mm Hg suggests a significant rise in LA pressure, caused by a severely stenotic mitral valve, and is an indication for intervention. Exercise testing also is helpful for detection of exercise-induced mitral regurgitation with myxomatous or ischemic mitral regurgitation. The mitral regurgitant jet would be of higher velocity than the TR jet, as MR reflects the LV-to-LA pressure gradient in systole (typically more than 100 mm Hg or faster than 5 m/s). Exercise to evaluate outflow obstruction may be helpful in patients with hypertrophic cardiomyopathy with a typical late-peaking systolic velocity curve.

ANSWER 12: B

Figure 11–34A shows tricuspid regurgitation, Figure 11–34B shows antegrade and retrograde pulmonic flow. This patient has severe pulmonic regurgitation, as shown by the dense diastolic regurgitant signal with a steep deceleration slope for the pulmonic valve velocity recording. The antegrade velocity across the pulmonic valve (*right,* Fig. 11–34B) with a velocity of 2.0 m/s indicates a maximum pressure gradient of only 16 mm Hg. The tricuspid regurgitant jet velocity of 2.5 m/s (*left,* Fig. 11–34A) reflects an RV to RA systolic pressure difference of 25 mm Hg (or RV systolic pressure of 30 mm Hg if RA pressure is 5 mm Hg). The TR velocity reflects the pressure difference; the density of the signal reflects the volume of TR. Because the density of the signal is slightly less intense than antegrade tricuspid flow, regurgitation is moderate, but not severe. Pulmonary pressures are normal, based on subtracting the systolic gradient across the pulmonic valve from the systolic RV pressure (30 − 16 = 14 mm Hg).

NOTES

12 Valve Regurgitation

BASIC PRINCIPLES

Vena Contracta (Fig. 12–1)

■ Narrowest width of the regurgitant jet, measured using color Doppler flow imaging

Key points:

❑ Optimal color flow images show flow acceleration proximal to the regurgitant valve and distal jet expansion in the receiving chamber, with the vena contracta being the narrow neck between them.

❑ Vena contracta measurements are most accurate when the flow signal is in the near field of the image (e.g., transthoracic parasternal long axis views) using a narrow sector width to optimize frame rate and zoom mode to increase image size.

❑ Small differences in vena contracta width correspond to substantial changes in regurgitant severity grade, so if a precise and accurate measurement is not possible, other approaches should be used.

Proximal Isovelocity Surface Area

■ Blood flow accelerates proximal to a regurgitant orifice.

■ The aliasing velocity on color Doppler flow imaging provides visualization of a contour where all the blood cells have the same velocity (isovelocity; Fig. 12–2).

■ The shape of this proximal isovelocity contour typically is a hemisphere, so the cross-sectional area (CSA) of this surface is $2\pi r^2$.

■ Volume flow rate is CSA times velocity (in this case the aliasing velocity):

$$\text{Instantaneous flow rate (cm}^3\text{/s)} = \text{CSA (cm}^2) \times V_{\text{aliasing}} \text{ (cm/s)}$$

Key points:

❑ The proximal isovelocity surface area (PISA) is best visualized from a window where the ultrasound beam is parallel to the flow direction, typically the apical long axis or four-chamber view.

❑ The aliasing velocity is decreased to 30 to 40 cm/s by shifting the Doppler baseline, which enhances PISA visualization.

❑ Both a narrow color sector and zoom mode are used for accurate measurement.

❑ PISA measures instantaneous flow rate (cm³/s); PISA must be integrated over the flow period to obtain flow volume (cm³ or ml).

❑ PISA may be inaccurate when the proximal flow field is not hemispherical in shape, so this approach is more useful for central jets than eccentric jets.

❑ It is more difficult to visualize the PISA when regurgitation is mild, and it is more difficult to visualize a PISA for aortic, compared with mitral, regurgitation.

❑ Identification of the valve plane by two-dimensional (2D) imaging is critical, because the PISA measurement is from the aliasing velocity to the valve orifice.

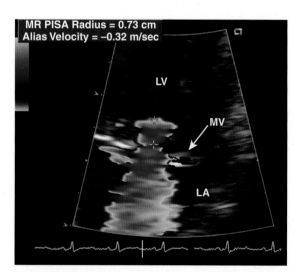

Figure 12–2 The proximal isovelocity surface area (PISA) is identified by the aliasing velocity (blue–red interface) proximal to the regurgitant valve seen in this zoomed image of the mitral valve (*MV*) in an apical four-chamber view. The PISA is assumed to be a hemispherical shape, although the image seen with color Doppler may be somewhat distorted, as in this example.

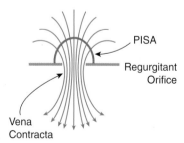

Figure 12–1 Schematic diagram showing the proximal jet geometry for valve regurgitation. Flow proximal to the regurgitant orifice increases in velocity as the flow stream narrows into the regurgitant orifice. There are multiple proximal isovelocity surface areas (PISAs) proximal to an orifice, with each PISA defined by a uniform blood velocity. The PISA seen with color flow depends on the aliasing velocity of the color scale. The flow stream continues to narrow beyond the orifice, with the narrowest flow region, the vena contracta, reflecting regurgitant volume.

Regurgitant Volume (Fig. 12–3)

- Regurgitant volume (RV) is the amount of blood that flows backward across the valve, measured in cm^3 or ml.
- RV can be calculated by subtracting the stroke volume (SV) across a competent valve (forward SV) from the antegrade volume flow rate across the regurgitant valve (total SV):

$$RV = Total\ SV - Forward\ SV$$

- Total SV also can be calculated by 2D echocardiographic measurement of left ventricular (LV) stroke volume using the apical biplane approach.

Key points:

- ❑ Transvalvular volume flow rate calculations are based on diameter (D) measurements (using a circular CSA) and the velocity time integral (VTI) of flow at that site:

$$SV = CSA \times VTI = \pi(D/2)^2 \times VTI$$

- ❑ Small errors in diameter measurement lead to large errors in calculated SV.
- ❑ The most common source of error is ensuring that diameter is measured at the same level as the VTI recording; this is particularly problematic for transmitral volume flow.
- ❑ When both aortic and mitral valves are regurgitant, pulmonary valve flow rate can be used for forward SV.
- ❑ 2D LV volumes provide total SV when image planes and endocardial definition are adequate, but volumes may be underestimated if apical views are foreshortened.

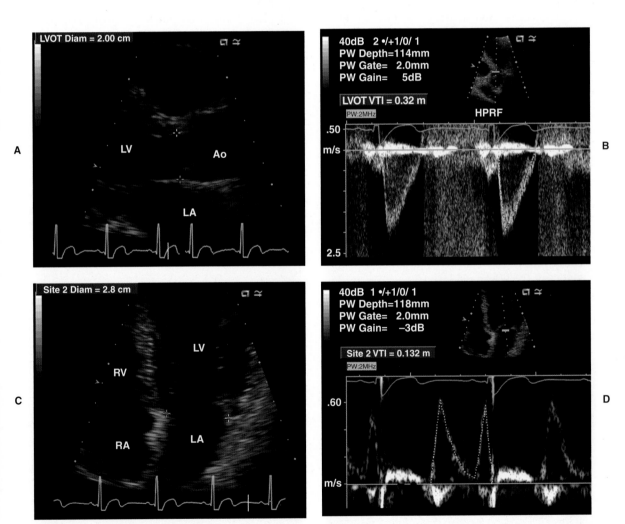

Figure 12–3 In this patient with aortic regurgitation, regurgitant volume is calculated as the difference between total stroke volume across the aortic valve and forward stroke volume across the mitral valve. The diameter (Diam) and velocity time integral (VTI) for transaortic (*A* and *B*) and transmitral (*C* and *D*) flow are shown. Transaortic (total) stroke volume (TSV) is left ventricular outflow tract cross-sectional area (CSA= πr^2 = 3.14[2 cm/2]^2 = 3.14 cm^2) times the velocity time integral (TSV = 3.14 cm^2 × 32 cm = 100 ml). Transmitral (forward) stroke volume (FSV) is π(2.8 cm/2)^2 × 13.2 cm = 81 ml. Then regurgitant stroke volume (RSV) is TSV − FSV, or 100 ml − 81 ml = 19 ml. Regurgitant fraction is 19 ml/100 ml × 100% = 19%. These findings suggest mild regurgitation.

Regurgitant Orifice Area

- Conceptually, regurgitant orifice area (ROA) is the size of the defect in the closed valve that allows valve regurgitation.
- The actual anatomy of the regurgitant orifice may be complex, sometimes with multiple sites of backflow across the valve.
- The continuity equation applies to both antegrade and retrograde flow across a valve.
- Thus ROA can be calculated from regurgitant SV and the VTI of the regurgitant jet (RJ) as:

$$\text{ROA (cm}^2) = \text{Regurgitant SV (cm}^3)/\text{VTI}_{RJ} \text{ (cm)}$$

Key points:

- ❏ ROA can be calculated using regurgitant SV calculated by any method.
- ❏ The continuous wave recording of the regurgitant jet is used to trace the velocity time integral (Fig. 12–4; refer to the RV calculation from Fig. 12–3).
- ❏ ROA also can be estimated using the PISA approach by dividing the PISA instantaneous volume flow rate by the maximum regurgitant jet velocity:

$$\text{ROA (cm}^2) = \text{PISA (cm}^3/\text{s})/\text{V}_{RJ} \text{ (cm/s)}$$

- ❏ The PISA-estimated ROA reflects the instantaneous ROA only and thus is most useful for regurgitation that extends equally throughout the flow period.
- ❏ In clinical practice, ROA should be calculated by more than one method, if possible, to ensure validity.

Distal Flow Reversals

- The direction of blood flow distal to a regurgitant valve is reversed from normal when regurgitation is severe.

- With severe mitral regurgitation (MR), there is systolic flow reversal in the pulmonary veins; with severe aortic regurgitation, there is holodiastolic flow reversal in the aorta (Fig. 12–5); and with severe tricuspid regurgitation, there is systolic flow reversal in the hepatic veins (Fig. 12–6).
- This qualitative indicator is integrated with other findings in classifying overall regurgitant severity.

Key points:

- ❏ These findings are more specific when flow reversal is more distal (e.g., abdominal compared with thoracic aorta for aortic regurgitation) and more severe (e.g., reversed versus blunted pulmonary vein systolic flow in MR).
- ❏ Flow reversal is sometimes seen even when regurgitation is not severe—for example, in hepatic and pulmonary veins in nonsinus rhythms or in the descending aorta with a patent ductus arteriosus.
- ❏ Flow reversal is best detected with low wall filter settings, gain reduced to avoid channel cross-talk, and the scale adjusted to the velocity range of interest.
- ❏ Normal patterns of flow sometimes are mistaken for flow reversal. In the descending aorta, early diastolic flow reversal is normal; in the hepatic veins, the atrial reversal can be prominent and may appear to extend into early systole.

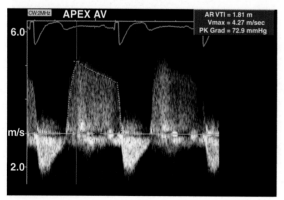

Figure 12–4 The velocity time integral (VTI) of aortic regurgitant flow in the same patient shown in Figure 12–3 is used to calculate regurgitant orifice area (ROA) as RSV/VTI = 19 cm³/181 cm = 0.10 cm² (where RSV is regurgitant stroke volume and VTI is the velocity time integral), again consistent with mild regurgitation.

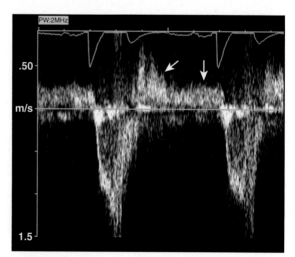

Figure 12–5 The Doppler flow signal in the descending thoracic aorta shows holodiastolic flow toward the transducer (reversal of flow, *arrows*) in this patient with moderate to severe aortic regurgitation. Holodiastolic flow reversal in the descending aorta also may be seen with other causes of diastolic flow exiting the proximal aorta, including a patent ductus arteriosus or a large arteriovenous fistula in an upper extremity.

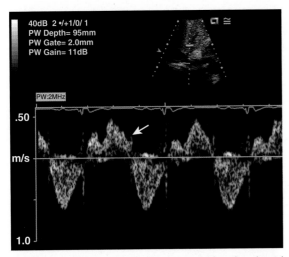

Figure 12–6 The hepatic vein flow signal, recorded from the subcostal window in the central hepatic vein, shows flow toward the transducer in systole (*arrow*), also termed systolic flow reversal, when severe tricuspid regurgitation is present.

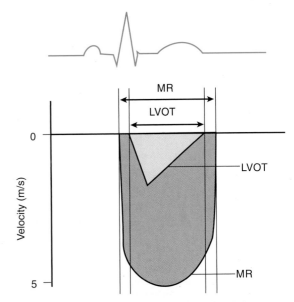

Figure 12–7 The shape of the continuous wave Doppler velocity curve reflects the instantaneous pressure differences between the aorta and left ventricle in diastole, with the relationship between pressures (*top*) and Doppler velocities (*bottom*) shown for chronic and acute aortic regurgitation.

Continuous Wave Doppler Signal (Fig. 12–7)

■ The shape of the continuous wave (CW) Doppler signal reflects the instantaneous pressure differences between the two chambers.
■ The density of the CW Doppler signal, relative to antegrade flow, reflects the volume of regurgitant flow.

Key points:

❐ The diastolic deceleration slope (or pressure half time) of the aortic regurgitant signal is steeper (shorter) with more severe aortic regurgitation.
❐ A late systolic decline in velocity with mitral regurgitation reflects a rise in left atrial (LA) pressure, suggestive of a V wave.

❐ The Doppler recording must be made with the ultrasound beam parallel to the direction of the regurgitant jet at the vena contracta.
❐ Optimal CW recordings of a regurgitant jet shows a smooth velocity curve with a dense signal along the outer edge of the spectral signal.
❐ Recordings are enhanced using gray-scale spectral analysis with the velocity scale adjusted to the range of interest, the wall filters increased to improve the signal-to-noise ratio, and gains lowered to prevent overestimation of velocities.

AORTIC REGURGITATION

THE ECHO EXAM: AORTIC REGURGITATION

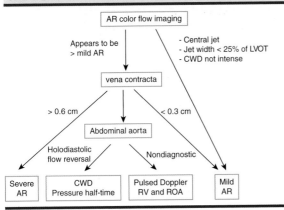

QUANTITATIVE EVALUATION OF AORTIC REGURGITANT SEVERITY

	MILD	SEVERE
Jet width/LVOT	< 25%	≥ 65%
Vena contracta (cm)	< 0.3	> 0.6
Pressure half time (ms)	> 500	< 200
Regurgitant volume (ml/beat)	< 30	≥ 60
Regurgitant fraction (%)	< 30	≥ 50
Regurgitant orifice area (cm²)	< 0.10	≥ 0.30

QUANTITATION OF AORTIC REGURGITATION SEVERITY

PARAMETER	MODALITY	VIEW	RECORDING	MEASUREMENTS
Vena contracta width	Color flow imaging	Parasternal long-axis	Angulate, decrease depth, narrow sector, zoom	Narrowest segment of regurgitant jet between proximal flow convergence and distal jet expansion
Descending aortic diastolic flow reversal	Pulsed Doppler	Subcostal and SSN	Sample volume 2-3 mm, decrease wall filters, adjust scale	
CW Doppler signal (intensity, slope, VTI)	CW Doppler	Apical	Careful positioning, and transducer angulation to obtain clear signal	Compare signal intensity of retrograde to antegrade flow, measure slope along edge of dense signal
Volume flow at 2 sites (RV, RF, ROA)	2D and pulsed Doppler	Parasternal (2D) and apical	LVOT diameter and VTI Mitral annulus diameter and VTI	Calculations in example

2D, *Two-dimensional;* CW, *continuous wave;* LVOT, *left ventricular outflow tract;* RF, *regurgitant fraction;* ROA, *regurgitant orifice area;* RV, *regurgitant volume;* SSN, *suprasternal notch;* VTI, *velocity time integral.*

AORTIC REGURGITATION: DIAGNOSTIC APPROACH

Etiology	Valve abnormality
	Aortic root disease
Severity of Regurgitation	Vena contracta width
	Descending aorta holosystolic flow reversal
	CW Doppler deceleration slope
	Calculation of RV, RF, and ROA
Co-existing Aortic Stenosis	Aortic jet velocity
Left Ventricular Response	LV dimensions or volumes
	LV ejection fraction
	dP/dt
Other Findings	Aortic coarctation (with bicuspid valve)

EXAMPLE

A 37-year-old man presents with an asymptomatic diastolic murmur. Echocardiography shows a bicuspid aortic valve with more than mild aortic regurgitation with:

Vena contracta width	5 mm
Descending aorta	Holodiastolic flow reversal in descending thoracic, but not proximal abdominal, aorta
CW Doppler	AR signal less dense than antegrade flow
	Pressure half time = 400 ms
	VTI_{AR} = 150 cm
LVOT diameter ($LVOT_D$)	2.8 cm
VTI_{LVOT}	24 cm
Mitral annulus diameter	3.1 cm
VTI_{MA}	12 cm

The vena contracta width indicates more than mild aortic regurgitation, but this could be moderate or severe.

Holodiastolic flow reversal in the proximal abdominal aorta would be consistent with severe AR. Flow reversal in the descending thoracic aorta indicates at least moderate AR but is less specific for severe AR.

CW Doppler signal density indicates at least moderate AR and a pressure half time >200 but <500 ms. is also consistent with moderate or severe aortic regurgitation.

Next, RV, RF, and ROA are calculated.

Using the LVOT and mitral annulus diameters (MA_D), the circular cross-sectional areas (CSA) of flow are calculated:

$$CSA_{LVOT} = \pi(\ LVOT_D\ /2)^2 = 3.14(2.8/2)^2 = 6.2\ cm^2$$

$$CSA_{MA} = \pi(\ MA_D\ /2)^2 = 3.14(3.1/2)^2 = 7.5\ cm^2$$

Stroke volume across each valve (cm^3 = ml), then is:

$$SV_{LVOT} = (CSA_{LVOT} \times VTI_{LVOT}) = 6.2\ cm^2 \times 24\ cm = 149\ cm^3$$

$$SV_{MA} = (CSA_{MA} \times VTI_{MA}) = 7.5\ cm^2 \times 12\ cm = 91\ cm^3$$

RV is calculated from transaortic flow (TSV, total stroke volume) and transmitral flow (FSV, forward stroke volume), as:

$$RV = TSV - FSV = 149\ ml - 91\ ml = 58\ ml$$

RF is:

$$RV = RSV/\ TSV \times 100\% = 58\ ml/149\ ml \times 100\% = 39\%$$

ROA is:

$$ROA = RSV/VTI_{AR} = 58\ cm^3/204\ cm = 0.28\ cm^2$$

The RV, RF, and ROA all are consistent with moderate (but nearly severe) aortic regurgitation.

AR, *Aortic regurgitation;* CW, *continuous wave;* LV, *left ventricular;* LVOT, *left ventricular outflow tract;* RF, *regurgitant fraction;* ROA, *regurgitant orifice area;* RV, *regurgitant volume;* VTI, *velocity time integral.*

Step-by-Step Approach

Step 1: Determine the Etiology of Regurgitation

■ Aortic regurgitation is due either to disease of the valve leaflets or abnormalities of the aortic root (Fig. 12–8).
■ Primary causes of aortic leaflet dysfunction include bicuspid valve, rheumatic disease, endocarditis, calcific disease, and some systemic diseases.
■ Aortic root enlargement resulting in aortic regurgitation may be due to Marfan syndrome, annuloaortic ectasia, hypertension, or aortic dissection.

Key points:

❏ Long and short axis images of the aortic valve allow identification of a bicuspid aortic valve (two leaflets in systole), rheumatic disease (commissural fusion), vegetations, and calcific changes.
❏ Leaflet perforation or fenestration cannot be visualized but is inferred from the location of the regurgitant jet orifice identified by color Doppler.
❏ When aortic regurgitation is more than mild, the aorta should be measured at several sites as detailed in Chapter 16. The transducer is moved cephalad to visualize the ascending aorta.
❏ Marfan syndrome is characterized by loss of the normal acute angle at the sinotubular junction.
❏ Systemic inflammatory diseases associated with aortic regurgitation cause dilation of the aorta and thickening of the posterior aortic root extending onto the base of the anterior mitral leaflet.

Step 2: Determine the Severity of Regurgitation

■ Regurgitant severity is evaluated using a stepwise approach with integration of several types of data.
■ In addition to Doppler measures of regurgitant severity, the cause of regurgitation and left ventricular (LV) size and systolic function are important parameters in clinical decision making.

Step 2A: Measurement of vena contracta width is the initial step in evaluation of aortic regurgitation (Figs. 12–9A and B).

Key Points:

❏ With aortic regurgitation, vena contracta usually is best measured in the parasternal long

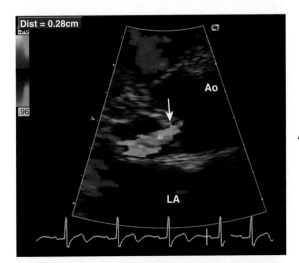

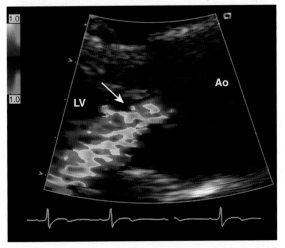

Figure 12–9 Examples of measuring vena contracta width with mild (A) and moderate (B) aortic regurgitation. Vena contracta width in aortic regurgitation is best recorded in the parasternal long axis view using zoom mode to focus on the aortic valve. The narrowest width of the regurgitant jet (arrows) is measured, ideally with the proximal flow acceleration and distal jet expansion regions seen. When regurgitation is mild, the proximal acceleration is difficult to visualize.

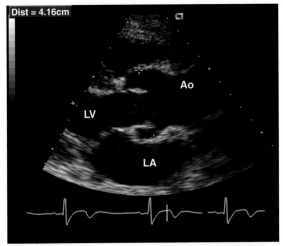

Figure 12–8 Parasternal long axis view in a patient with aortic regurgitation showing dilated sinuses of Valsalva that may be the cause of valve dysfunction.

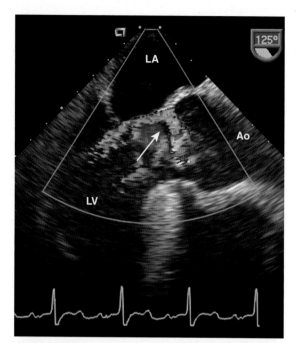

Figure 12–10 Transesophageal echocardiography long axis view of the aortic valve in diastole showing a narrow eccentric jet of aortic regurgitation. The jet originates in the central part of the valve (note proximal acceleration region, *arrow*) but extends along the ventricular side of the noncoronary cusp and then down the anterior mitral valve leaflet. Vena contracta width is measured at the narrowest diameter of the jet; in this case, vena contracta width is parallel to the valve leaflet closure plane.

axis view on transthoracic echocardiography (TTE) or the long axis view at about 120 degrees rotation on transesophageal echocardiography (TEE).

☐ Vena contracta is measured as the smallest width of the jet, taking care with eccentric jets to prevent an oblique diameter measurement (Fig. 12–10).

☐ A vena contracta width of smaller than 0.3 cm indicates mild regurgitation; a vena contracta width of larger than 0.6 cm indicates severe regurgitation.

☐ Further evaluation is needed when vena contracta is 0.3 to 0.6 cm, when images of the vena contracta are suboptimal, or when further quantitation is needed for clinical decision making.

Step 2B: The next step is evaluation of diastolic flow reversal in the descending aorta.

Key points:

☐ Holodiastolic flow reversal in the proximal abdominal aorta is highly specific for severe aortic regurgitation (Fig. 12–11).

☐ Holodiastolic flow reversal in the descending thoracic aorta is seen in some patients with moderate, as well as those with severe, aortic regurgitation.

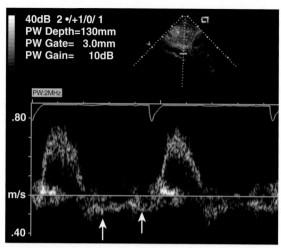

Figure 12–11 With severe aortic regurgitation, flow in the proximal abdominal aorta, recorded from the subcostal window, shows antegrade flow in systole with retrograde flow throughout diastole (*arrows*), reflecting severe backflow across the aortic valve.

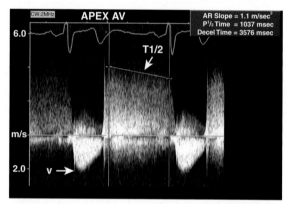

Figure 12–12 CW Doppler evaluation of aortic regurgitation provides information based on (1) the velocity of antegrade flow (*v*) reflecting both the volume of flow and coexisting valve stenosis, (2) the relative density of the regurgitant signal compared with the density of antegrade flow, and (3) the time course of the velocity signal. In this example, the diastolic slope is flat, with a pressure half time of longer than 1000 msec, and the signal is much less dense than antegrade flow; both of these features are consistent with mild regurgitation. Both T½ and P½ are used to refer to the pressure half time.

☐ Early diastolic flow reversal in the descending aorta is normal and should not be mistaken for aortic regurgitation.

☐ If holodiastolic aortic flow reversal is seen without color Doppler evidence of severe aortic regurgitation, consider other causes of diastolic flow in the aorta, such as a patent ductus arteriosus.

Step 2C: CW Doppler evaluation of aortic regurgitation is a standard part of the evaluation (Fig. 12–12).

Key points:

☐ Aortic regurgitation usually is best recorded from an apical approach using CW Doppler,

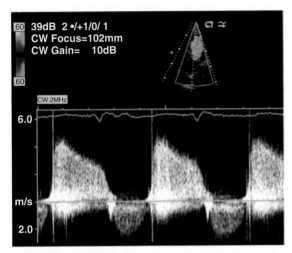

Figure 12–13 In this patient with severe aortic regurgitation, the CW Doppler signal in diastole is as (or more) dense as the antegrade flow signal in systole.

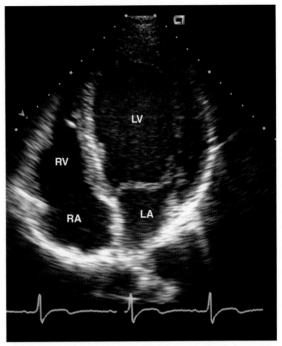

Figure 12–14 In this patient with severe aortic regurgitation, the apical four-chamber view shows a dilated left ventricle (LV) with increased sphericity (rounded shape of the apex).

because this window often allows parallel alignment between the ultrasound beam and regurgitant jet.

- ❑ In cases with an eccentric, posteriorly directed aortic regurgitant jet, the best intercept angle may be obtained from the parasternal window.
- ❑ On TEE, a transgastric apical view may allow recording of the aortic regurgitant jet, but it may not be possible to obtain a parallel intercept angle.
- ❑ The density of the aortic regurgitant velocity signal compared with the density of the antegrade signal provides a qualitative measure of regurgitant severity (Fig. 12–13).
- ❑ In general, a steep diastolic deceleration slope (pressure half time of less than 200 msec) is consistent with severe regurgitation, whereas a flat slope (more than 500 msec) indicates mild regurgitation. However, some patients with compensated severe regurgitation have a long pressure half time.
- ❑ Pressure half time is measured using the same approach as measurement of pressure half time in mitral stenosis.

Step 2D: When further quantitation is needed, RV and ROA can be calculated.

Key points:

- ❑ The most common approach is to calculate total SV across the aortic valve and then subtract forward SV (calculated across the mitral or pulmonic valve) to determine RV.
- ❑ ROA is calculated by dividing RV by the VTI of the CW aortic regurgitation velocity curve.
- ❑ The PISA often is difficult to visualize with aortic regurgitation.

- ❑ Methods to calculate RV based on antegrade and retrograde flow in the descending aorta have been described but are not routinely used.

Step 3: Evaluate Antegrade Aortic Flow and Stenosis

- ■ Many patients with aortic regurgitation also have some degree of aortic stenosis.
- ■ However, antegrade aortic velocity is increased in patients with severe regurgitation because of the increased antegrade volume flow rate across the aortic valve in systole.
- ■ Thus in addition to velocity and mean pressure gradient, aortic valve area should be calculated using the continuity equation as described in Chapter 11.

Step 4: Evaluate the Consequences of Chronic Ventricular Pressure and Volume Overload

- ■ The left ventricle dilates in response to the chronic load imposed by aortic regurgitation, with the extent of LV dilation reflecting the severity of regurgitation (Fig. 12–14).
- ■ Some patients develop irreversible LV dysfunction in the absence of symptoms.
- ■ The most important parameters to measure on echocardiography in patients with chronic severe aortic regurgitation are LV size and ejection fraction.

Key points:

- ☐ LV end-diastolic and end-systolic dimensions and volumes should be measured and compared side-by-side with previous examinations.
- ☐ Indexing dimensions and volumes to body surface area is especially important in women and smaller patients.
- ☐ With severe aortic regurgitation, LV volumes are increased in direct proportion to the RV;

the SV calculated using the biplane apical approach is the total SV (forward SV plus regurgitant SV).

- ☐ The ventricle becomes more spherical in patients with aortic regurgitation, so it is especially important to ensure that ventricular dimensions are measured at the same position on sequential examinations in each patient.

MITRAL REGURGITATION

THE ECHO EXAM: MITRAL REGURGITATION

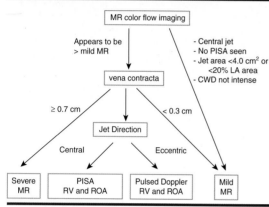

QUANTITATIVE EVALUATION OF MITRAL REGURGITANT SEVERITY (ASE GUIDELINES)

MITRAL REGURGATION	MILD	SEVERE
Jet area (cm²)	< 4 cm² or < 20% LA area	> 40% LA area
Vena contracta (cm)	< 0.3	≥ 0.7
Regurgitant volume (ml)	< 30	≥ 60
Regurgitant fraction (%)	< 30	≥ 50
Regurgitant orifice area (cm²)	< 0.20	≥ 0.40

LA, *Left atrial.*

QUANTITATION OF MITRAL REGURGITATION SEVERITY

PARAMETER	MODALITY	VIEW(S)	RECORDING	MEASUREMENTS
Vena contracta width	Color flow imaging	Parasternal long axis	Angulate, decrease depth, narrow sector, zoom	Narrowest segment of regurgitant jet between proximal flow convergence and distal jet expansion
Color flow imaging	Color flow imaging	Parasternal and apical	Narrow sector, decrease depth	Central vs. eccentric, anterior vs. posterior
CW Doppler signal	CW Doppler	Apical	Careful positioning and transducer angulation to obtain clear signal	Compare signal intensity of retrograde to antegrade flow
Proximal isovelocity surface area	Color flow imaging	A4C or A long axis	Decrease depth, narrow sector, zoom, adjust aliasing velocity	Adjust aliasing velocity so PISA is hemispherical, measure from orifice to aliasing boundary
Volume flow at 2 sites	2D and pulsed Doppler	Parasternal (2D) and apical	LVOT diameter and VTI Mitral annulus diameter and VTI	See calculations for aortic regurgitation example, with substitution of transmitral flow for TSV and transaortic flow for FSV
Pulmonary vein systolic flow reversal	Pulsed Doppler	A4C on TTE but TEE often needed	Pulmonary vein flow in all 4 veins	Qualitative

2D, *Two-dimensional;* A4C, *apical four-chamber;* CW, *continuous wave;* FSV, *forward stroke volume;* LVOT, *left ventricular outflow tract;* PISA, *proximal isovelocity surface area;* TEE, *transesophageal echocardiography;* TSV, *total stroke volume;* TTE, *transthoracic echocardiography;* VTI, *velocity time integral.*

MITRAL REGURGITATION: DIAGNOSTIC APPROACH

Etiology	Primary valve disease
	Secondary (functional)
Severity of Regurgitation	Vena contracta width
	Jet direction (central, eccentric)
	CW Doppler signal
	Calculation of RV, RF, and ROA
	Central jet: PISA method
	Eccentric jet:
	Volume flow at 2 sites
	Pulmonary vein flow reversal
Left Ventricular Response	LV dimensions or volumes
	LV ejection fraction
	dP/dt
Pulmonary Vasculature	Pulmonary systolic pressure
	Right ventricular size and systolic function
Other Findings	Left atrial size

EXAMPLE

A 52-year-old man with a dilated cardiomyopathy presents with worsening heart failure symptoms. Echocardiography shows a dilated left ventricle with an ejection fraction of 32% and a central jet of mitral regurgitation with:

Vena Contracta Width	8 mm
CW Doppler	MR signal as dense as antegrade flow with no evidence for a V wave
	dP/dt = 840 mm Hg/s
	Maximum MR velocity = 4.6 m/s
	VTI_{MR} = 150 cm
PISA Radius	1.2 cm
	Aliasing velocity = 30 cm/s
Right Superior Pulmonary Vein	Systolic flow reversal

The vena contracta width indicates severe mitral regurgitation.

CW Doppler signal density indicates moderate to severe MR, and the absence of a V wave suggests a chronic disease process. The dP/dt is less than 1000 mm Hg/s, consistent with decreased LV contractility.

Color flow indicates a central jet, so the PISA method can be used to quantitate regurgitant severity.

The *PISA* is calculated from the radius measurement as:

$$PISA = 2\pi r^2 = 2\pi(1.0 \text{ cm})^2 = 6.3 \text{ cm}^2$$

The maximum *instantaneous regurgitant volume (RV_{inst})* is calculated from PISA and the aliasing velocity ($V_{aliasing}$) as:

$$RV_{inst} = PISA \times V_{aliasing} = 6.3 \text{ cm}^2 \times 30 \text{ cm/s} = 189 \text{ cm}^3/s$$

Maximum ROA (instantaneous) then is calculated from the RV and MR jet velocity (where 4.6 m/s = 460 cm/s):

$$ROA_{max} = RV_{max} /V_{MR} = (189 \text{ cm}^3/s)/460 \text{ cm/s} = 0.41 \text{ cm}^2$$

This ROA is consistent with severe mitral regurgitation.

RV over the systolic flow period can be estimated as:

$$RV = ROA \times VTI_{MR} = 0.41 \text{ cm}^2 \times 150 \text{ cm} = 62 \text{ cm}^3 \text{ or ml}$$

This regurgitant volume also is consistent with severe mitral regurgitation.

If the jet is eccentric, quantitation should be performed using trans-aortic (forward) stroke volume and transmitral (total) stroke volume calculations, as illustrated for aortic regurgitation.

AR, *Aortic regurgitation;* CW, *continuous wave;* LV, *left ventricular;* LVOT, *left ventricular outflow tract;* MR, *mitral regurgitation;* PISA, *proximal isovelocity surface area;* RF, *regurgitant fraction;* ROA, *regurgitant orifice area;* RV, *regurgitant volume;* VTI, *velocity time integral.*

Step-by-Step Approach

Step 1: Determine the Etiology of Regurgitation

■ MR may be primary (caused by abnormalities of the valve leaflets and chordae) or functional (secondary to LV dilation or dysfunction with normal leaflets).

■ Primary causes of mitral leaflet and chordal dysfunction include myxomatous mitral valve disease (mitral valve prolapse), rheumatic disease, mitral annular calcification, and endocarditis (Fig. 12–15).

■ LV dilation results in functional MR because of annular dilation and malalignment of the papillary muscles, resulting in tethering or "tenting" of the valve leaflets in systole.

■ Ischemic MR may be due to papillary muscle dysfunction, regional dysfunction of the inferior-lateral wall, or diffuse LV dysfunction and dilation. MR may be intermittent if reversible ischemia results in inadequate leaflet closure.

Key points:

❑ Mitral valve anatomy is evaluated in multiple TTE views, including long axis, short axis, and four-chamber image planes. If better definition of valve anatomy is needed for clinical decision making, TEE imaging may be helpful (Fig. 12–16).

❑ Imaging of the mitral valve allows identification of myxomatous valve disease, rheumatic disease (commissural fusion), vegetations, and calcific changes.

❑ With myxomatous mitral valve disease, the degree of thickening, redundancy, and prolapse of each leaflet is described.

❑ The tip of a flail leaflet segment points toward the roof of the left atrium in systole; a severely prolapsing segment is curved so that the tip points toward the LV apex (Fig. 12–17).

❑ Restricted leaflet motion is characteristic of functional MR. The area defined by the tented leaflets and the annular plane at end-

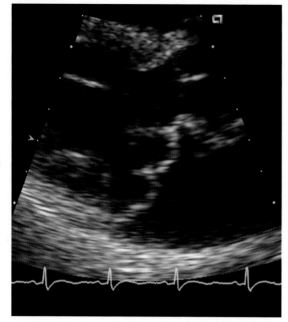
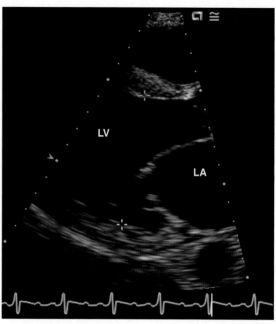

Figure 12–15 An example of primary mitral regurgitation caused by myxomatous mitral valve disease (A) with prolapse of both mitral leaflets on this end-systolic frame. An example of functional mitral regurgitation (B) caused by leaflet tethering in a patient with a dilated cardiomyopathy.

systole provides an index of the severity of restricted motion (Fig. 12–18).

Step 2: Determine the Severity of Regurgitation

- Regurgitant severity is evaluated using a step-wise approach with integration of several types of data.
- In addition to Doppler measures of regurgitant severity, the cause of regurgitation, LV size and systolic function, and LA size and pulmonary pressures are important parameters in clinical decision making.

Step 2A: Measurement of vena contracta width is the initial step in evaluation of MR (Fig. 12–19).

Key points:

- ❏ With MR, vena contracta usually is best measured in the parasternal long axis view on TTE or the long axis view at about 120 degrees rotation on TEE.
- ❏ Vena contracta is measured as the smallest width of the jet, taking care with eccentric jets to prevent an oblique diameter measurement. Both the proximal acceleration region and the distal jet expansion should be visualized to ensure the narrowest segment of the jet is measured.
- ❏ A vena contracta width of smaller than 0.3 cm indicates mild regurgitation; a vena con-

tracta width of 0.7 cm or greater indicates severe regurgitation.
- ❏ Further evaluation is needed when vena contracta is between 0.3 and 0.7 cm, when images of the vena contracta are suboptimal, or when further quantitation is needed for clinical decision making.

Step 2B: Evaluation of jet direction determines the next step in evaluation of mitral regurgitant severity.

- Central jets typically are seen with functional MR caused by LV dilation.
- Ischemic MR often results in an eccentric posteriorly directed jet.
- Mitral valve prolapse often results in an eccentric regurgitant jet with the jet directed away from the affected leaflet (Fig. 12–20).

Key points:

- ❏ With holosystolic regurgitation and a central jet, the PISA approach to quantitation of severity is appropriate; use of the PISA approach with late systolic MR or an eccentric jet is problematic.
- ❏ With an eccentric jet or late systolic MR, pulsed Doppler measurement of RV and ROA is appropriate.
- ❏ The duration of MR in systole can be visualized on frame-by-frame review of the cardiac cycle or can be inferred from the CW Doppler MR jet signal.

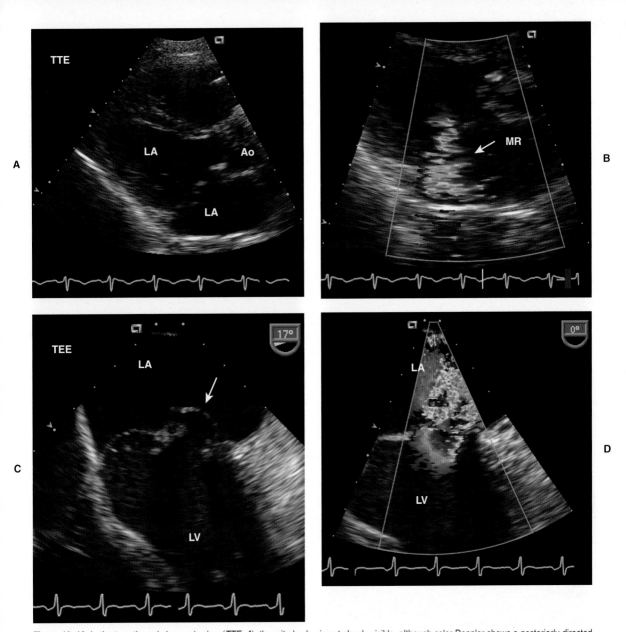

Figure 12–16 In the transthoracic long axis view (*TTE, A*), the mitral valve is not clearly visible, although color Doppler shows a posteriorly directed mitral regurgitant (*MR, B*) jet. Transesophageal images (*TEE, C*) show severe prolapse of the posterior mitral leaflet (*arrow*) with severe mitral regurgitation and a wide vena contracta (*D*). The mitral leaflet curves into the left atrium (*LA*), but the tip of the leaflet points toward the left ventricular apex, so these findings are consistent with severe prolapse, but not a flail segment, in this view.

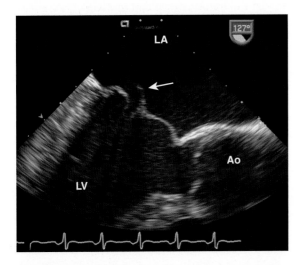

Figure 12–17 This transesophageal echocardiography view of the mitral valve in a long axis view shows the posterior mitral leaflet closure on the atrial side of the valve in systole. The tip of the central scallop of the posterior leaflet (*arrow*), seen in this view, points toward the roof of the left atrium (*LA*), consistent with a flail leaflet segment.

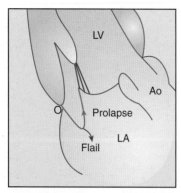

Figure 12–18 The term "prolapse" of the mitral leaflet indicates that the chordal connections of the leaflet to the papillary muscle are intact, so, regardless of the severity of prolapse, the tip of the leaflet still points toward the left ventricular apex. With chordal rupture, the mitral leaflet segment becomes "flail," and the tip of the flail segment points toward the roof of the left atrium.

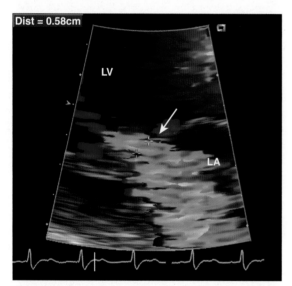

Figure 12–19 Vena contracta width for mitral regurgitation is best measured in a parasternal long axis view using zoom mode to maximize the size of the image of the proximal jet geometry. The vena contracta is the narrow neck between the proximal acceleration on the ventricular side of the valve and jet expansion in the left atrium.

Step 2C: When clinically indicated, RV and ROA are calculated.

Key points:

- With late systolic MR or eccentric jets, total SV is calculated across the mitral valve (SV_{MR}), and then forward SV (calculated across the LV outflow tract [SV_{LVOT}] or pulmonic valve) is subtracted to obtain RV (Fig. 12–21):

$$RV_{MR} = SV_{MR} - SV_{LVOT}$$

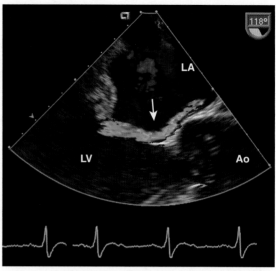

Figure 12–20 In the same patient as Figure 12–17, color Doppler in the transesophageal echocardiography long axis view shows an eccentric anteriorly directed mitral regurgitant jet. With myxomatous mitral valve disease, the direction of the jet typically is opposite the affected leaflet. This anteriorly directed jet confirms that regurgitation is primarily due to involvement of the posterior valve leaflet.

- The 2D biplane total LV SV (SV_{2D}) can be used instead of transmitral flow to calculate regurgitant volume:

$$RV_{MR} = SV_{2D} - SV_{LVOT}$$

- ROA is calculated by dividing RV by the velocity time integral (VTI_{MR}) of the CW Doppler MR velocity curve during systole:

$$ROA = RV/VTI_{MR}$$

- The PISA approach provides instantaneous flow rate, which is divided by the peak MR velocity (V_{MR}) to estimate ROA:

$$ROA = (PISA \times V_{aliasing})/V_{MR}$$

- The RV can be estimated using the PISA method by multiplying the ROA by the VTI of the mitral regurgitant jet (RJ):

$$RV = ROA \times VTI_{RJ}$$

- The PISA images are optimized using an aliasing velocity of 20 to 40 cm/s. The radius (r) of the PISA is the distance between the edge of the color corresponding to the aliasing velocity and the closed leaflets in systole (Fig. 12–22).
- Recording images for PISA measurement with and without color facilitates correct identification of the valve orifice plane.
- A quick estimate of ROA can be obtained by setting the aliasing velocity at close to 40 cm/s and assuming an MR maximum velocity of 5 m/s; then $ROA \approx r^2/2$.

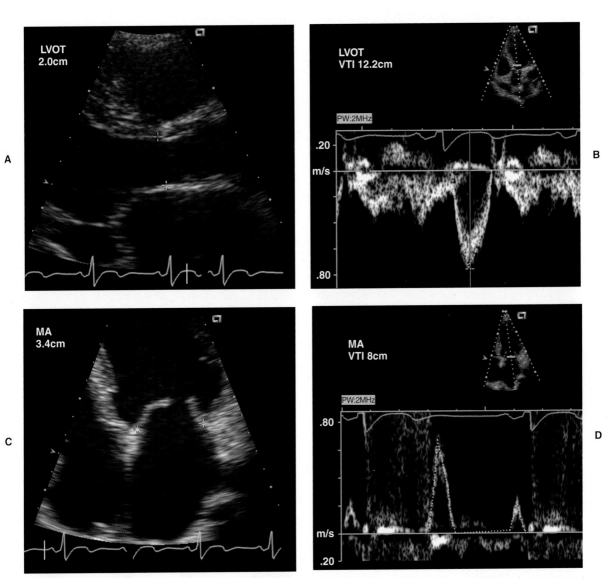

Figure 12–21 Calculation of regurgitant volume in a patient with mitral regurgitation (secondary to a dilated cardiomyopathy) is based on measurement of mitral annular (*MA*) and LV outflow tract (*LVOT*) diameters (D, *A* and *C*) and velocity time integrals (VTI, *B* and *D*). Total (transmitral) stroke volume (TSV) is mitral annular cross-sectional area (CSA = πr^2 = 3.14[3.4/2]^2 = 9.1 cm^2) multiplied by the velocity time integral (TSV = 9.1 cm^2 × 8 cm = 73 ml). Transaortic (forward) stroke volume (FSV) is $\pi(2.0/2)^2$ × 12.2 cm = 38 ml. Then regurgitant stroke volume (RSV) is TSV − FSV, or 73 ml − 38 ml = 35 ml. Regurgitant fraction is 35 ml/73 ml × 100% = 48%. These findings suggest moderate regurgitation.

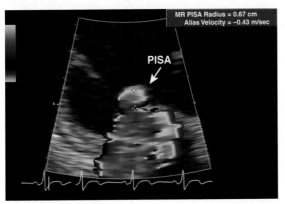

Figure 12–22 The proximal isovelocity surface area (*PISA*) is best visualized from the apical window in a long axis (as in this example) or four-chamber view. Zoom mode is used to maximize the image size of the PISA, with a velocity scale without variance and with the baseline moved so that the aliasing velocity is about 40 cm/s. In this example, the instantaneous flow rate is calculated as the surface area of the PISA ($2\pi r^2$ = 2 × 3.14 × (0.67)^2 = 2.8 cm^2 times the aliasing velocity of 43 cm/s, which equals 121 cm^3/s. If the mitral regurgitant maximum velocity is 5 m/s (500 cm/s), then regurgitant orifice area (ROA) is 121 cm^3/s / 500 cm/s = 0.24 cm^2.

Step 2D: Additional simple measures of regurgitant severity include pulmonary vein systolic flow reversal and the density of the CW Doppler signal.

- Reversal or blunting of the normal pattern of pulmonary venous inflow into the left atrium in systole is seen in most patients with severe MR (Fig. 12–23).
- The density of the CW Doppler MR curve, compared with the density of antegrade flow, indicates relative MR severity (Fig. 12–24).

Key points:

- ❐ The specific location of systolic flow reversal depends on jet direction, so TEE imaging may be needed to evaluate all four pulmonary veins; the absence of systolic flow reversal on TTE does not exclude severe regurgitation.
- ❐ Systolic flow reversal may be present even when regurgitation is not severe in patients with atrial arrhythmias or other factors that affect normal atrial filling patterns.
- ❐ The CW Doppler MR jet usually is best recorded from an apical approach on TTE or a four-chamber view on TEE, because these windows allow parallel alignment between the ultrasound beam and regurgitant jet.
- ❐ In cases with an eccentric, posteriorly directed regurgitant jet, the best intercept angle may be obtained from the parasternal window, or occasionally from a suprasternal approach.

Step 3: Evaluate Antegrade Mitral Flow and Stenosis

- Patients with rheumatic MR often have some degree of mitral stenosis.

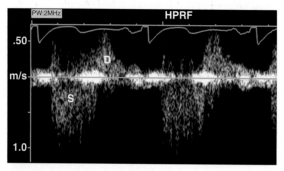

Figure 12–23 Pulmonary vein flow recorded on transthoracic echocardiography from the apical four-chamber view in the right superior pulmonary vein. Signal strength often is suboptimal, as in this example; even so, the flow into the left atrium in diastole (*D*) can be distinguished from the systolic (*S*) flow reversal due to severe mitral regurgitation.

- All patients with severe MR have an elevated antegrade mitral velocity because of the increased antegrade volume flow rate across the mitral valve in diastole.
- Mitral stenosis is distinguished from a high volume flow rate by the mitral pressure half time.

Step 4: Evaluate the Consequences of Chronic Ventricular Volume Overload

- The left ventricle dilates in response to the chronic load imposed by MR. However, the extent of LV dilation is much less than is seen with aortic regurgitation, because aortic regurgitation results in pressure and volume overload, whereas MR predominantly imposes a volume overload.
- Some patients develop irreversible LV dysfunction in the absence of symptoms, so the most important parameters to measure on echocardiography in patients with chronic severe MR are LV size and ejection fraction.

Key points:

- ❐ LV end-diastole and end-systolic dimensions and volumes should be measured and compared side-by-side with previous examinations. Even a slight increase in systolic size is clinically significant because the threshold for intervention is an end-systolic dimension of only 40 mm.

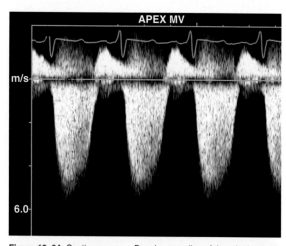

Figure 12–24 Continuous wave Doppler recording of the mitral regurgitant velocity is evaluated for (1) the velocity and deceleration curve of the antegrade flow in diastole, (2) the relative density of the retrograde flow compared with antegrade flow, and (3) the shape and timing of the regurgitant velocity curve. In this example, the antegrade flow is normal velocity (less than 1 m/s), with a steep deceleration curve indicating the absence of mitral stenosis. The regurgitant signal is almost as dense as antegrade flow and is holosystolic, consistent with severe regurgitation. In addition, the fall-off in velocity in late systole suggests that left atrial pressure is elevated in late systole, consistent with a V wave and acute regurgitation.

- Indexing dimensions and volumes to body surface area is especially important in women and smaller patients.
- With severe MR, LV volumes are increased in direct proportion to the regurgitant volume; the SV calculated using the biplane apical approach is the total SV (forward SV plus regurgitant SV).
- The ejection fraction measurement is accurate in patients with MR. However, even a small decline in ejection fraction (<60%) has important clinical implications, so precise measurement is essential.
- Measurement of LV dP/dt (rate of rise in pressure) from the MR jet is useful (see Chapter 6).

Step 5: Evaluate Other Consequences of Mitral Regurgitation

- LA enlargement is assessed as described in Chapter 2.
- Pulmonary systolic pressures are estimated as described in Chapter 6.
- Right ventricular (RV) size and systolic function are evaluated as described in Chapter 6.

PULMONIC REGURGITATION

Step-by-Step Approach

Step 1: Determine the Etiology of Regurgitation

- A small amount of pulmonic regurgitation is seen in most individuals (Fig. 12–25).
- Pathologic regurgitation most often is due to congenital heart disease, such as a repaired tetralogy of Fallot.

Key points:
- Imaging the pulmonic valve is difficult in adult patients.
- Thickened deformed leaflets may be seen with congenital pulmonic valve disease (Fig. 12–26).

Step 2: Evaluate the Severity of Pulmonic Regurgitation

- Vena contracta width is helpful for evaluation of pulmonic regurgitation.
- The density and shape of the CW Doppler waveform are diagnostic (Fig. 12–27).
- Further quantitation of pulmonic regurgitation is rarely performed using echocardiography.

Key points:
- Pulmonic regurgitation is low velocity (if pulmonary diastolic pressure is normal), so the color Doppler display may show uniform laminar flow in diastole in the RV outflow tract (Fig. 12–28).
- The CW Doppler curve is especially helpful for detection of severe pulmonic regurgitation, showing a dense signal with a steep deceleration slope that reaches the baseline at end-diastole (Fig. 12–29).

Step 3: Evaluate the Consequences of Right Ventricular Volume Overload

- Severe pulmonic regurgitation results in RV dilation and eventual systolic dysfunction.

Key points:
- Evaluation of RV size and systolic function by echocardiography is largely based on qualitative evaluation of 2D images using a scale of normal, mild, moderate, and severely abnormal.
- Sequential studies are helpful in distinguishing residual RV dilation or dysfunction after repair of tetralogy of Fallot from progressive postoperative changes.
- Cardiac magnetic resonance imaging allows quantitation of RV volumes and ejection fraction.

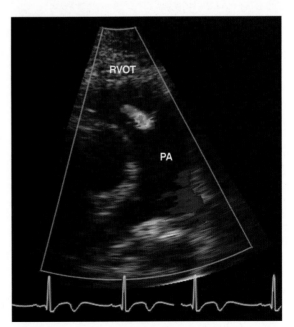

Figure 12–25 Color Doppler image of pulmonic regurgitation in a parasternal short axis view in diastole. The vena contracta is narrow, reflecting mild regurgitation. *RVOT,* Right ventricular outflow tract; *PA,* pulmonary artery.

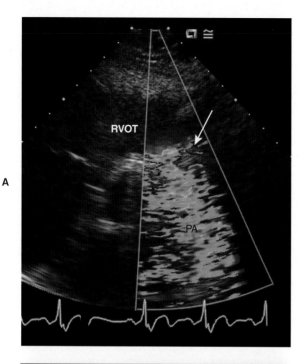

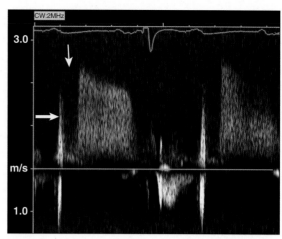

Figure 12–27 Continuous wave Doppler recording of pulmonic regurgitation. The signal is much less dense than antegrade flow, consistent with mild regurgitation. A prominent pulmonic closing click (*arrow*) is followed by an area of signal drop-out, probably caused by initial competence of the valve in early diastole, followed by the typical low velocity diastolic curve of pulmonic regurgitation. The velocity time course reflects the pulmonary artery–to–right ventricular pressure difference in diastole. Low velocity flow is consistent with a small pressure gradient, and thus normal pulmonary diastolic pressures.

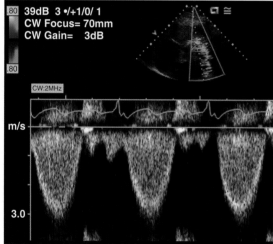

Figure 12–26 This patient with congenital pulmonic stenosis has thickened valve leaflets with a systolic increase in velocity at the leaflet level (*A*). Continuous wave Doppler shows moderate stenosis with a jet velocity of 3.2 m/s, but little regurgitation is detected (*B*). *RVOT*, Right ventricular outflow tract.

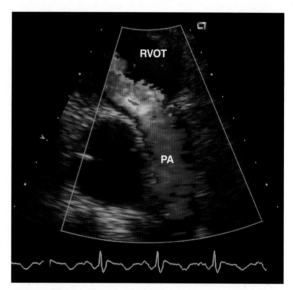

Figure 12–28 Color Doppler evaluation of the pulmonic valve in a parasternal short axis view shows laminar flow filling the right ventricular outflow tract (*RVOT*) in diastole, consistent with severe pulmonic regurgitation. Because flow velocities are low, there is little variance, so regurgitation may be missed on cine images but is evidenced on a frame-by-frame review. *PA,* Pulmonary artery.

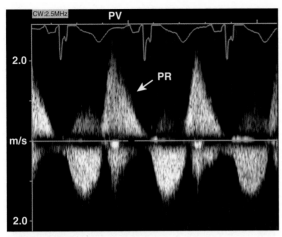

Figure 12–29 Continuous wave Doppler recording of pulmonary flow in a patient with severe pulmonic regurgitation (*PR*). The density of retrograde flow across the valve (above the baseline) is equal to the density of antegrade flow in systole. In addition, the end-diastolic velocity of the pulmonic regurgitation approaches zero, indicating equalization of diastolic pressures in the pulmonary artery and right ventricle.

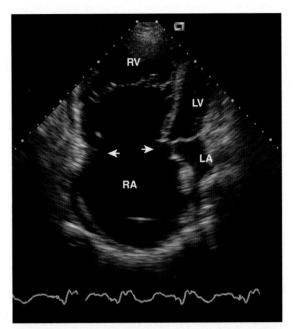

Figure 12–30 Apical four-chamber view in a patient with Epstein's anomaly of the tricuspid valve. The tricuspid valve leaflets are apically displaced, so the portion of the right ventricle (*RV*) between the leaflets and the tricuspid annulus (*arrow*) has a right atrial pressure. Severe tricuspid regurgitation results in severe right atrial and right ventricular enlargement. This patient has an intact atrial septum.

TRICUSPID REGURGITATION

Step-by-Step Approach

Step 1: Evaluate the Etiology of Tricuspid Regurgitation

- Tricuspid regurgitation may be due to primary valve disease or may be secondary to annular dilation.
- Primary causes of tricuspid regurgitation include endocarditis, Ebstein's anomaly, rheumatic disease, carcinoid, and myxomatous disease.
- Secondary tricuspid regurgitation is seen with pulmonary hypertension of any cause, including pulmonary hypertension due to mitral valve disease, pulmonary parenchymal disease, and primary pulmonary hypertension.

Key points:

- ❏ Tricuspid valve vegetations are diagnosed on TTE or TEE.
- ❏ With Ebstein's anomaly, there is apical displacement (insertion of tricuspid leaflet more than 10 mm apical from mitral valve leaflets) of one or more valve leaflets (Fig. 12–30).
- ❏ Carcinoid results in short, thick, and immobile valve leaflets.
- ❏ Rheumatic tricuspid disease occurs in 20% to 30% of patients with rheumatic mitral disease.

- ❏ The diagnosis of secondary tricuspid regurgitation is based on the presence of pulmonary hypertension and the absence of structural abnormalities of the leaflets.

Step 2: Evaluate the Severity of Tricuspid Regurgitation

- Vena contracta width is the key step in evaluation of tricuspid regurgitant severity.
- Density of the CW Doppler velocity curve, relative to antegrade flow, is also helpful.
- Systolic flow reversal in the hepatic veins is seen with severe tricuspid regurgitation.

Key points:

- ❏ A vena contracta of larger than 0.7 cm is specific for severe tricuspid regurgitation (Fig. 12–31).
- ❏ Vena contracta width is best measured in the parasternal short axis or RV inflow view.
- ❏ A dense CW Doppler signal is seen with severe tricuspid regurgitation, but velocity reflects the RV to right atrial (RA) systolic pressure gradient, not regurgitant severity (Fig. 12–32).
- ❏ Evaluation of hepatic vein flow patterns is problematic unless sinus rhythm is present.

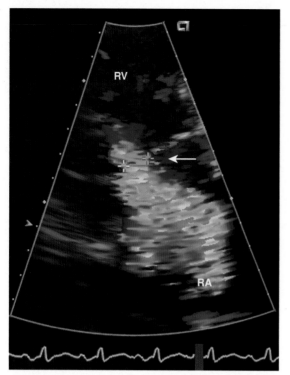

Figure 12–31 The vena contracta in the tricuspid regurgitant jet is visualized in the right ventricular inflow view from the parasternal window using the zoom mode to maximize resolution of the proximal jet geometry. The vena contract width of 4 mm is consistent with moderate regurgitation. Evaluation of the vena contracta is more accurate than visualization of the size of the flow disturbance in the right atrium for quantitation of tricuspid regurgitation.

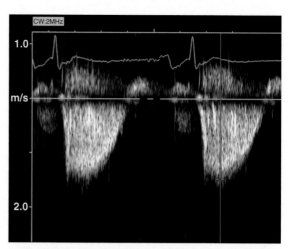

Figure 12–32 This continuous wave Doppler recording shows severe tricuspid regurgitation with a dense systolic signal. The velocity is low because pulmonary pressures are normal and right atrial pressure is elevated because of severe tricuspid regurgitation.

Step 3: Evaluate the Consequences of Right Ventricular Volume Overload

- Severe chronic tricuspid regurgitation is associated with RV enlargement.
- RV systolic function may be normal or may be reduced with chronic tricuspid regurgitation.
- RV size and systolic function are evaluated qualitatively, as described in Chapter 6.
- RA size is increased with chronic tricuspid regurgitation.

NOTES

SELF-ASSESSMENT QUESTIONS

QUESTION 1

A 26-year-old man is referred for evaluation of a cardiac murmur. The number of aortic valve leaflets was difficult to visualize, but the valve may be bicuspid. The antegrade velocity across the valve is normal, and LV size and systolic function are normal. Color Doppler of the valve in a parasternal long axis view is shown in Figure 12–33.

The most appropriate comment in the echo report regarding the findings in this image is:

    A. Normal finding.
    B. Doppler artifact.
    C. Calculation of ROA is needed.
    D. Periodic echocardiography is indicated.
    E. Urgent TEE is needed.

QUESTION 2

A 28-year-old pregnant woman is referred for echocardiography to evaluate a murmur. The anatomy and Doppler flows for all four cardiac valves are normal. The flow in the proximal abdominal aorta is shown in Figure 12–34.

These findings are most consistent with:

    A. Normal physiologic changes of pregnancy
    B. Severe aortic regurgitation
    C. Aortic dissection
    D. Patent ductus arteriosus
    E. Peripartum cardiomyopathy

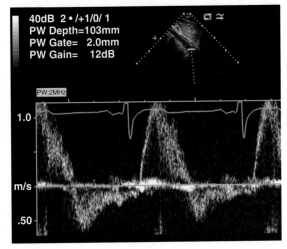

Figure 12–34

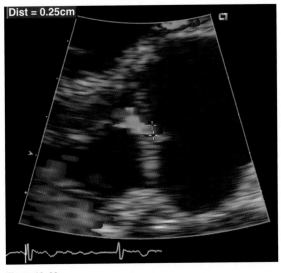

Figure 12–33

QUESTION 3

A 32-year-old asymptomatic man referred for evaluation of a murmur has a bicuspid aortic valve. Aortic regurgitation is present with a vena contracta width of 6 mm. The CW Doppler regurgitant velocity curve is shown in Figure 12–35.

The pressure half time of the aortic regurgitant jet is: _____msec.

This is consistent with (mild/moderate/severe) aortic regurgitation.

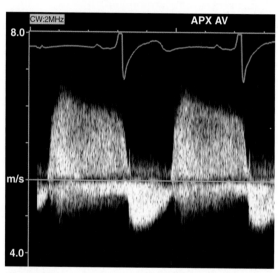

Figure 12–35

QUESTION 4

In the 32-year-old man in Question 3, the following measurements are made:

LV outflow tract diameter: 2.8 cm   VTI: 24 cm
Mitral annulus diameter: 3.2 cm   VTI: 12 cm
CW Doppler: aortic regurgitant   VTI: 220 cm
LV end-diastolic volume (EDV): 214 ml
LV end-systolic volume (ESV): 80 ml
Body surface area: 2.1 m²
Heart rate: 72 beats per minute (bpm)

Calculate:
Ejection fraction: _____
Total stroke volume: _____
Forward stroke volume: _____
Regurgitant stroke volume: _____
Regurgitant fraction: _____
Regurgitant orifice area:_____
   Overall regurgitant severity is:

A. Mild
B. Moderate
C. Severe

QUESTION 5

A 28-year-old man with a bicuspid aortic valve returns for annual evaluation. He is asymptomatic and runs daily for 45 minutes with no change in his exercise tolerance over the past year. Last year his echocardiogram showed aortic regurgitation with a vena contracta of 9 mm and holodiastolic flow reversal in the proximal abdominal aorta. At that time his LV dimensions were 68 at end-diastole and 52 at end-systole with an ejection fraction of 62%. Six months ago his LV end-diastolic dimension had increased to 74 mm with an end-systolic dimension of 54 mm. Now his LV dimensions are 78 at end-diastole and 56 at end-systole with an ejection fraction of 56%. What other information would be most helpful for clinical decision making at this point?

A. Regurgitant orifice area
B. LV dP/dt calculated from the mitral regurgitant jet
C. LV myocardial strain rate analysis
D. Anatomy and size of the ascending aorta
E. Doppler exercise stress test

QUESTION 6

A 54-year-old man with myxomatous valve disease has an eccentric, anteriorly directed late systolic mitral regurgitant jet. The vena contracta width is 5 mm, LA anterior-posterior dimension is 44 mm, LV end-diastolic dimension is 56 mm with an end-systolic dimension of 38 mm, and the biplane apical ejection fraction is 68%. The 2D LV stroke volume is 120 ml.

The most appropriate measurement at this point is:

A. Radius of the proximal isovelocity surface area
B. Indexed end-systolic LV volume
C. LV dP/dt from the mitral regurgitant jet
D. Pulmonary vein peak systolic velocity
E. LV outflow tract stroke volume

QUESTION 7

In a 58-year-old man with an eccentric mitral regurgitant jet, the following data are obtained:

LV outflow tract diameter: 2.4 cm   VTI: 18 cm
Mitral annulus diameter: 3.6 cm   VTI: 12 cm
CW Doppler: mitral regurgitant   VTI: 118 cm
LV end-diastolic volume (EDV): 175 ml
LV end-systolic volume (ESV): 55 ml
Body surface area: 2.3 m^2
Heart rate: 84 bpm

Calculate:

Ejection fraction: _____
Total stroke volume: _____
Forward stroke volume: _____
Regurgitant stroke volume: _____
Regurgitant fraction: _____
Regurgitant orifice area:_____
   Overall regurgitant severity is:

   A. Mild
   B. Moderate
   C. Severe

QUESTION 8

A 56-year-old man with a dilated cardiomyopathy has central mitral regurgitation caused by leaflet tenting. The vena contracta width is 6 mm, and the CW Doppler signal is moderately intense with a slow rate of velocity increase in early systole and a steep falloff in velocity in late systole.

Based on the data shown in Figure 12–36, calculate:

Proximal isovelocity surface area: _____
Instantaneous mitral regurgitant flow rate: _____
_____
Regurgitant orifice area: _____
Regurgitant volume: _____

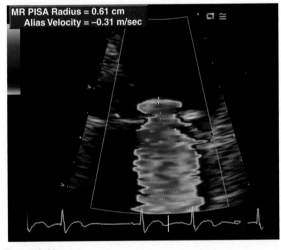

A

MR PISA Radius = 0.61 cm
Alias Velocity = –0.31 m/sec

Figure 12–36

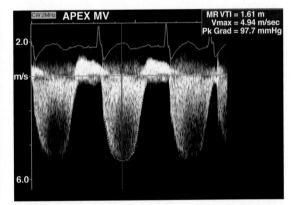

B

APEX MV
CW:2MHz
2.0
m/s
6.0
MR VTI = 1.61 m
Vmax = 4.94 m/sec
Pk Grad = 97.7 mmHg

QUESTION 9

Identify the most likely cause of mitral regurgitation for the three patients shown in Figure 12–37 (*3A* and *3B* are from the same patient). Each answer may be used once, more than once, or not at all.

A. Myxomatous mitral valve disease
B. Rheumatic valve disease
C. Dilated cardiomyopathy
D. Ischemic mitral regurgitation
E. Endocarditis

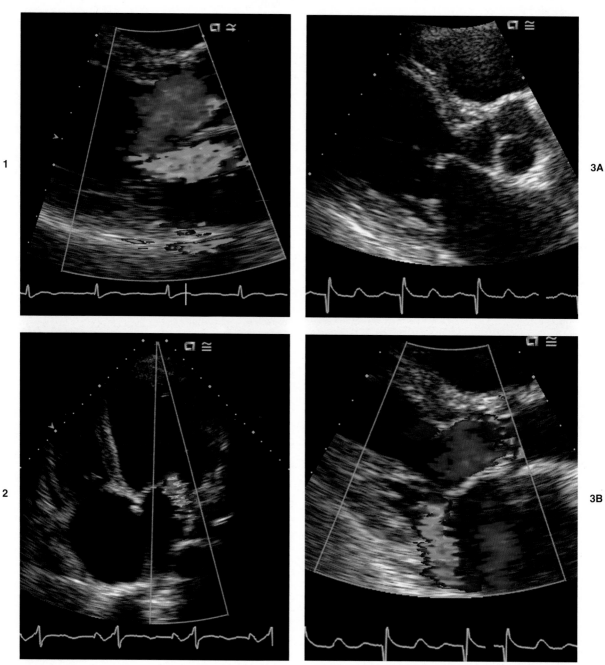

Figure 12–37

QUESTION 10

A 64-year-old woman with myxomatous valve disease has bileaflet prolapse with a vena contracta of 5 mm, a regurgitant volume of 42 ml, a regurgitant fraction of 40%, and a regurgitant orifice area of 0.3 cm^2. She complains of exertional dyspnea. Exercise testing is performed, and she achieves 112% of her maximum predicted heart rate with a better than expected exercise duration for her age and gender. At rest her tricuspid regurgitant jet velocity is 2.4 m/s, increasing to 3.1 m/s immediately post-exercise.

These findings are consistent with:

A. Normal exercise response for age
B. Increased severity of mitral regurgitation with exercise
C. Increased severity of tricuspid regurgitation with exercise
D. Primary pulmonary disease
E. Nonparallel intercept angle post-exercise

QUESTION 11

The velocity curve in Figure 12–38 demonstrates a late diastolic dip in velocity that most likely is due to:

A. Severe pulmonic regurgitation
B. RA contraction
C. RV contraction
D. Pulmonary hypertension
E. Pulmonic stenosis

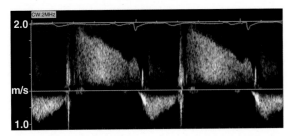

Figure 12–38

QUESTION 12

In a patient with a repaired tetralogy of Fallot, the right ventricle is enlarged but has normal systolic function. The velocity curve shown in Figure 12–39 is obtained.

This finding is most consistent with:

A. Residual ventricular septal defect
B. Severe pulmonary hypertension
C. Severe pulmonary stenosis
D. Severe pulmonary regurgitation
E. Severe tricuspid regurgitation

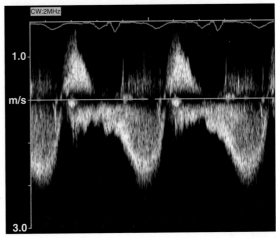

Figure 12–39

QUESTION 13

A 38-year-old woman is referred for evaluation of dyspnea. The Doppler curve shown in Figure 12–40 is recorded.

This finding is most consistent with *severe*:

A. Tricuspid regurgitation
B. Tricuspid stenosis
C. Pulmonary hypertension
D. Pulmonary regurgitation

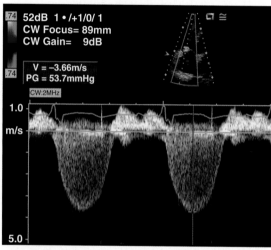

Figure 12–40

QUESTION 14

A 48-year-old woman with severe rheumatic mitral stenosis is referred for echocardiography prior to percutaneous mitral valvuloplasty. Evaluation of the tricuspid valve shows severe tricuspid regurgitation. Which of the following features would be most helpful in distinguishing tricuspid regurgitation secondary to pulmonary hypertension versus rheumatic involvement of the tricuspid valve in this patient?

A. Vena contracta width
B. Density of the CW Doppler velocity curve
C. Distance of the tricuspid annulus from the mitral annulus
D. Diastolic flattening of the ventricular septum
E. 2D evaluation of the tricuspid valve chordae

NOTES

ANSWERS

ANSWER 1: D

The flow signal is consistent with aortic regurgitation with no findings to suggest a Doppler artifact. Aortic regurgitation also was documented with CW Doppler. This color flow image shows a vena contracta of 2 mm, indicating mild regurgitation, so further quantitation is not necessary. However, the presence of aortic regurgitation, particularly with an anatomically abnormal valve, is definitely pathologic. Periodic evaluation is indicated, but with mild regurgitation and a normal left ventricle, an appropriate examination interval is 1 to 3 years. Transesophageal echocardiography would provide better images of valve anatomy but is unlikely to change patient management at this point.

ANSWER 2: D

There is holodiastolic flow reversal in the proximal abdominal aorta, a finding that usually is associated with severe aortic regurgitation. When diastolic flow reversal is present in the absence of aortic regurgitation (as shown by direct evaluation of the valve flows), other causes for diastolic "run-off" in the aorta should be considered, most commonly a patent ductus arteriosus with diastolic flow from the higher pressure aorta (diastolic pressure about 60 mm Hg) into the lower pressure pulmonary artery (diastolic pressure less than 20 mm Hg). Aortic dissection would result in a linear flap in the aortic lumen with differential flow in the true and false lumens, but not diastolic flow reversal. The physiologic changes of pregnancy include an increased cardiac output resulting from placental flow; this increases antegrade systolic velocities and does not affect diastolic flow in the aorta. Peripartum cardiomyopathy results in a low forward cardiac output but does not affect diastolic flow in the aorta.

ANSWER 3

The pressure half time is 360 msec. To determine the pressure half time, place a line along the diastolic slope of the CW Doppler spectral tracing. Then measure the horizontal distance (time in milliseconds) between the peak velocity in early diastole and the point on the line equal to the peak velocity divided by 1.4. This time interval is the pressure half time. A pressure half time of 360 msec is consistent with moderate regurgitation. The density of the aortic regurgitant signal relative to the density of the antegrade signal also is consistent with moderate regurgitation. The CW Doppler data is integrated with other echo findings (vena contracta width, descending aortic flow reversal, valve anatomy, LV size and function) in the final assessment of regurgitant severity. Further evaluation with measurement of regurgitant stroke volume, fraction, and orifice area may be helpful in some patients with moderate regurgitation.

ANSWER 4

Ejection fraction is:

$$EF = (EDV - ESV)/EDV \times 100\% = (214 - 80)/214 \times 100\% = 63\%$$

Total stroke volume is equivalent to LV stroke volume for both aortic and mitral regurgitation. For aortic regurgitation, total stroke volume also can be calculated in the LV outflow tract as:

$$SV_{total} = CSA_{LVOT} \times VTI_{LVOT} = \pi(2.8\ cm/2)^2 \times 24\ cm = 148\ cm^3 = 148\ ml$$

Forward stroke volume is equal to transpulmonary or transmitral flow. So, in this case,

$$SV_{forward} = CSA_{MA} \times VTI_{MA} = \pi(3.2\ cm/2)^2 \times 12\ cm = 96\ cm^3 = 96\ ml$$

$$Regurgitant\ volume = SV_{total} - SV_{forward} = 148\ ml - 96\ ml = 52\ ml$$

$$Regurgitant\ fraction = RV/TSV \times 100\% = 52\ ml/148\ ml = 35\%$$

$$Regurgitant\ orifice\ area = RV/VTI_{AR} = 52\ cm^3/220\ cm = 0.24\ cm^2$$

These numbers are consistent with moderate aortic regurgitation.

As a final step, the results should be examined for internal consistency. The 2D total stroke volume of 134 ml should be equal to the LV outflow tract stroke volume of 148 ml; however, this difference is within the limits of clinical measurement error. In addition, the overall estimate of regurgitant severity is similar whether the Doppler or 2D stroke volume is used in the calculations. With the 2D total stroke volume, regurgitant volume is 38 ml, regurgitant fraction is 28%, and regurgitant orifice area is 0.17 cm².

Often the 2D stroke volume underestimates total stroke volume because of foreshortened apical images. However, in this example, the indexed LV volumes (102 ml/m² for EDV and 38 ml/m² for ESV) are moderately increased, consistent with LV dilation caused by aortic regurgitation. Another check of internal consistency is to look at the cardiac output. At a heart rate of 72 bpm, the forward cardiac output based on Doppler data is 6.9 L/min, or a cardiac index of 3.3 L/min/m^2, which is normal for an asymptomatic ambulatory patient.

ANSWER 5: D

The presence of a bicuspid aortic valve is associated with aortic root dilation in some patients. This patient meets definite criteria for aortic valve replacement because he has severe aortic regurgitation by several criteria and his LV end-systolic dimension is larger than 55 mm. Surgical planning includes deciding whether he should have aortic valve replacement alone or the ascending aorta should be replaced as well.

Measurement of regurgitant orifice area is not necessary because the simpler measures of vena contracta width and aortic flow reversal are diagnostic of severe aortic regurgitation. LV dP/dt might be helpful in patients with valve disease to evaluate for evidence of decreased contractility, but this patient needs surgery anyway. LV myocardial strain rate analysis has not been shown to be helpful in evaluation of patients with valve disease. An exercise stress test is not needed because surgery is indicated even in an asymptomatic patient with this degree of LV dilation.

ANSWER 6: E

The vena contracta is between 3 and 7 mm, indicating that further evaluation of mitral regurgitant severity is needed for clinical decision making in this patient with anatomic mitral valve disease. Measurement of the LV outflow tract stroke volume (forward stroke volume) will allow calculation of regurgitant volume and fraction, in conjunction with the 2D LV total stroke volume. The jet is eccentric and only occurs in late systole, so using the proximal isovelocity surface area approach to quantitate regurgitant severity is not appropriate. Indexing LV end-systolic volume to body size is helpful when the degree of LV dilation is a concern, but LV dimensions are normal in this patient. If quantitative measures indicate that regurgitation is severe, LV dP/dt might help in evaluation of ventricular contractility, particularly when ejection fraction is borderline. The presence of blunted or reversed systolic flow in the pulmonary veins is a helpful qualitative measure of regurgitant severity but would not separate moderate from severe regurgitation in this patient, because flow reversal often is not seen in all four pulmonary veins and therefore requires TEE for complete evaluation.

ANSWER 7

Ejection fraction is:

$$EF = (EDV - ESV)/EDV \times 100\% = (175 - 55)/175 \times 100\% = 69\%$$

Total stroke volume also can be calculated across the mitral annulus as:

$$SV_{total} = CSA_{MA} \times VTI_{MA} = \pi(3.6 \text{ cm}/2)^2 \times 12 \text{ cm} = 122 \text{ cm}^3 = 122 \text{ ml}$$

With mitral regurgitation, forward stroke volume is calculated in the LV outflow tract as:

$$SV_{forward} = CSA_{LVOT} \times VTI_{LVOT} = \pi(2.4 \text{ cm}/2)^2 \times 18 \text{ cm} = 81 \text{ cm}^3 = 81 \text{ ml}$$

$$\text{Regurgitant volume} = SV_{total} - SV_{forward} = 122 \text{ ml} - 81 \text{ ml} = 41 \text{ ml}$$

$$\text{Regurgitant fraction} = RV/TSV \times 100\% = 41 \text{ ml}/122 \text{ ml} = 34\%$$

$$\text{Regurgitant orifice area} = RV/VTI_{MR} = 41 \text{ cm}^3/118 \text{ cm} = 0.34 \text{ cm}^2$$

These numbers are consistent with moderate mitral regurgitation.

As a final step, the results should be examined for internal consistency. Total stroke volume is equivalent to 2D LV stroke volume and this case shows a total stroke volume of 122 ml by Doppler versus 120 ml by 2D measurement. Notice that LV volumes with chronic mitral regurgitation are smaller than with chronic aortic regurgitation. The mechanism for this difference is that mitral regurgitation is ejected into the low pressure left atrium, so that the primary effect on the ventricle is an increase in volume flow. In contrast, aortic regurgitation requires ejection into the high pressure aorta, which imposes both a pressure and volume overload on the ventricle. It also is helpful to consider the indexed ventricular volumes in patients with chronic regurgitation. This patient has a mildly increased end-diastolic volume index (76 ml/m^2) and a normal end-systolic volume index (24 ml/m^2), as would be expected with only moderate mitral regurgitation. His resting cardiac output (based on the forward stroke volume) is 81 ml times 84 bpm, or 6.8 L/m with a cardiac index (divide by body surface area) of 3.0 L/min.

ANSWER 8

The PISA is calculated from the radius of the hemisphere defined by the aliasing velocity–the distance from the aliasing boundary to the mitral orifice–as the surface area of a hemisphere: $2\pi r^2$, so the PISA is $2 \times 3.14 \times (0.6 \text{ cm})^2 = 2.34 \text{ cm}$.

This surface area is multiplied by the aliasing velocity (31 cm/s) to obtain the instantaneous regurgitant flow rate:

$$\text{Instantaneous flow rate} = (PISA \times V_{aliasing}) = 2.34 \text{ cm} \times 31 \text{ cm/s} = 72 \text{ cm}^3/s$$

ROA is calculated by dividing the instantaneous regurgitant flow rate by the maximum mitral regurgitant velocity (4.9 m/s or 490 cm/s), so:

$$ROA = RV/V_{MR} = 72 \text{ cm}^3/s \ / \ 490 \text{ cm/s} = 0.15 \text{ cm}^2$$

This calculation assumes that the maximum flow rate and maximum velocity occur at the same point in time. Then, if the orifice area is constant throughout systole, RV is:

$$RV = ROA \times VTI_{RJ} = 0.15 \text{ cm}^2 \times 161 \text{ cm} = 24 \text{ ml}$$

This regurgitant orifice area and regurgitant volume are consistent with mild mitral regurgitation. The simplified method for calculation of ROA also can be used in this case. The aliasing velocity is close to 40 cm/s, and the maximum mitral regurgitant jet is close to 5 m/s, so:

$$ROA \ r^2/2 = 0.6^2/2 = 0.18 \text{ cm}^2$$

ANSWER 9

The first patient has myxomatous mitral valve disease (Answer A) in a parasternal long axis view. Although the prolapsing posterior leaflet is a bit difficult to see on this image, the anteriorly directed jet is most consistent with posterior leaflet prolapse.

The second patient has a dilated cardiomyopathy (Answer C), with the four-chamber view showing enlargement of all four chambers (note scale). A central or laterally directed jet is typical with dilated cardiomyopathy and leaflet tethering, as illustrated here. This is difficult to distinguish from ischemic mitral regurgitation on a single image, but there are no obvious areas of infarction in this view, and the cine images showed global hypokinesis.

The third patient has rheumatic mitral valve disease (Answer B). The end-systolic color Doppler image shows a thickened anterior leaflet, but the appearance and jet direction are not diagnostic. However, the diastolic image clearly demonstrates diastolic doming of the mitral leaflets due to commissural fusion, which is pathognomonic for rheumatic valve disease.

ANSWER 10: A

Assuming an RA pressure of 5 mm Hg, the tricuspid regurgitant jet velocity indicates that pulmonary systolic pressure rose from 28 mm Hg at rest (mildly elevated) to 43 mm Hg with exercise. This is a normal rise in pulmonary pressures with exercise. Similarly, the normal rise is systemic blood pressure with exercise; there also is a normal increase in pulmonary pressures. In young normal individuals, systolic pulmonary pressure rises from about 18 mm Hg at rest to 28 mm Hg at peak exercise, with a gradual increase in the rise in pressures with aging, so an increase from about 25 to 45 mm Hg is typical at age 60 years.

If mitral regurgitant severity increased with exercise, there would be a greater (excessive) rise in pulmonary pressures because of the elevation of LA pressure. An increase in tricuspid regurgitation severity would increase the density of the CW Doppler curve but would not affect the maximum velocity. Primary pulmonary disease may be associated with an excessive rise in pulmonary pressures with exercise, but the patient has only mild pulmonary hypertension at rest (most likely secondary to her mitral valve disease) and a normal exercise response. A nonparallel intercept angle post-exercise would result in underestimation of jet velocity (and pulmonary pressures). If the tricuspid jet velocity was recorded from the same window on the baseline and post-exercise studies, a change in intercept angle is unlikely.

ANSWER 11: B

This pulmonic regurgitant velocity curve shows a dip in the diastolic deceleration slope that occurs after the P wave on the ECG. With atrial contraction, the slight rise in RV diastolic pressure results in a slight decrease in the pulmonary artery–to–RV pressure difference, hence a slight decrease in the pulmonic regurgitant velocity. Thus this diastolic dip is referred to as the A wave and corresponds to the A wave seen on an M-mode tracing of pulmonic valve motion.

Severe pulmonic regurgitation shows a dense velocity curve (compared with antegrade flow) with an end-diastolic velocity close to zero. RV contraction in systole does not affect the diastolic pulmonic regurgitant velocity. Pulmonary hypertension is associated with a higher velocity in late diastole corresponding to the diastolic pressure difference from the pulmonary artery to the right ventricle. Assuming an RV diastolic pressure of 5 mm Hg, the late diastolic pulmonic regurgitant velocity of less than 1 m/s suggests a pulmonary diastolic pressure of less than 10 mm Hg. With pulmonic stenosis, the antegrade velocity in systole is elevated. In addition, the A wave is more prominent, because with RV hypertrophy and diastolic dysfunction, RA contraction results in excessive elevation of RV diastolic pressure.

ANSWER 12: D

The CW Doppler recording of flow of RV outflow shows normal velocity of antegrade flow in the pulmonary artery with an equally dense diastolic velocity signal consistent with severe pulmonary regurgitation. A residual ventricular septal defect would be associated with a less dense high velocity flow signal from the high pressure left ventricle to lower pressure RV in systole. Severe pulmonary hypertension would be associated with a high velocity tricuspid regurgitant signal and a higher velocity in the pulmonary regurgitant signal, reflecting the pressure gradient between the pulmonary artery and right ventricle in diastole. Severe pulmonic stenosis would result in a high velocity antegrade signal in the pulmonary artery in systole reflecting the pressure gradient across the valve. Severe tricuspid regurgitation would be associated with a dense signal for retrograde flow across the tricuspid valve in systole.

ANSWER 13: C

The Doppler tracing shows a high velocity systolic flow curve and a low velocity diastolic flow curve consistent with flow across the tricuspid valve. The antegrade flow in diastole is much denser than the retrograde flow in systole, indicating only mild tricuspid regurgitation. The nor-mal velocity with steep deceleration slope of antegrade flow in diastole shows that there is no tricuspid stenosis. The velocity in the regurgitant jet of 3.7 (3.66) m/s indicates an RV-to-RA systolic pressure difference of 55 mm Hg, so estimated RV systolic pressure is at least 60 mm Hg (assuming a normal RA pressure). In the absence of pulmonic stenosis, RV and pulmonary systolic pressure are equal, so this Doppler tracing is most consistent with severe pulmonary hypertension. If severe pulmonic regurgitation were present, the Doppler curve across the pulmonic valve would show a dense diastolic flow signal.

ANSWER 14: E

Pulmonary systolic pressure usually is elevated when rheumatic mitral stenosis is present. Tricuspid regurgitation often is secondary to pulmonary hypertension with RV and annular dilation and is likely to improve with the decline in pulmonary pressures after relief of mitral valve obstruction. In contrast, some patients have tricuspid regurgitation caused by rheumatic involvement of the tricuspid leaflets; in these patients regurgitation is likely to persist after intervention for mitral stenosis. The best way to identify rheumatic involvement of the tricuspid valve is evidence of chordal fusion and thickening or leaflet thickening and shortening on 2D images of the valve. Both vena contracta width and the density of the CW Doppler curve are useful for evaluation of regurgitation severity, but not for determining the cause of regurgitation. There is an increased distance of the tricuspid annulus from the mitral annulus with Ebstein's anomaly but not with rheumatic disease. The pattern of ventricular septal motion reflects the degree of right-sided volume and pressure overload but does not distinguish the cause of disease.

NOTES

13 Prosthetic Valves

THE ECHO EXAM

BASIC PRINCIPLES

STEP-BY-STEP APPROACH
Review the Clinical and Operative Data
Obtain Images of the Prosthetic Valve
Record Prosthetic Valve Doppler Data
Evaluate for Prosthetic Valve Stenosis
Evaluate for Prosthetic Valve Regurgitation
Evaluate Left Ventricular Geometry
and Function
Measure Pulmonary Pressures and Evaluate
Right Heart Function

SPECIFIC VALVE TYPES
Bioprosthetic Aortic Valves
Valved Conduits or Valve Resuspension
Mechanical Aortic Valves
Mitral Valve Repair
Bioprosthetic Mitral Valves
Mechanical Mitral Valves
Tricuspid Valve Prostheses and Rings
Pulmonic Valve Replacements

SELF-ASSESSMENT QUESTIONS

THE ECHO EXAM: PROSTHETIC VALVES

TRANSTHORACIC EXAMINATION

IMAGING
Valve leaflet thickness and motion
Left ventricle size, wall thickness, and systolic function

DOPPLER
Antegrade prosthetic valve velocity
Evaluate for stenosis
Search carefully for regurgitation
Pulmonary artery pressures

TRANSTHORACIC DOPPLER EVALUATION OF PROSTHETIC VALVES

COMPONENTS	MODALITY	VIEW	RECORDING	MEASUREMENTS
Antegrade flow velocity	Pulsed or CW Doppler	Apical	Antegrade transmitral or transaortic velocity	Peak velocity (compare with normal values for valve type and size)
Measures of valve stenosis	Pulsed and CW Doppler	Apical	Careful positioning to obtain highest velocity signal	Mean gradient Aortic valves: ratio of LVOT to aortic velocity Mitral valve: pressure half time
Valve regurgitation	Color imaging and CW Doppler	Parasternal, apical, and SSN	Jet origin, direction, and size on color CW Doppler of each valve Pulmonary vein flow Descending aorta flow	Vena contracta width Intensity of CW Doppler signal Pulmonary vein systolic flow reversal (MR) Descending aorta flow reversal (AR)
Pulmonary pressures	CW Doppler	RV inflow and apical	TR-jet velocity IVC size and variation	Calculate PAP as $4v^2$ of TR jet plus estimated right atrial pressure

AR, *Aortic regurgitation;* CW, *continuous wave;* IVC, *inferior vena cava;* LVOT, *left ventricular outflow tract;* MR, *mitral regurgitation;* PAP, *pulmonary artery pressure;* RV, *right ventricular;* SSN, *suprasternal notch;* TR, *tricuspid regurgitation.*

TRANSESOPHAGEAL EXAMINATION

IMAGING
Valve leaflet thickness and motion
Examine atrial side of mitral prostheses
Left ventricle size, wall thickness, and systolic function

DOPPLER
Antegrade prosthetic valve velocity
Evaluate for stenosis
Search carefully for regurgitation
Pulmonary artery pressures

TRANSESOPHAGEAL EVALUATION OF PROSTHETIC VALVES

COMPONENTS	MODALITY	VIEW	RECORDING	LIMITATIONS
Valve Imaging	2D echo	High esophageal	Mitral valve in high esophageal four-chamber view Aortic valve in high esophageal long and short axis views	Aortic valve prosthesis may shadow anterior segments of the aortic valve. With both aortic and mitral prostheses, the aortic shadow may obscure the mitral prosthesis.
Antegrade flow velocity	Pulsed or CW Doppler	High esophageal or transgastric apical	Antegrade transmitral or trans-aortic velocity	Alignment of Doppler beam with trans-aortic valve flow may be problematic; compare with TTE data.
Measures of valve stenosis	Pulsed and CW Doppler	High esophageal or transgastric apical	Careful positioning to obtain highest velocity signal	Mean gradient Aortic valves: ratio of LVOT to aortic velocity (alignment may be suboptimal) Mitral valve: pressure half time
Valve regurgitation	Color imaging and CW Doppler	High esophageal with rotational scan	Document origin of jet and proximal flow acceleration, and jet size and direction	Measure vena contracta, record pulmonary venous flow pattern, search carefully for eccentric jets.
Pulmonary pressures	CW Doppler 2D echo	RV inflow and apical Subcostal	TR-jet velocity IVC size and variation	Calculate PAP as $4v^2$ of TR jet plus estimated right atrial pressure. May be difficult to align Doppler beam parallel to TR jet; correlate with TTE data.

2D, *Two-dimensional;* CW, *continuous wave;* IVC, *inferior vena cava;* LVOT, *left ventricular outflow tract;* PAP, *pulmonary artery pressure;* RV, *right ventricular;* TR, *tricuspid regurgitation;* TTE, *transthoracic echocardiography.*

ECHOCARDIOGRAPHIC SIGNS OF PROSTHETIC VALVE DYSFUNCTION

Increased antegrade velocity across the valve
Decreased valve area (continuity equation or $T_{1/2}$)
Increased regurgitation on color flow
Increased intensity of continuous wave Doppler regurgitant signal
Progressive chamber dilation
Persistent left ventricular hypertrophy
Recurrent pulmonary hypertension

EXAMPLE
A 62-year-old man who had a mechanical mitral valve replacement 2 years ago for myxomatous mitral valve disease presents with increasing heart failure symptoms and a systolic murmur. He is in chronic atrial fibrillation.

Transthoracic echocardiography shows:

LA anterior-posterior dimension	5.7 cm
LV dimensions (systole/diastole)	6.2/3.8 cm
Ejection fraction	56%
Transmitral E velocity	1.8 m/s
Mitral pressure half time	100 msec
TR jet velocity	3.2 m/s
IVC size and variation	Normal

Color flow imaging shows ghosting and reverberations in the left atrial region, but no definite regurgitant jet can be identified. Continuous wave Doppler shows a mitral regurgitant signal that is incomplete in duration and not as dense as antegrade flow.

This transthoracic study is difficult to interpret without a previous study for comparison. The left atrial and left ventricular dilation and the borderline ejection fraction may be residual from before the valve surgery or could represent progressive changes after valve replacement.

Pulmonary artery pressure (PAP) is moderately elevated at:

$$PAP = 4(V_{TR})^2 + RAP = 4(3.2)^2 + 10 = 41 + 10 = 51 \text{ mm Hg}$$

Again, pulmonary hypertension may be residual or recurrent after valve surgery but the presence of pulmonary hypertension suggests the possibility of significant prosthetic mitral regurgitation. Although a clear regurgitant jet is not demonstrated because of shadowing and reverberations from the valve prosthesis, the high antegrade flow velocity with a short pressure half time and detection of regurgitation with continuous wave Doppler indicate that further evaluation is needed.

Transesophageal echocardiography demonstrates a paravalvular mitral regurgitant jet with a proximal acceleration region seen at the lateral aspect of the annulus, a vena contracta width of 7 mm, and an eccentric jet directed along the posterior-lateral left atrial wall. The left pulmonary veins show definite systolic flow reversal; the right pulmonary veins show blunting of the normal systolic flow pattern. These findings are consistent with severe para-prosthetic regurgitation.

On transesophageal imaging, the left ventricle was not well visualized because of shadowing and reverberations from the mitral prosthesis; although transgastric short axis views were obtained, ejection fraction could not be calculated. The maximum TR jet obtained on transesophageal echocardiography was 2.9 m/s. Because a higher jet was obtained on transthoracic imaging, the TEE jet most likely underestimates pulmonary pressures.

In summary, this patient has severe para-prosthetic mitral regurgitation with left atrial and left ventricular dilation, moderate pulmonary hypertension, and a borderline ejection fraction. As is typical with prosthetic valves, the combination of transthoracic and transesophageal echocardiography was needed for diagnosis.

IVC, *Inferior vena cava;* LA, *left atrial;* LV, *left ventricular;* RAP, *right atrial pressure;* TEE, *transesophageal echocardiography;* TR, *tricuspid regurgitation.*

BASIC PRINCIPLES

- Evaluation of prosthetic valves by echocardiography is based on the same principles as evaluation of native valve disease.
- Fluid dynamics (and Doppler flows) depend on the specific valve type and size (Fig. 13–1).
- Dysfunction of mechanical valves usually is due to valve thrombosis resulting in systemic embolism, incomplete closure (regurgitation), or inadequate opening (stenosis).
- Dysfunction of tissue valves usually is due to leaflet degeneration (regurgitation) or calcification (stenosis).
- All prosthetic valves are at risk of endocarditis, which often primarily affects the annular ring rather than the valve leaflets.

Key points:

- ❐ The most common mechanical valve now implanted is a bileaflet design with two semicircular disks that open to form a central slit-like orifice and two larger lateral openings.
- ❐ Other types of mechanical valves include a single disk valve that "tilts" to open, either on a central strut or with hinges in the annular ring. Ball-cage valves may still be seen in some patients.
- ❐ There are several types of tissue valves; they are classified as stented, stentless, and combined valve-root prostheses (including homograft valves).

- ❐ On echocardiography, mechanical valves result in ultrasound reverberations and shadowing that limit direct visualization of valve function.
- ❐ A stented tissue valve is recognized by the three valve struts; a stentless tissue valve may be indistinguishable from a normal native valve.
- ❐ Percutaneously implanted valves (in development) have three tissue leaflets mounted in an expandable cylinder. Once deployed, the echocardiographic appearance is similar to a stentless tissue valve.

STEP-BY-STEP APPROACH

Step 1: Review the Clinical and Operative Data

- Information on the operative procedure is reviewed before the echocardiographic examination.
- The valve type and size, obtained from the medical record or the patient's valve ID card, are included on the echocardiographic report.
- Blood pressure and heart rate at the time of the echocardiogram are recorded.

Key points:

- ❐ Information in the operative report helps guide the echocardiographic image acquisition and improves the final interpretation.

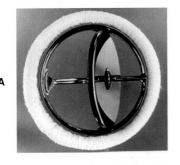
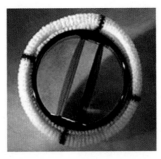
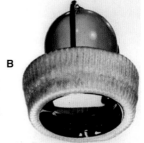
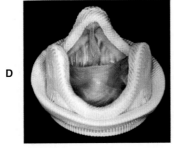
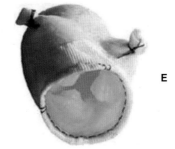

Figure 13–1 Major types of prosthetic heart valves: (A) tilting disc, (B) bileaflet, (C) ball, (D) stented bioprosthesis, and (E) stentless bioprosthesis *From: Yoganathan AP and Travis BR. In Otto CM, ed: The Practice of Clinical Echocardiography, 3rd ed, Philadelphia: Elsevier, 2007.*

- With aortic valve surgery, key features are valve replacement versus resuspension, concurrent replacement of the aortic root either above the sinotubular junction or including the sinuses of Valsalva, and surgical coronary reimplantation (with aortic root surgery).
- With mitral valve surgery, key features are valve repair or replacement, preservation of the mitral leaflets and chords with valve replacement, amputation of the left atrial (LA) appendage, and whether a concurrent atrial ablation (e.g., maze) procedure was done.
- The valve type and size determine the expected hemodynamics and are important for distinguishing normal prosthetic Doppler data from prosthetic valve stenosis or regurgitation.

- On early postoperative studies, unexpected findings are discussed directly with the surgeon to correlate with observations during the surgical procedure.

Step 2: Obtain Images of the Prosthetic Valve

- Prosthetic aortic valves are imaged in parasternal long and short axis views (Fig. 13–2).
- Prosthetic mitral valves are imaged in parasternal long and short axis and in apical four-chamber and long axis views (Fig. 13–3).
- Transesophageal echocardiography (TEE) imaging is needed to evaluate the LA side of mechanical mitral prosthetic valves, because of shadowing from the transthoracic approach, when valve dysfunction is suspected (Fig. 13–4).

A 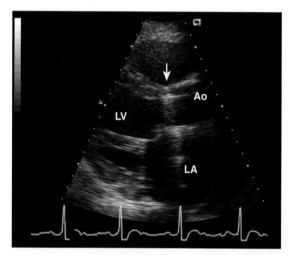 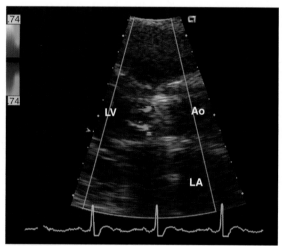 B

Figure 13–2 Parasternal long axis view of a mechanical aortic valve showing the reverberations along the ultrasound beam path (*A, arrow*) with color Doppler (*B*) showing the normal small eccentric aortic regurgitant jets with a bileaflet valve.

A 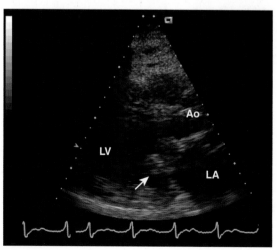 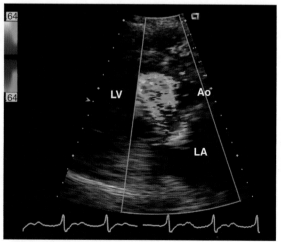 B

Figure 13–3 Parasternal long axis view (*A*) of a stented tissue mitral valve prosthesis with the typical appearance of the struts (*arrow*) protruding into the left ventricle (*LV*) and with color Doppler (*B*) showing the inflow stream directed toward the ventricular septum.

- TEE also often provides better images of the posterior aspect of aortic valve prostheses.

Key points:

◻ Transthoracic imaging of mechanical valves is limited by reverberations and shadowing. Even so, the leaflets and annular region may be adequately evaluated by this approach for most baseline or follow-up studies in clinically stable patients.

◻ Tissue valves have a trileaflet structure similar to a native aortic valve. Mitral tissue valves are stented to provide support for the leaflets, and the leaflets are easily visible in both parasternal and apical views (Fig. 13–5).

◻ With aortic tissue valves, support is provided either by stents, by attachment directly to the aortic wall (stentless valves), or by implanting an intact valve and root (sometimes called a "mini-root" approach). The aortic tissue prosthesis is highly visible in long and short axis views.

◻ When prosthetic valve dysfunction is suspected on clinical grounds or based on transthoracic echocardiography (TTE) findings, both TTE and TEE are recommended.

Step 3: Record Prosthetic Valve Doppler Data

- Antegrade velocities across the prosthetic valve are recorded with pulsed and continuous wave (CW) Doppler.
- Prosthetic valve regurgitation is evaluated using CW and color Doppler.

Key points:

◻ Both tissue and mechanical valves are inherently stenotic compared with normal native valves.

◻ The normal antegrade velocity and pressure gradient depends on the specific valve type, valve size, heart rate, and cardiac output (Table 13–1).

◻ Ideally, Doppler data are compared with the patient's own baseline postoperative examination, done when the patient has fully recovered from surgery and is clinically stable.

◻ If a baseline examination is not available, recorded data are compared with published data for that valve type and size.

◻ A small amount of regurgitation is normal with most prosthetic valves.

Step 3A: Evaluate for Prosthetic Valve Stenosis

- Maximum and mean gradients are calculated with the Bernoulli equation from transvalvular velocities (Fig. 13–6).
- Continuity equation valve area can be calculated for aortic valve prostheses (Fig. 13–7).
- The mitral pressure half time is measured for prosthetic valves in the mitral position (Fig. 13–8).

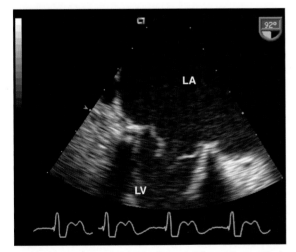

Figure 13–4 Transesophageal view of a stented tissue mitral prosthesis showing the clear visualization of the valve leaflets within the struts. With the transducer on the atrial side of the valve, the acoustic shadow and reverberations obscure the left ventricle (*LV*) but not the left atrial (*LA*) side of the valve, resulting in improved detection of prosthetic valve dysfunction.

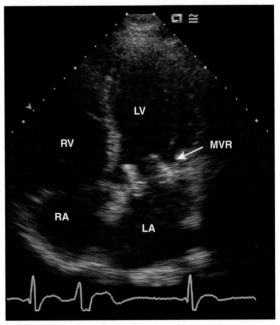

Figure 13–5 Stented tissue mitral valve replacement (*MVR*) in apical four-chamber view showing the typical orientation of the stents angled toward the ventricular septum.

TABLE 13–1

NORMAL REFERENCE VALUES OF EFFECTIVE ORIFICE AREAS FOR PROSTHETIC VALVES

	ORIFICE AREA (cm²) BY PROSTHETIC VALVE SIZE, mm					
	19	21	23	25	27	29
Stented bioprosthetic valves						
Medtronic intact	0.85	1.02	1.27	1.40	1.66	2.04
Medtronic Mosaic	1.20	1.22	1.38	1.65	1.80	2.00
Hancock II	...	1.18	1.33	1.46	1.55	1.60
Carpentier-Edwards Perimount	1.10	1.30	1.50	1.80	1.80	...
St. Jude Medical X-cell	...	...	...	...	...	...
Stentless bioprosthetic valves						
Medtronic freestyle	1.15	1.35	1.48	2.00	2.32	...
St. Jude Medical Toronto SPV	...	1.30	1.50	1.70	2.00	2.50
Mechanical valves						
St. Jude Medical Standard	1.04	1.38	1.52	2.08	2.65	3.23
St. Jude Medical Regent	1.50	2.00	5.40	2.50	3.60	4.80
MCRI On-X	1.50	1.70	2.00	2.40	3.20	3.20
Carbomedics	1.00	1.54	1.63	1.98	2.41	2.63
Björk Shiley CC	...	...	...	...	...	...

Effective orifice area is expressed in cm² as mean values available in the literature.
From Blais C, Dumesnil JG, Baillot R, et al : Circulation 108:983, 2003.

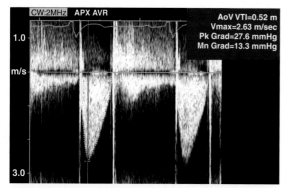

Figure 13–6 Continuous wave Doppler of antegrade flow across a bileaflet mechanical aortic valve. The antegrade velocity of 2.6 m/s is normal for a 25-mm valve size, with the typical triangular shape of the velocity curve and prominent valve opening and closing clicks. Mean gradient is calculated by tracing the curve and averaging the instantaneous gradients, as with a native aortic valve.

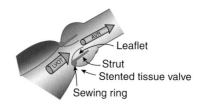

$$SV_{LVOT} = SV_{AVR}$$
$$CSA_{LVOT} \times VTI_{LVOT} = EOA \times VTI_{AVR}$$
$$EOA = (CSA_{LVOT} \times VTI_{LVOT})/VTI_{AVR}$$

Figure 13–7 Schematic drawing of the continuity equation with a stented tissue aortic valve replacement (AVR). Stroke volume (SV) proximal to the valve in the left ventricular outflow tract (LVOT) equals SV through the AVR. SV at each site is equal to the cross-sectional area (CSA) of flow times the velocity time integral (VTI) of flow at that site. LVOT flow is measured with pulsed Doppler from an apical approach; CSA$_{LVOT}$ is calculated as a circle from a mid-systolic LVOT diameter measurement; and the VTI of flow through the valve prosthesis is measured with CW Doppler, usually from the apical approach. This equation then is solved for the aortic prosthetic effective orifice area (EOA).

Key points:

❏ Left ventricular (LV) outflow tract diameter is measured from the two-dimensional (2D) images for calculation of valve area. The valve size may differ from the subaortic anatomy and thus cannot be substituted for this diameter measurement.

❏ When measurement of outflow tract diameter is difficult, the ratio of the velocity proximal to the valve and in the orifice is used as a measure of stenosis severity.

❏ With bileaflet mechanical valves, the small central orifice often results in high velocities because of local acceleration, which should not be mistaken for prosthetic valve stenosis.

❏ The mitral pressure half time is used to calculate valve area, as for native mitral stenosis. Often the pressure half time itself is reported.

❏ "Patient–prosthesis mismatch" describes a normally functioning prosthetic valve that has a valve area inadequate for the patient's body size (Fig. 13–9).

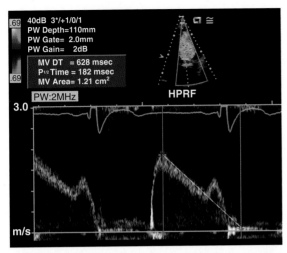

Figure 13–8 High pulse repetition frequency (HPRF) Doppler recording of antegrade flow across a tissue mitral prosthesis is consistent with mild stenosis with a pressure half time of 182 msec and estimated functional valve area of 1.2 cm².

Step 3B: Evaluate for Prosthetic Valve Regurgitation

- Prosthetic valve regurgitation is evaluated using CW and color Doppler (Fig. 13–10).
- Evaluation of prosthetic mitral regurgitation requires TEE; transthoracic imaging is nondiagnostic because of shadowing and reverberation by the valve prostheses.
- A small amount of prosthetic regurgitation is normal; moderate to severe prosthetic or any degree of paraprosthetic regurgitation is pathologic.

Key points:

- ❑ Prosthetic regurgitation often is first detected with CW Doppler because of the high signal-to-noise ratio, excellent tissue penetration, and wide beam geometry of CW Doppler (Fig. 13–11).
- ❑ Normal prosthetic regurgitation has a weak CW Doppler signal and typically is brief in duration.
- ❑ A dense or holosystolic (or diastolic) CW Doppler signal is an indication for further evaluation (Fig. 13–12).

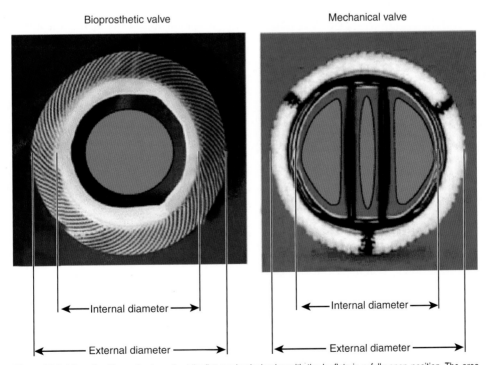

Figure 13–9 View of a bioprosthesis and a bileaflet mechanical valve with the leaflets in a fully open position. The area highlighted in purple is the effective orifice area (*EOA*). Patient–prosthesis mismatch is present when the EOA is smaller than needed to maintain a normal cardiac output at rest and with exercise without an excessive increase in transvalvular pressure gradient. *From Pibarot P, Dumesnil JG:* Heart *92(8):1022-1029, 2006.*

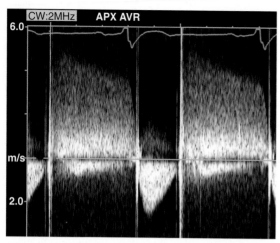

Figure 13–10 Prosthetic aortic valve regurgitation recorded with continuous wave Doppler from an apical approach shows prominent valve clicks. The diastolic aortic regurgitant signal is much less dense than the antegrade systolic signal, consistent with mild regurgitation.

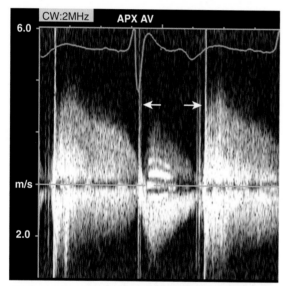

Figure 13–11 Transthoracic apical continuous wave Doppler of an aortic valve prosthesis. Prominent linear signals due to valve opening and closing are seen (*arrows*). The dense bands in systole are a common artifact, but the moderately dense signal of aortic regurgitation is consistent with at least moderate regurgitation. The signal is seen on both sides of the baseline, suggesting a nonparallel intercept angle, likely due to an eccentric jet direction.

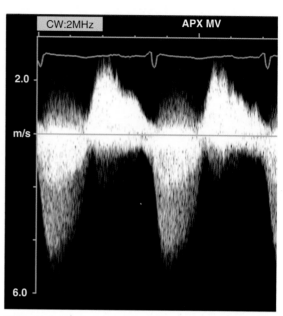

Figure 13–12 Transthoracic apical continuous wave Doppler after mitral valve repair. The antegrade flow velocity is increased to more than 2 m/s, and a systolic signal is present. The systolic signal is consistent with mitral regurgitation (not left ventricular outflow) based on the timing of flow. The density of the signal suggests that more than trivial regurgitation is present. Transesophageal echocardiography is needed for further evaluation to prevent shadowing by the annular ring.

larger vena contracta and jet area, and lasts longer during the cardiac cycle.

❏ Significant prosthetic regurgitation, especially of the mitral valve, may not be detectable on transthoracic imaging.

Step 4: Evaluate Left Ventricular Geometry and Function

■ After valve surgery, LV dilation and hypertrophy may regress, but many patients have persistent abnormalities.

■ Systolic ventricular dysfunction often improves after valve surgery, but diastolic dysfunction may be evident for many years.

■ Left ventricular geometry and systolic and diastolic function are evaluated in patients with prior heart valve surgery, as detailed in Chapters 6 and 7.

Key points:

❏ After aortic valve replacement for aortic stenosis, LV hypertrophy regresses and systolic function improves, but diastolic dysfunction may be chronic.

❏ After valve replacement for aortic or mitral regurgitation, LV dilation and systolic dysfunction improve in most patients, but a subset have irreversible LV dilation and systolic dysfunction.

❏ Normal prosthetic regurgitation on color Doppler is spatially localized adjacent to the valve, has a small vena contracta and jet area, is through the prosthesis (not paravalvular), and is brief in duration.

❏ The exact pattern of normal prosthetic regurgitation depends on the valve type (e.g., central with bioprosthetic valves, two eccentric jets with bileaflet mechanical valves).

❏ Pathologic prosthetic valve regurgitation on color Doppler often is paravalvular, has a

- ❏ In patients with isolated mitral stenosis, LV size and systolic function usually are normal both before and after valve surgery.
- ❏ Comparison of the early postoperative study with the preoperative exam helps distinguish residual ventricular abnormalities from new ventricular dysfunction.

Step 5: Measure Pulmonary Pressures and Evaluate Right Heart Function

- There is an immediate decrease in pulmonary pressures after valve surgery that is directly related to the fall in LA pressure (e.g., the passive component of pulmonary hypertension).
- The late decrease in pulmonary pressures is variable and depends on the extent of irreversible changes in the pulmonary vasculature.
- Pulmonary pressures and right heart function are evaluated in patients with prior heart valve surgery as detailed in Chapter 6.

Key points:

- ❏ Measurement of pulmonary pressures on the early postoperative study serves as the baseline for subsequent studies.
- ❏ After mitral valve surgery, recurrent pulmonary hypertension might be due to prosthetic regurgitation, which otherwise might be missed on TTE.
- ❏ Right ventricular systolic function usually improves when pulmonary pressures decline after valve surgery.

SPECIFIC VALVE TYPES

Bioprosthetic Aortic Valves

- Tissue aortic valves have three thin leaflets, similar to a native aortic valve.
- With stented tissue valves, the three stents are seen in both long and short axis views.
- The flow profile and hemodynamics are similar to a native valve, with only a small degree of central regurgitation.

Key points:

- ❏ Aortic tissue valves are well visualized in long and short axis views both on transthoracic imaging from a parasternal window and on TEE from a high esophageal window.
- ❏ Both TTE and TEE may be needed for complete evaluation when endocarditis is suspected, because each approach visualizes the part of the valve that is obscured by the ring shadow from the other approach.

- ❏ Antegrade flow across the valve is recorded from the apical window using CW Doppler. Alignment with flow is usually not optimal on a TEE study.
- ❏ Valve regurgitation is evaluated by color Doppler in the short and long axis views of the valve, with measurement of vena contracta, as described in Chapter 12 for native valves, when possible (Fig. 13–13).
- ❏ Valve regurgitation also is evaluated with CW Doppler from the apical view, with the velocity scale, gain, and filters adjusted to demonstrate the regurgitant flow signal (Fig. 13–14).

Valved Conduits or Valve Resuspension

- The native aortic valve may be sutured inside a tube graft replacement of the aortic root (called valve resuspension or the David procedure; Fig. 13–15).

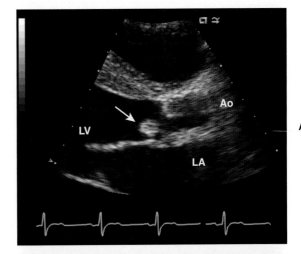

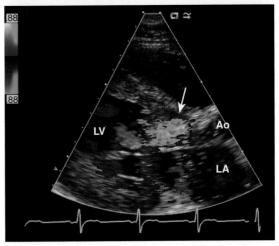

Figure 13–13 *A,* This bioprosthetic aortic valve has a flail leaflet (*arrow*), with (*B*) color Doppler showing regurgitation that fills the left ventricular (*LV*) outflow tract in diastole, consistent with severe regurgitation.

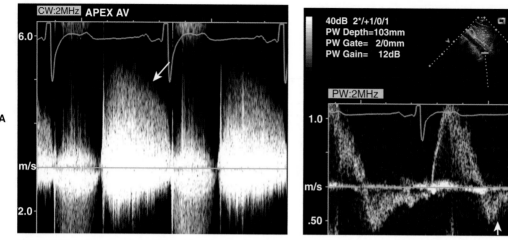

Figure 13–14 In the same patient as Figure 13–13, the continuous wave Doppler signal (A) confirms severe regurgitation with an equal signal density for antegrade systolic and retrograde diastolic aortic flow. Pulsed Doppler recording in the proximal abdominal aorta (B) shows holodiastolic flow reversal, again consistent with severe aortic regurgitation.

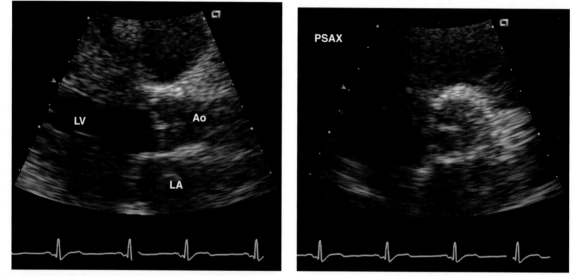

Figure 13–15 The native aortic valve has been resuspended within an aortic tube graft replacement, resulting in normal-appearing leaflets in long (A) and short (PSAX, B) axis views, with increased echogenicity of the aortic walls.

■ A combined tissue aortic valve with an attached segment of aorta (either a homograft or heterograft) may be used when endocarditis is present or there is involvement of the aorta.

■ When aortic root replacement includes the sinuses of Valsalva, the right and left coronary ostium are reimplanted into the prosthetic aorta (Fig. 13–16).

Key points:

❑ The structure and dimensions of the aorta at each level (annulus, sinuses, sinotubular junction, and mid-ascending aorta) are measured in patients with aortic valve surgery.

❑ The coronary reimplantation sites are best seen on TEE imaging (Fig. 13–17).

❑ Postoperative echocardiographic findings may include periaortic edema, hematoma, or surgical material. Review of the images with the surgical team is helpful in distinguishing expected postoperative findings from infection or bleeding (Fig. 13–18).

❑ With valve resuspension or any other subcoronary stentless valve implantation, the height and symmetry of the commissures affects valve function, so these valves are imaged using a higher frequency transducer and zoom mode.

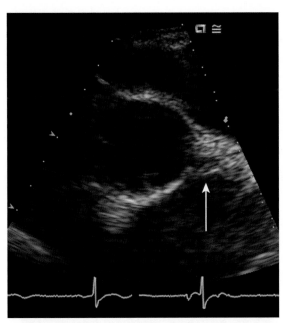

Figure 13–16 Transthoracic short axis view just superior to the aortic valve, showing the reimplanted left main coronary artery (*arrow*) in a 32-year-old man with Marfan syndrome and root replacement.

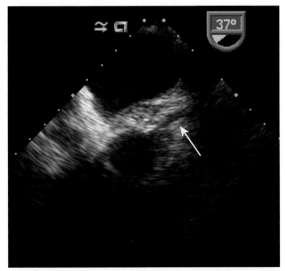

Figure 13–17 Transesophageal echocardiographic image in a short axis view of the aorta just superior to the aortic valve showing the reimplanted left main coronary (*arrow*) after valve resuspension surgery.

Mechanical Aortic Valves

■ Both stenosis and regurgitation of a mechanical valve in the aortic position can be evaluated on transthoracic imaging.

■ TEE is needed when the indication for echocardiography is bacteremia, fever, or embolic events.

■ A mechanical valve may be used in a composite aortic root and valve replacement with coro-

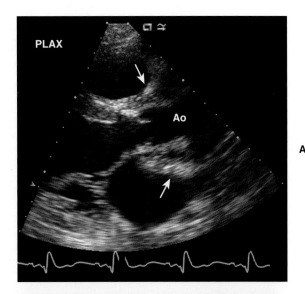

A

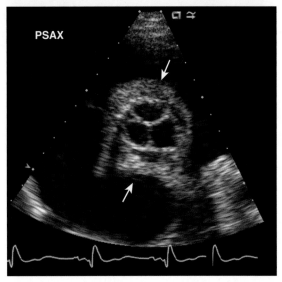

B

Figure 13–18 Replacement of the ascending aorta and resuspension of the aortic valve complicated by periaortic postoperative hematoma and tissue edema (*arrows*), seen in parasternal long axis (*PLAX, A*) and short axis views (*PSAX, B*)

nary reimplantation (the Bentall or modified Bentall procedure).

Key points:

❑ An aortic mechanical prosthesis is best imaged in long and short axis views from the parasternal transthoracic or high esophageal windows (Fig. 13–19).

❑ Infection typically involves the paravalvular region, so imaging includes evaluation of the aortic wall thickness, identification of the coronary ostium, and visualization of the paravalvular region.

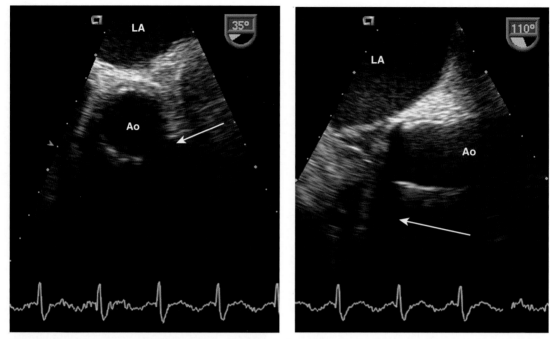

Figure 13–19 Transesophageal short axis (*A*) and long axis (*B*) images of a mechanical aortic valve. In short axis, the circular sewing ring with minor irregularity at the suture sites is seen. The posterior aspect of the sewing ring shadows the anterior aspect (*arrow*). Similarly, in the long axis view, the valve itself casts shadows and reverberations (*arrow*) that obscure the left ventricular outflow tract and anterior aspect of the valve. Evaluation of an aortic valve prosthesis typically requires both transthoracic and transesophageal imaging.

❐ Antegrade velocity is recorded using CW Doppler from the apical window. Prominent valve opening and closing clicks often are seen.

❐ A high antegrade velocity (and small calculated valve area) for a bileaflet valve in the aortic position may be due either to normal valve function (with a high velocity in the central slit-like orifice), patient–prosthesis mismatch, or valve stenosis. These conditions are differentiated based on clinical information, other echocardiographic findings, and, in some cases, other diagnostic evaluation such as fluoroscopy of valve motion (Fig. 13–20).

❐ Prosthetic aortic valve regurgitation is evaluated with color Doppler in short and long axis views of the valve (TTE or TEE) with identification of jet origin (valvular or paravalvular) and vena contracta width.

❐ Normal regurgitation of a bileaflet mechanical valve typically consists of two or more eccentric small jets that originate at the closure points of the valve occluders with the sewing ring.

❐ CW Doppler is used to evaluate prosthetic aortic regurgitation based on the density and time course of the diastolic regurgitant signal.

❐ Diastolic flow reversal in the descending aorta, as with native valve regurgitation, is

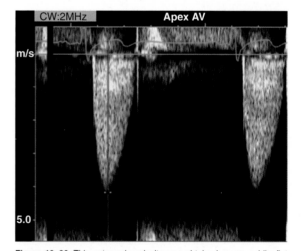

Figure 13–20 This antegrade velocity was obtained across a bileaflet mechanical aortic valve replacement in an asymptomatic 23-year-old man. Fluoroscopy immediately after the echo study showed normal leaflet occluder motion.

also useful for evaluation of prosthetic aortic regurgitation.

Mitral Valve Repair

■ The most common mitral valve repair includes resection of a segment of the posterior leaflet,

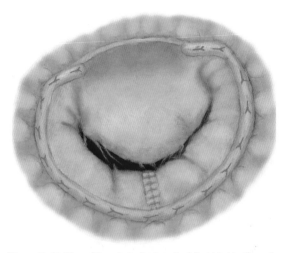

Figure 13–21 View of the mitral valve from the left atrial side after valve repair, showing the suture in the posterior leaflet at the site of resection of the prolapsed segment and the annuloplasty ring. *From Stewart WJ and Griffin BP. In Otto CM, ed:* The Practice of Clinical Echocardiography, *3rd ed, Philadelphia: Elsevier, 2007.*

with a suture line in the mid-segment of the posterior leaflet and placement of an annuloplasty ring (Fig. 13–21).

■ Other procedures used for mitral valve repair include transfer of a segment of the anterior leaflet to the posterior leaflet, use of artificial chords, suturing of the anterior and posterior leaflets together in their mid-segments (Alfieri repair), and a variety of other techniques.

■ Percutaneous approaches to mitral valve repair in development include deployment of a device in the coronary sinus to mimic an annuloplasty ring and a clip or suture to mimic an Alfieri-type repair.

Key points:

❏ Knowledge of details of the repair procedure is helpful for interpreting the echocardiographic findings.

❏ The mitral annuloplasty ring causes shadows and reverberations that may obscure mitral regurgitation from the transthoracic approach; TEE is indicated when regurgitation is suspected (Fig. 13–22).

❏ Mitral valve repair may be associated with a mild degree of functional stenosis, which is evaluated based on mean pressure gradient and pressure half time valve area, as for a native valve.

❏ With a successful repair, there is no more than trace to mild (1+) residual mitral regurgitation.

❏ Recurrent mitral regurgitation after valve repair is evaluated as for a native valve.

❏ An infrequent complication of mitral valve repair is subaortic obstruction caused by systolic anterior motion of the mitral leaflets. This complication is related to the size and rigidity of the annuloplasty ring.

Bioprosthetic Mitral Valves

■ Bioprosthetic mitral valves are stented, with the stents typically oriented slightly toward the ventricular septum.

■ Imaging and Doppler evaluation of a bioprosthetic mitral valve are similar to evaluation of a native valve.

■ Shadowing and reverberations from the sewing ring and stents decrease the accuracy of TTE for evaluation of valve dysfunction; TEE is more accurate when a prosthetic mitral valve is present (Fig. 13–23).

Key points:

❏ With a prosthetic mitral valve, inflow into the left ventricle is directed toward the ventricular septum, the opposite of the normal diastolic vortex in the left ventricle.

❏ Recording of antegrade flows and calculation of pressure gradient and valve area are no different from those for a native mitral valve.

❏ Although the apical window usually provides a parallel alignment for Doppler recordings, in some cases, the mitral inflow can be recorded from a parasternal window, depending on the orientation of the valve inflow stream.

❏ Prosthetic regurgitation is evaluated with CW and color Doppler, as for a native valve, but TEE is considered when valve dysfunction is suspected because significant regurgitation may not be detected from the transthoracic approach.

❏ A small amount of central regurgitation is normal for a bioprosthetic valve.

Mechanical Mitral Valves

■ The valve occluders are best seen from the apical transthoracic or high esophageal window, using zoom mode to focus on the mitral valve (Fig. 13–24).

■ Antegrade flow across the valve is recorded from the apical window, using pulsed or CW Doppler, depending on the maximum transvalvular velocity.

■ Evaluation for regurgitation requires TEE because the left atrium is shadowed by the prosthesis itself, both from the parasternal and apical windows.

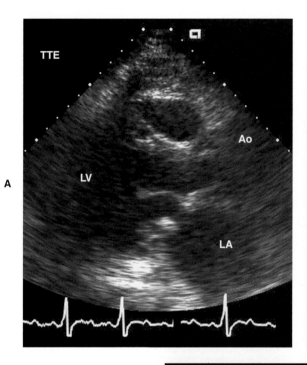

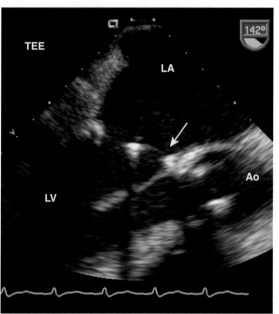

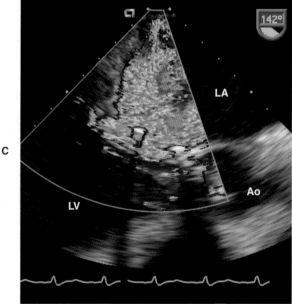

Figure 13–22 *A,* Evaluation by transthoracic imaging (*TTE*) after mitral valve repair may have limited image quality, and shadowing by the valve ring may obscure Doppler evaluation of regurgitation. *B,* Transesophageal imaging (*TEE*) offers better image quality, and the shadows from the annuloplasty ring now are projected toward the left ventricle. Note the abnormal position of the annuloplasty ring on the TEE view. *C,* Color Doppler confirmed severe mitral regurgitation, which was not evident on transthoracic imaging.

Key points:

❏ Adjustments in the rotation of the image plane from the standard views may be needed to show both leaflets, from both the transthoracic and transesophageal approach.

❏ CW Doppler is especially important for detection of mechanical mitral valve regurgitation because the broad CW beam may detect a regurgitant signal that is obscured by shadowing on color Doppler flow imaging (Fig. 13–25).

❏ Other clues that suggest mitral prosthetic regurgitation on transthoracic imaging include a high antegrade velocity across the mitral valve and recurrent (or persistent) pulmonary hypertension.

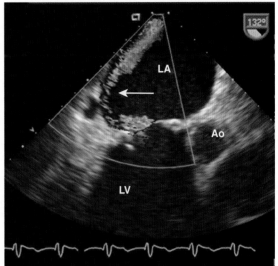

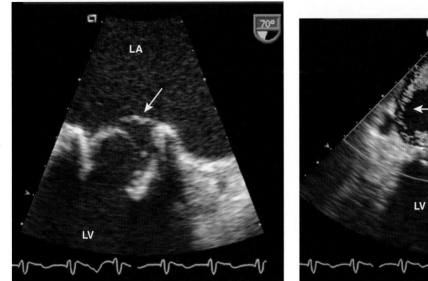

Figure 13–23 A stented bioprosthetic mitral valve with a flail leaflet (*A*) and an eccentric jet of severe mitral regurgitation by color flow Doppler (*B*), seen on transesophageal, but not transthoracic, imaging.

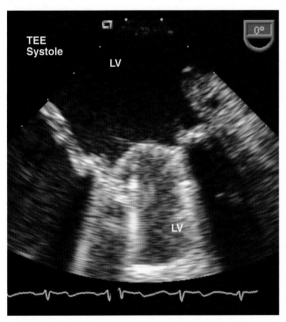

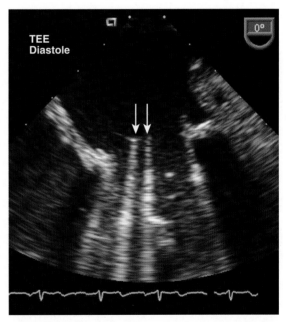

Figure 13–24 Transesophageal echocardiography (*TEE*) images of a bileaflet mechanical mitral valve in systole (*A*) and diastole (*B*), showing the two parallel (*arrows*) open occluders in diastole.

- ❏ TEE provides superior imaging of the posterior aspects of the prosthetic mitral valve and is more accurate than transthoracic imaging for diagnosis of prosthetic regurgitation.
- ❏ Clear definition of the leaflets and annular ring allows visualization of the normal regurgitant jets that originate at the closure plane of the occluders with the sewing ring.
- ❏ Paravalvular regurgitation originates outside the sewing ring, often has an identifiable

proximal isovelocity surface area (PISA) on the ventricular side of the valve, and typically has a very eccentric jet direction in the left atrium (Fig. 13–26).
- ❏ Pulmonary venous flow patterns in patients with mechanical mitral valves are affected by atrial rhythm, atrial mechanical function, and mitral valve hemodynamics, as well as by the presence of mitral regurgitation.

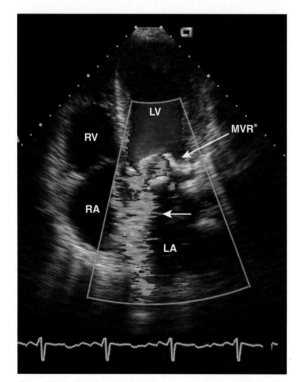

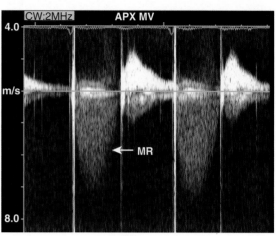

Figure 13–25 *A,* On transthoracic echocardiography (*TTE*), the mechanical mitral valve results in reverberations (*Reverb.*) and shadows obscuring the left atrium in the apical four-chamber view. *B,* However, with continuous wave Doppler, a systolic signal (*arrow*) consistent with mitral regurgitation (*MR*) is detected. *ICU,* Intensive care unit; *MVR,* mitral valve replacement.

Figure 13–26 Transthoracic apical four-chamber view in a patient with a tissue mitral prosthesis (*MVR*) and paravalvular regurgitation shows a very eccentric jet (*arrow*) that hugs the atrial septum and was missed on initial parasternal images.

□ Paravalvular regurgitation may be clinically important regardless of hemodynamic severity because it may be a sign of infection or may be a cause of hemolytic anemia.

Tricuspid Valve Prostheses and Rings

■ Tricuspid valve replacement is uncommon; either a stented bioprosthetic or mechanical valve is used (Fig. 13–27).

■ In patients undergoing mitral valve surgery, a tricuspid annuloplasty ring often is placed if severe tricuspid regurgitation is present.

■ Evaluation of a prosthetic tricuspid valve is similar to evaluation of a mitral valve replacement.

Key points:

□ Tricuspid valve prostheses often can be fully evaluated on transthoracic imaging because the valve is close to the chest wall and because the right atrium can be evaluated from the parasternal window, without shadowing by the valve prosthesis.

□ TEE imaging is helpful when transthoracic images are nondiagnostic.

□ Antegrade flows are recorded using pulsed or CW Doppler from the apical window for calculation of pressure gradients and pressure half time valve area.

□ Prosthetic tricuspid regurgitation is evaluated by standard approaches using CW and color Doppler.

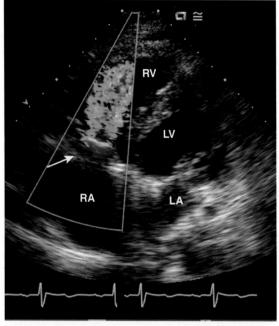

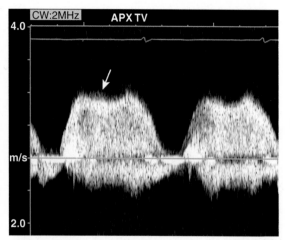

Figure 13–27 *A,* Apical view of a tissue tricuspid valve with color Doppler showing proximal acceleration (*arrow*) and a stenotic jet inflow signal. *B,* Continuous wave Doppler shows a high velocity and long pressure half time, consistent with severe prosthetic stenosis.

Pulmonic Valve Replacements

- Most pulmonic valve replacements are seen in patients with congenital heart disease.
- Pulmonic valve substitutes include homografts and bioprosthetic valves, either in a conduit or isolated. Percutaneously implanted bioprosthetic valves are in development.
- Mechanical valves are occasionally used in the pulmonic position.

Key points:

- ❑ Visualization of prosthetic pulmonic valves from either TTE or TEE approaches often is limited in adults. Alternate diagnostic procedures, such as cardiac magnetic resonance imaging or cardiac catheterization and angiography, often are needed.
- ❑ Antegrade velocity is recorded with pulsed or CW Doppler in the parasternal short axis or right ventricular outflow view (Fig. 13–28).
- ❑ Pulsed and color Doppler are used to document the level of obstruction. Many of these patients also have subvalvular or supravalvular pulmonic stenosis, and stenosis can occur at the distal anastomosis site of the conduit or in the branch pulmonary arteries.
- ❑ Severe prosthetic regurgitation is seen as to-and-fro flow on color Doppler; because the pressure difference is low, there may be little evidence of a flow disturbance.
- ❑ On CW Doppler, severe prosthetic pulmonic regurgitation is seen as a diastolic signal with

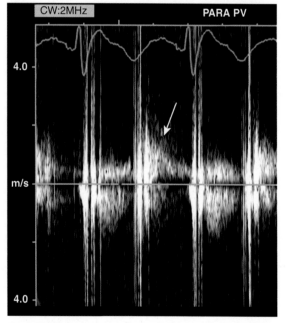

Figure 13–28 Continuous wave Doppler interrogation of a mechanical pulmonic valve replacement with the transducer in a high parasternal position. The scale has been set with a wide velocity range to examine both for stenosis and regurgitation. In this case, the antegrade velocity is only mildly increased, prominent valve clicks are present, and there is a diastolic signal (*arrow*) most consistent with tricuspid inflow (note timing relative to antegrade pulmonary flow).

a density equal to antegrade flow and a steep slope, often reaching the baseline before the end of diastole.

QUESTION 1

This transesophageal image (Fig. 13–29) shows:

A. Aortic dissection
B. Mechanical aortic valve replacement
C. Left ventricular thrombus
D. Tissue mitral prosthesis
E. Stentless tissue aortic valve

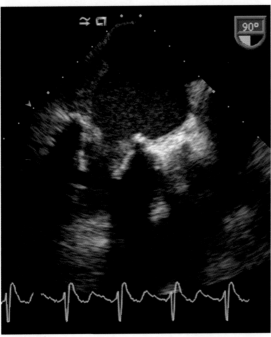

Figure 13–29

QUESTION 2

A 48-year-old woman with a mechanical mitral prosthesis returns for annual follow up. Her level of anticoagulation has been subtherapeutic intermittently, and she complains of increasing dyspnea on exertion.

The Doppler tracing shown in Figure 13–30 is obtained. Based on this data, the next best step in management is:

A. Surgical consultation
B. Cardioversion
C. Transesophageal echocardiography
D. Coronary angiography
E. Pharmacologic nuclear stress study

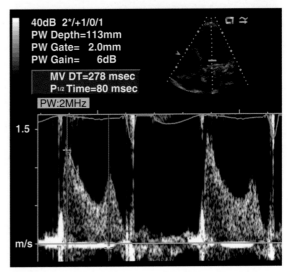

Figure 13–30

QUESTION 3

This transesophageal image (Fig. 13–31) shows:

    A. Flail aortic valve leaflet
    B. Mechanical valve prosthesis
    C. Normal aortic valve
    D. Stented tissue prosthesis
    E. Aortic root graft with valve resuspension

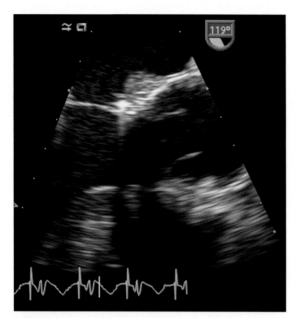

Figure 13–31

QUESTION 4

A 24-year-old man underwent surgical repair of tetralogy of Fallot as a child, with closure of the ventricular septal defect and implantation of a valved conduit from the right ventricle to pulmonary artery. This Doppler tracing (Fig. 13–32) was recorded on his routine annual evaluation. This finding is most consistent with:

    A. Severe pulmonic regurgitation
    B. Moderate pulmonary hypertension
    C. Residual ventricular septal defect
    D. Mild aortic regurgitation
    E. Moderate tricuspid regurgitation

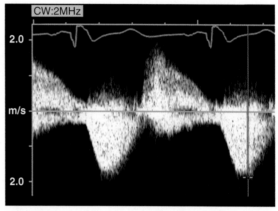

Figure 13–32

QUESTION 5

A 48-year-old woman has persistent heart failure symptoms after aortic valve replacement. On the parasternal views, color Doppler shows a flow disturbance at the anterior aspect of the valve sewing ring, adjacent to the right ventricular outflow tract and ventricular septum. The CW Doppler signal at that site was recorded to help identify the origin of the abnormal flow signal. Based on this Doppler signal (Fig. 13–33), the most likely diagnosis is:

A. Aortic rupture and pseudoaneurysm
B. Coronary blood flow
C. Aortic-to-right ventricular fistula
D. Ventricular septal defect
E. Paravalvular aortic regurgitation

QUESTION 6

A 72-year-old man with prior bileaflet mechanical aortic valve replacement presented with a new murmur and fever. This echocardiographic image (Fig. 13–34) is consistent with:

A. Ventricular septal defect
B. Normal prosthetic valve function
C. Paravalvular regurgitation
D. Coronary blood flow
E. Artifact

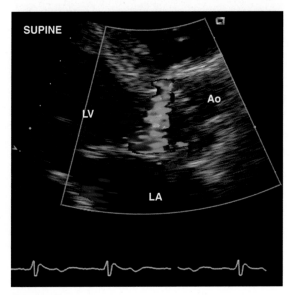

Figure 13–34

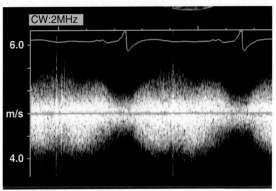

Figure 13–33

QUESTION 7

This TEE image (Fig. 13–35) in a patient with an aortic homograft valve implanted 10 years ago is consistent with:

    A. Aneurysm of the aortic mitral intervalvular fibrosa
    B. Paravalvular abscess
    C. Normal postoperative changes
    D. Aortic dissection
    E. Lipomatous hypertrophy of the interatrial septum

QUESTION 8

A patient with a 10-year-old prosthetic heart valve is referred for echocardiography. This Doppler tracing (Fig. 13–36) shows all of the following *except*:

    A. Atrial fibrillation
    B. Mitral regurgitation
    C. Mechanical valve
    D. Hypertension
    E. Aortic stenosis

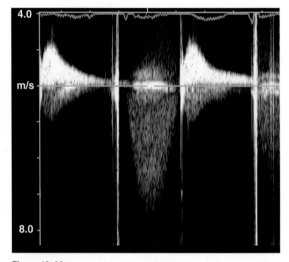

Figure 13–36

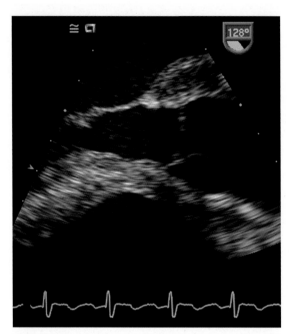

Figure 13–35

QUESTION 9

A patient is referred for echocardiography. He has a median sternotomy scar and knows he has a heart valve but is not sure which one. Based on this echocardiographic image (Fig. 13–37), which type of valve does the patient most likely have?

A. Stentless
B. Homograft
C. Stented bioprosthesis
D. Mechanical
E. Valve resuspension

QUESTION 10

A patient is seen for evaluation with a history of tricuspid valve replacement 20 years ago. What is the most likely explanation for the 2D and color Doppler patterns seen in Figure 13–38?

A. Prosthetic valve stenosis
B. Pacer lead entrapped in valve
C. Ball cage valve
D. Disk escape
E. Valve dehiscence

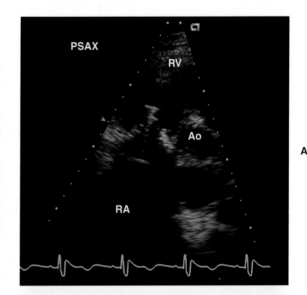

A

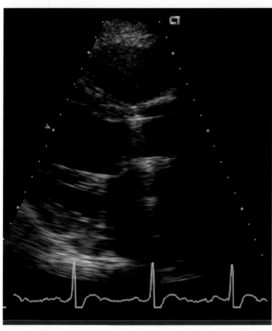

Figure 13–37

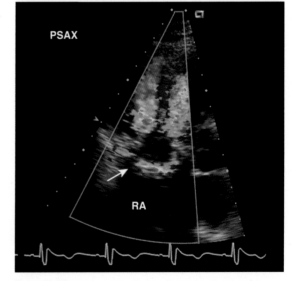

B

Figure 13–38

QUESTION 11

Another patient who has had valve surgery but does not know what type is referred for echocardiography and you obtain this image (Fig. 13–39).

The most likely valve type is:

A. Stentless
B. Homograft
C. Stented bioprosthesis
D. Mechanical
E. Valve resuspension

QUESTION 12

This TEE image (Fig. 13–40) is most consistent with:

A. Coronary fistula
B. Paravalvular abscess
C. Aortic pseudoaneurysm
D. Aortic valve prosthesis
E. Transposed great vessels

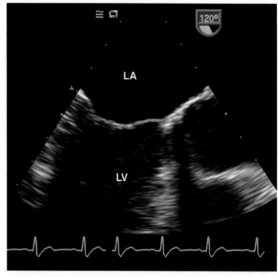

Figure 13–40

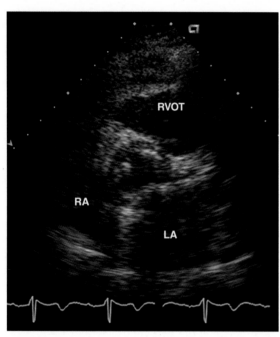

Figure 13–39

ANSWERS

ANSWER 1: D

This two-chamber view shows a porcine mitral prosthesis with the typical appearance of the struts, although the leaflets are not well seen. The valve casts prominent shadows and reverberations that obscure the left ventricle. A laminated thrombus is seen along the atrial wall. The aorta is obscured by the valve shadowing and is not clearly visible in this view. Most mechanical valves have a low profile and do not protrude into the LV chamber. TEE is not sensitive for diagnosis of LV thrombus because the LV apex often is foreshortened and is in the far field of the image. A stentless aortic valve would look similar to a native aortic valve, other than increased thickness of the aortic wall. Stentless valves cannot be implanted in the mitral position.

ANSWER 2: C

This Doppler tracing shows a normal transmitral inflow pattern for a mechanical valve. Prominent valve clicks are present, and the antegrade mitral velocity is within normal limits with a normal deceleration slope. There are no findings to suggest valve thrombosis to prompt surgical consultation. She is in sinus rhythm based on the mitral A velocity, so cardioversion is not needed. Coronary angiography or a nuclear stress study would be helpful if coronary disease were suspected, but her exertional symptoms would be better evaluated by stress echocardiography with rest and exercise recording of the tricuspid regurgitant jet velocity for estimation of pulmonary pressures. TEE is the most appropriate next step to evaluate for prosthetic regurgitation. Clues on the transthoracic study might include an increased antegrade velocity compared with previous studies, a hyperdynamic left ventricle, or elevated pulmonary pressures. However, transthoracic imaging is not sensitive for detection of prosthetic mitral regurgitation, so TEE is reasonable in this patient with new symptoms and inadequate anticoagulation.

ANSWER 3: E

This image shows a long axis view of the aortic valve and root. The walls of the aorta are bright, with thickening and shadowing in the LV outflow tract region, suggestive of an ascending aortic tube graft replacement (in this case for Marfan syndrome). The aortic leaflets are thin and are seen open in mid-systole, so this image is consistent with valve suspension.

Diagnosis of a flail leaflet would require a diastolic image. A mechanical valve would not have normal native leaflets and would have shadows and reverberations. A normal aortic valve would not have the shadowing in the subaortic region. There are no stents to suggest a stented valve prosthesis, although a stentless tissue valve might have this appearance.

ANSWER 4: A

This CW Doppler tracing shows flow across the pulmonic valve. The antegrade flow is only slightly increased in velocity at 1.8 m/s, consistent with no significant stenosis. However, there is a dense diastolic signal that reaches the baseline before end-diastole, which is consistent with severe pulmonic regurgitation.

This signal cannot be tricuspid valve flow because sinus rhythm is present and there is no A velocity in diastole, which would be expected with tricuspid inflow. The onset of systolic flow also is later after the QRS than would be seen with tricuspid regurgitation. Aortic regurgitation would have a higher diastolic velocity, reflecting the diastolic pressure difference between the aorta and left ventricle. Similarly, a residual ventricular septal defect would have a high velocity flow signal in systole because of the high pressure gradient between the two ventricles.

ANSWER 5: C

The Doppler spectrum shows a high velocity (4 m/s) flow that is present in both systole and diastole, with the lowest velocity at end-diastole and the highest at end-systole. This finding is most consistent with an aortic–to-right ventricular fistula, and this diagnosis was confirmed at catheterization and repeat cardiac surgery. The high velocity flow in systole reflects the difference between aortic and right ventricular pressure in systole, with persistent, but decelerating, flow in diastole reflecting the diastolic aortic pressure decline.

Flow into a contained aortic rupture, or pseudoaneurysm, typically is low velocity to-and-fro flow into the contained space. Coronary blood flow occurs predominantly in diastole, with little systolic flow. A ventricular septal defect is characterized by high velocity systolic flow; although diastolic flow may be seen, it is very low in velocity, paralleling the diastolic pressure difference between the two ventricles. Aortic regurgitation occurs only in diastole; any associated systolic signal caused by antegrade flow would have a clear onset and end compared with the diastolic signal.

ANSWER 6: C

This parasternal long axis image shows an eccentric color jet that originates from the anterior aspect of the valve sewing ring and extends across the outflow tract to the anterior mitral valve leaflet, consistent with paravalvular regurgitation, which raises the concern of prosthetic valve endocarditis in the clinical setting of fevers and a new murmur.

A ventricular septal defect would be directed into the right ventricular outflow tract. Normal prosthetic regurgitation originates within the valve ring and typically has a uniform color. Coronary blood flow would be seen in the septum but not extending into the ventricular chamber. An artifact is unlikely because the color signal does not extend over tissue boundaries, although this would be better appreciated on the real time images.

ANSWER 7: B

In this TEE long axis view of the aortic valve, there is marked thickening in both the anterior and posterior aspects of the aortic root, with areas of echodensity and echolucency suggestive of a paravalvular abscess. Although early after surgery this appearance might be nonspecific, these findings are not expected 10 years later. An aneurysm of the aortic mitral intervalvular fibrosa would be seen as an echolucent chamber between the aortic and mitral valves with communication into the left ventricle at the base of the anterior mitral leaflet. An aortic dissection typically would have an intimal flap; this image might mimic an aortic intramural hematoma, but both dissection and intramural hematoma would be unlikely with a homograft aortic root. The atrial septum is not seen in this view, and lipomatous hypertrophy does not extend into the posterior aortic root.

ANSWER 8: E

This Doppler tracing of flow across a bileaflet mechanical mitral valve replacement shows the absence of an atrial contribution to filling, consistent with atrial fibrillation; prominent valve clicks consistent with a mechanical valve; and a systolic signal consistent with the presence of mitral regurgitation. LV systolic pressure (and thus systemic blood pressure) is higher than 200 mm Hg based on the 7 m/s mitral regurgitant jet. Using the Bernoulli equation, this indicates an LV to LA systolic pressure difference of 196 mm Hg. LV systolic pressure would be this pressure difference plus LA pressure. This signal cannot be aortic stenosis because the diastolic signal is clearly not aortic regurgitation (based on velocity and time course), and the systolic signal extends right up to the onset of mitral inflow. The first beat shows an apparent delay between the end of mitral inflow and the onset of mitral regurgitation, but this delay is not seen on the second beat.

ANSWER 9: D

In this parasternal long axis image, the aortic valve is not well seen. However, the increased echogenicity and reverberations originating from the aortic valve region are diagnostic for a low profile mechanical valve. A stented bioprosthesis (porcine valve or bovine pericardial) would have the characteristic stents protruding into the aortic sinuses. The stentless tissue valve and homograft valve both would be characterized by increased thickness and echogenicity of the ascending aorta, but the valve leaflets would appear similar to a native valve and there would be no reverberations. With valve resuspension, there may be shadowing caused by the prosthetic material used to stabilize the annulus, but reverberations would not be seen.

ANSWER 10: C

These images show a normally functioning ball cage valve in the tricuspid position. These valves are not commonly used currently but still may be seen in some patients. On the 2D image, the cage protrudes into the right ventricle, with the bright echo in the middle of the right ventricle caused by the leading edge of the ball at its greatest excursion. Color Doppler demonstrates the ball as the circular area without color in the center of the flow stream that goes around the ball occluder. Given the unusual appearance of the 2D images, other considerations might include a calcified stenotic valve, a pacer lead, or prolapse of a valve prosthesis into the right ventricle caused by annular dehiscence. However, the color flow pattern is diagnostic.

ANSWER 11: C

This short axis view of the aortic valve shows the characteristic appearance of the three stents seen with bioprosthetic stented valves.

ANSWER 12: D

This TEE long axis image shows the left atrium with the mitral valve closed in systole. A section of the ascending aorta is seen, but aortic valve region is completely black, with an apparent extension into an echo-free space anterior to the aorta that might be misinterpreted as an abscess or pseudo-aneurysm. In fact, this is a mechanical aortic valve with prominent shadowing of the anterior part of the valve by the posterior sewing ring. The echo free space anterior to the aorta is partly artifact because of shadowing, with a section of the right ventricular outflow tract seen superiorly. The right coronary artery arises in the region shadowed by the valve prosthesis, but this image does not show evidence for a coronary fistula. If transposition of the great vessels was present, the aorta would be anterior to the pulmonary artery.

NOTES

14 Endocarditis

THE ECHO EXAM: ENDOCARDITIS

DUKE CRITERIA (SHORT VERSION)

DEFINITE ENDOCARDITIS:

2 major or
1 major + 3 minor or
5 minor criteria

Major Criteria:

Bacteremia with a typical organism
Echo evidence of endocarditis

Minor Criteria:

Predisposing condition
Fever
Vascular phenomenon
Immunologic phenomenon
Other microbiologic evidence

ECHOCARDIOGRAPHIC APPROACH

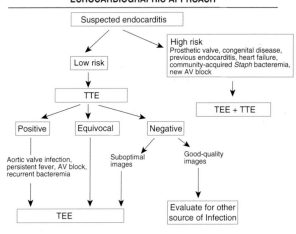

DETECTION OF VALVULAR VEGETATIONS

Start with standard views
Scan carefully between image planes
Use high frequency transducer
Optimize image quality
Look for indirect signs (valve regurgitation, echolucent space, etc.)
TEE whenever risk is high or TTE is nondiagnostic

TEE, *Transesophageal echocardiography;* TTE, *transthoracic echocardiography.*

DIFFICULT ISSUES IN ECHO EVALUATION FOR ENDOCARDITIS

Active versus healed vegetation
Nonbacterial thrombotic endocarditis (NBTE)
Abnormal underlying valve anatomy
Prosthetic valve
Detection of abscess
Need for clinical and microbiologic correlation

EXAMPLE:

A 28-year-old man with a known bicuspid aortic valve presents with a 2-week history of fevers and fatigue. Physical examination shows a blood pressure of 120/40 mm Hg and a harsh diastolic murmur at the left sternal border. Blood cultures (three sets) are positive for *Streptococcus viridans.* With a predisposing factor, fevers, and positive blood cultures with a typical organism, the pre-test likelihood of endocarditis is very high (more than 90%).

Transthoracic echocardiography shows a bicuspid aortic valve with a mass on the ventricular side of the leaflets with independent motion. Left ventricular size and systolic function are normal. Color flow Doppler shows aortic regurgitation with an eccentric jet and a vena contracta width of 7 mm, continuous wave Doppler shows a dense signal with a deceleration slope of 120 msec, and there is holodiastolic flow reversal in the proximal abdominal aorta.

The TTE findings are diagnostic for endocarditis, so this patient now has two major Duke criteria and a diagnosis of *definite endocarditis.* With his bicuspid aortic valve, there may have been some degree of underlying aortic regurgitation. However, the normal left ventricular size and the steep deceleration slope of the continuous wave aortic regurgitant jet are consistent with superimposed *acute* aortic regurgitation. Aortic regurgitation is *severe,* as evidenced by a wide vena contracta and holodiastolic flow reversal in the aorta.

The following day, a prolonged PR interval (first-degree atrioventricular block) is noted on the electrocardiogram, and TEE is performed. The TEE shows an echolucent area in the aortic annulus region consistent with abscess, and the patient is referred for prompt surgical intervention.

BASIC PRINCIPLES

■ Echocardiographic evaluation for endocarditis uses an integrated approach with transthoracic echocardiography (TTE) and transesophageal echocardiography (TEE), depending on the clinical setting and the initial echocardiographic findings.

■ The modified Duke criteria for infective endocarditis are the current clinical standard.

■ The primary goals of the echocardiographic examination in a patient with suspected or known endocarditis are to:

❑ Detect and describe valvular vegetations
❑ Quantitate the degree of valve dysfunction
❑ Identify paravalvular abscess or other complications
❑ Evaluate the hemodynamic effects of valve dysfunction on ventricular size and function and on pulmonary pressures

❏ Provide prognostic data on the clinical course and the need for surgical intervention

Key points:

❏ Definite endocarditis is present when blood cultures are positive and diagnostic findings are present on echocardiography; these are called "major criteria" for the diagnosis of endocarditis.

❏ Diagnostic echocardiographic findings for endocarditis include the following:
  ❏ Typical vegetation on a valve or prosthetic material
  ❏ Paravalvular abscess
  ❏ New prosthetic valve dehiscence
  ❏ New valvular regurgitation

❏ In the absence of the major criteria (blood cultures and echocardiographic findings), the minor criteria for diagnosis of endocarditis are:
  ❏ Predisposing heart condition or intravenous drug use
  ❏ Fever
  ❏ Vascular phenomenon (arterial emboli, mycotic aneurysm, conjunctival hemorrhage, etc.)
  ❏ Immunologic phenomenon (glomerulonephritis, rheumatoid factor, etc.)
  ❏ Other microbiologic evidence

❏ Definite endocarditis is based on the presence of two major *or* one major plus three minor *or* all five minor criteria. Possible endocarditis is based on one major plus one minor *or* three minor criterion.

STEP-BY-STEP APPROACH

Step 1: Review the Clinical Data

■ Key clinical data in the patient undergoing echocardiography for suspected endocarditis are:
  ❏ Blood culture results
  ❏ History of underlying cardiac disease or intravenous drug use
  ❏ Other evidence of endocarditis (fever, embolic events, PR interval prolongation, etc.)
  ❏ Any contraindication to TEE

■ The clinical data helps focus the echocardiographic examination so that particular attention is directed toward:
  ❏ Detection of right-sided vegetations in patients with a history of intravenous drug use
  ❏ Comparison of the current study with previous examinations in patients with underlying valve pathology
  ❏ Additional imaging, often with TEE, of prosthetic valves and pacer leads

Key points:

❏ The sensitivity of echocardiography for detection of valve vegetations depends as much on the diligence of the exam as on image quality, so a pretest estimate of the likelihood of disease is helpful to the sonographer.

❏ Review of any previous imaging studies before performing the exam allows quick recognition of new abnormalities.

❏ Clinical data is critical for interpretation of echocardiographic data. The images of a cardiac tumor, thrombus, or an infected vegetation are similar—the final diagnosis is based on integration of echocardiographic and clinical data.

❏ Clinical data determine the urgency and most appropriate initial diagnostic modality as well as the need for any subsequent studies.

Step 2: Choose Transthoracic or Transesophageal Echocardiography (Table 14–1)

■ Most centers perform TTE first in patients with suspected endocarditis.

■ Transthoracic imaging is followed by TEE if transthoracic images are nondiagnostic, if a prosthetic valve is present, or if the patient has a high risk of endocarditis.

■ TEE also is an appropriate initial diagnostic approach in patients with a prosthetic valve or other intracardiac devices (such as pacer leads).

■ In a patient with suspected or known endocarditis, TEE is recommended if clinical data suggest the possibility of paravalvular abscess.

Key points:

❏ TEE is more sensitive for detection of valve vegetations compared with transthoracic imaging (a sensitivity of about 90% compared with about 70%; Fig. 14–1).

❏ TEE is more sensitive for detection of paravalvular abscess compared with transthoracic imaging (sensitivity of more than 90% compared with about 50%).

❏ TEE is the preferred approach for detection of vegetations and evaluation of valve dysfunction in patients with prosthetic valves or other intracardiac devices (such as pacer leads; Fig. 14–2).

❏ Transthoracic imaging provides more reliable measurements of left ventricular (LV) size and ejection fraction, because images of the left ventricle are often oblique or foreshortened on TEE views.

❏ Transthoracic imaging provides more accurate Doppler evaluation of stenotic valves

TABLE 14-1

ACC/AHA 2006 RECOMMENDATIONS FOR ECHOCARDIOGRAPHY IN INFECTIVE ENDOCARDITIS

	TRANSTHORACIC ECHO (TTE)	TRANSESOPHAGEAL ECHO (TEE)
SUSPECTED ENDOCARDITIS		
1. Detection of valvular vegetations (with or without positive blood cultures)	Recommended	
2. Known valve disease with positive blood cultures and nondiagnostic TTE		Recommended
3. Persistent staphylococcal bacteremia without a known source		Reasonable
4. Nosocomial staphylococcal bacteremia		May be considered
KNOWN ENDOCARDITIS		
1. Evaluation of valve hemodynamics	Recommended	Recommended if TTE nondiagnostic
2. Detection and assessment of complications (abscess, perforation, shunt)	Recommended	Recommended
3. Reassessment of valve function in high risk patients (e.g., virulent organism, clinical deterioration, persistent or recurrent fever, new murmur, persistent bacteremia)	Recommended	
PROSTHETIC VALVE ENDOCARDITIS		
1. Diagnosis and complications	TEE is preferred approach	Recommended
2. Patient with a prosthetic valve and a persistent fever without bacteremia or a new murmur	Reasonable	
3. Reevaluation of prosthetic valve endocarditis during antibiotic therapy in the absence of clinical deterioration	May be considered	
PERIOPERATIVE MANAGEMENT		
1. Preoperative evaluation in patients with known infective endocarditis		Recommended
2. Intraoperative TEE in patients undergoing valve surgery for infective endocarditis		Recommended

Recommended, *Class I;* reasonable, *Class IIa;* may be considered, *Class IIb.*

Derived from ACC/AHA 2006 guidelines for the management of patients with valvular heart disease: a report of the American College of Cardiology/American Heart Association Task Force on Practice Guidelines (writing Committee to Revise the 1998 guidelines for the management of patients with valvular heart disease) developed in collaboration with the Society of Cardiovascular Anesthesiologists, endorsed by the Society for Cardiovascular Angiography and Interventions and the Society of Thoracic Surgeons. J Am Coll Cardiol 48(3):e1-148, 2006.

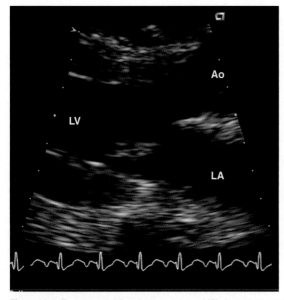

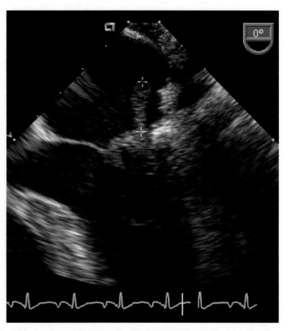

Figure 14-1 Transthoracic (*A*) and transesophageal (*B*) views of the mitral valve in a patient with bacteremia. The large mobile mitral valve vegetation is easily seen on the transesophageal image but was barely visible on the transthoracic study. This typical vegetation is attached to the upstream side of the valve (atrial side of mitral valve), is not as echodense as the valve tissue, is irregular in shape, and has a chaotic pattern of motion that is separate from the normal motion of the valve tissue.

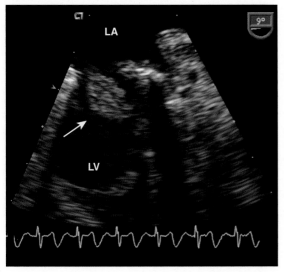
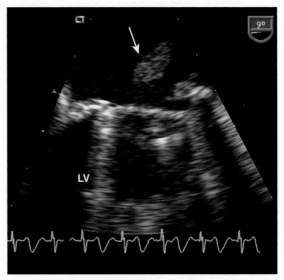

Figure 14–2 In this patient with endocarditis of a mechanical bileaflet mitral valve, the transthoracic study did not show valve vegetations because of shadowing and reverberations by the prosthesis. These transesophageal images show a large irregular mass, consistent with a vegetation, attached to the valve that prolapsed into the left ventricle (*LV*) in diastole (*A*) and the left atrium (*LA*) in systole (*B*).

and estimation of pulmonary pressures, because TEE often results in a nonparallel intercept angle between the Doppler beam and high velocity jet.

❑ When TEE is contraindicated, a repeat transthoracic study in 5 to 10 days has additive value, with the prevalence of diagnostic findings increasing from 20% on the initial study to 40% on the repeat examination, when endocarditis is suspected on clinical grounds.

Step 3: Examine Valve Anatomy to Detect Valvular Vegetations

■ Valvular vegetations on echocardiography are seen as an abnormal, irregular mass attached to the valve apparatus (Fig. 14–3).

■ Valve vegetations typically are attached to the upstream side of the valve leaflet (e.g., atrial side of the mitral or tricuspid valve, LV side of aortic valve; Fig. 14–4).

■ Motion of a vegetation typically is chaotic, with a spatial range in excess of normal valve excursion and a temporal pattern of rapid oscillations (Fig. 14–5).

Key points:

❑ In addition to standard views of each valve, the image plane is slowly moved from side to side (or in a rotational sweep on TEE), because vegetations often are seen only in oblique views.

❑ Zoom mode, a narrow sector, high transducer frequency, and harmonic imaging are

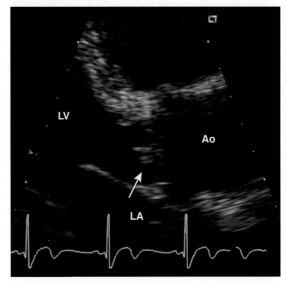

Figure 14–3 Small linear mobile echo densities on the ventricular side of the aortic valve in diastole may be a vegetation or a normal variant called Lambl's excrescences, small fibrous strands typically attached near the tip of each valve cusp, that are more prevalent with increased age. This patient had positive blood cultures and associated aortic regurgitation, with a clinical course consistent with endocarditis.

used to enhance details of valve anatomy (Fig. 14–6).

❑ An M-mode recording through a suspected vegetation seen on two-dimensional (2D) imaging helps distinguish vegetation from an artifact or valve tissue, based on the pattern and speed of motion of the structure.

❑ Vegetations may be missed on TTE; transesophageal imaging has a higher sensitivity

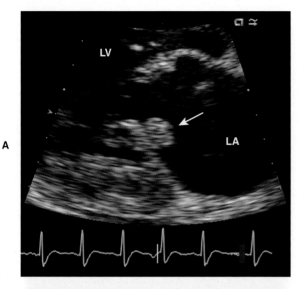

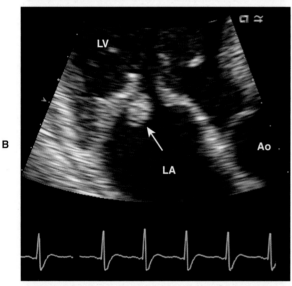

Figure 14–4 Parasternal (*A*) and apical (*B*) long axis zoomed images of the mitral valve show an echodensity on the atrial side of the posterior leaflet, consistent with a vegetation.

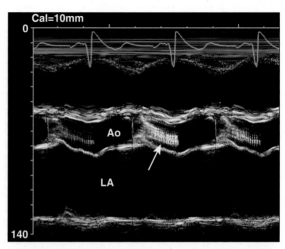

Figure 14–5 M-mode tracing of the aortic valve used to evaluate the motion of a small linear echodensity in a patient referred for possible endocarditis. The M-mode shows fine oscillations of the mass in diastole, suggesting a vegetation rather than nonspecific leaflet thickening.

for detection of vegetation because of improved image quality.

❑ Other valve masses may be mistaken for an infected vegetation, including (Fig. 14–7):
  ❑ Papillary fibroelastoma
  ❑ Partial flail mitral leaflet or chord
  ❑ Nonbacterial thrombotic endocarditis
  ❑ Valve thrombus (especially with prosthetic valves)
  ❑ Normal valve variants (such as Lambl's excrescence)
  ❑ Ultrasound artifacts

❑ Valve vegetations tend to decrease in size and increase in echogenicity with effective

therapy. However, some vegetations may still be present years after active infection.

Step 4: Evaluate Valve Dysfunction Resulting from Endocarditis

■ Vegetations are associated with distortion of valve anatomy and destruction of valve tissue, typically resulting in valve regurgitation (Fig. 14–8).
■ The presence and severity of valve dysfunction are evaluated no differently from evaluation in a patient with valve disease of any cause (see Chapters 11 and 12).
■ Valve regurgitation in a patient with endocarditis often is acute, rather than chronic, in duration.

Key points:

❑ Vegetations may impede complete valve closure, resulting in regurgitation at the coaptation plane with either native or prosthetic valves.
❑ Valve destruction results in regurgitation from leaflet perforation or deformity of the leaflet edge.
❑ Regurgitation of prosthetic valves often is paravalvular, resulting from infection in the annulus with valve dehiscence (Fig. 14–9).
❑ About 10% of patients with endocarditis do not have significant valve regurgitation because the vegetation is located at the leaflet base, which does not impair valve function.
❑ Rarely, a large vegetation causes stenosis from obstruction of the native or prosthetic valve orifice by the vegetation mass.

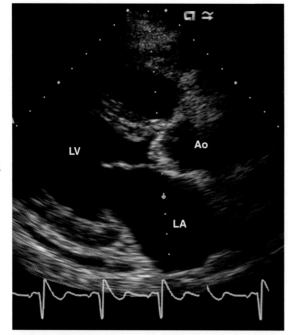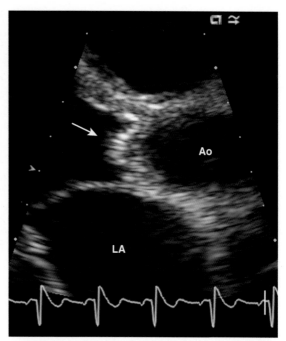

A

B

Figure 14–6 *A*, This long axis view at a standard depth shows a thickened prolapsing aortic valve in diastole. *B*, Using zoom mode, it is seen in more detail, with real time images showing independent rapid oscillating motion of the prolapsing tissue, suggestive of a vegetation.

❏ Prosthetic valve stenosis can result from a small infected vegetation or thrombus impinging on normal disc prosthetic valve infections excursion.

Step 5: Evaluate for the Possibility of a Paravalvular Abscess or Fistula

■ A paravalvular abscess is present in 20% to 60% of native aortic valve endocarditis cases and in about 15% of mitral valve infections (Fig. 14–10).
■ Paravalvular infection is typical with prosthetic valve endocarditis; paravalvular infection is present in more than 60% of cases.
■ On echocardiography, a paravalvular abscess may be echolucent or echodense. A paravalvular aortic abscess often communicates with the aortic lumen, appearing as an aneurysm of the sinus of Valsalva (Fig. 14–11).
■ Rupture of paravalvular infection into adjacent chambers results in an infected fistula (Fig. 14–12).

Key points:

❏ TEE is indicated when a paravalvular abscess is suspected, because the sensitivity of transthoracic imaging is low.
❏ Aortic paravalvular infection often is recognized based on distortion of the normal contours of the sinuses of Valsalva.

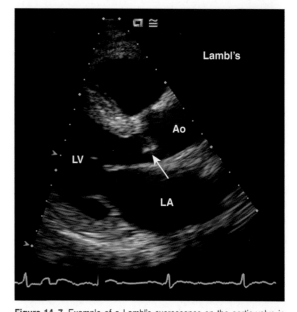

Figure 14–7 Example of a Lambl's excrescence on the aortic valve in diastole. These can be difficult to distinguish from vegetations but often are smaller, more linear and echodense, are not associated with valve dysfunction, and do not change in size or appearance on sequential studies.

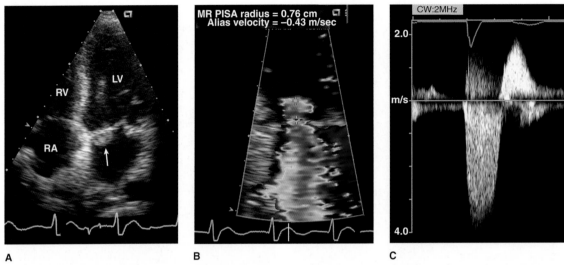

A

B

C

Figure 14–8 *A,* A large mass is seen on the left atrial side of the mitral valve consistent with a valvular vegetation. Although the mass is distant from the coaptation point, color Doppler shows significant regurgitation, which is quantitated with standard approaches, including the proximal isovelocity surface area method (*B*) and the continuous wave Doppler signal (*C*).

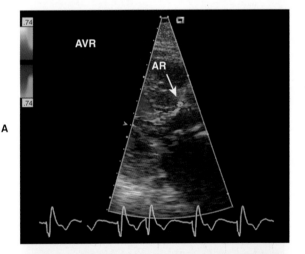

A

B

Figure 14–9 *A,* An eccentric jet of aortic regurgitation that originates anterior to the valve sewing ring is seen in a parasternal long axis view. *B,* Although signal quality is suboptimal, the continuous wave Doppler signal recorded from the apical window shows a similar density of antegrade and retrograde aortic flow, suggesting significant regurgitation may be present.

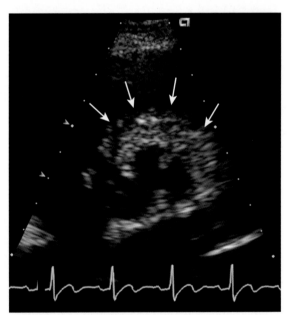

Figure 14–10 A paravalvular abscess can be difficult to detect on transthoracic imaging. In this parasternal short axis view, there is increased echogenicity in the para-aortic region that may be due to abscess formation.

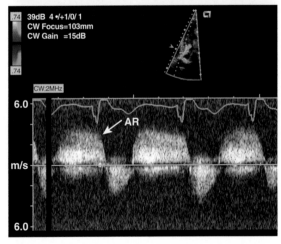

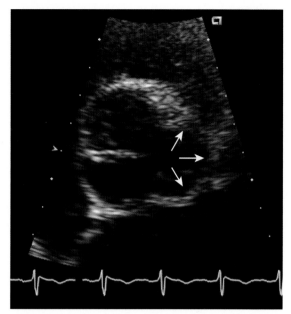

Figure 14–11 Infection of the sinuses of Valsalva also can present as an asymmetric dilation of the sinus, as seen with the left coronary sinus of Valsalva in this image. Comparison with previous images and trans-esophageal imaging both are helpful in distinguishing an infected sinus from a benign congenital dilation of the sinus.

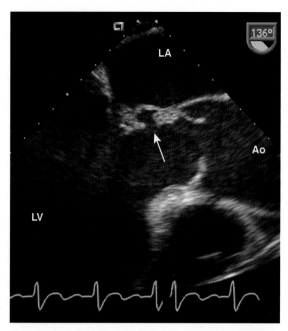

Figure 14–13 In this patient with aortic valve endocarditis, infection has extended into the base of the adjacent anterior mitral leaflet with thickening and a small perforation.

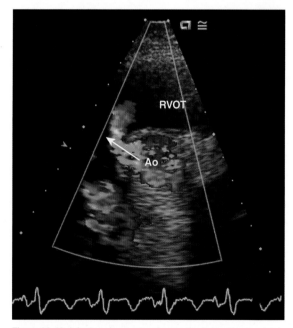

Figure 14–12 Infection of an aortic valve prosthesis resulting in a fistula from the aorta (*Ao*) to the right ventricular outflow tract (*RVOT*) seen on transthoracic echocardiography in a parasternal short axis view. The appearance is similar to a ventricular septal defect, but Doppler interrogation showed both diastolic and systolic flow more consistent with aortic–to–right ventricular flow.

❏ Paravalvular aortic infection may extend into the base of the anterior mitral leaflet, resulting in mitral leaflet perforation (Fig. 14–13).

❏ An aortic paravalvular abscess may rupture into the left ventricle (resulting in severe aortic regurgitation) or into the left atrium, right atrium, or right ventricular outflow tract (resulting in a fistula).

❏ With prosthetic aortic valves, infection may result in an aneurysm of the aortic–mitral intervalvular fibrosa (a space between the aortic and mitral valve that communicates with the left ventricle; Fig. 14–14).

❏ A mitral paravalvular abscess may extend into the pericardium, resulting in purulent pericarditis.

Step 6: Measure the Hemodynamic Consequences of Valve Dysfunction

■ Valve dysfunction resulting from endocarditis may result in ventricular dilation and dysfunction or in pulmonary hypertension.

■ However, because regurgitation often is acute, evidence of chronic volume overload may be absent even when regurgitation is severe.

Key points:

❏ Evaluation of a patient with endocarditis includes measurement of LV dimensions, volumes, and ejection fraction, as detailed in Chapter 6.

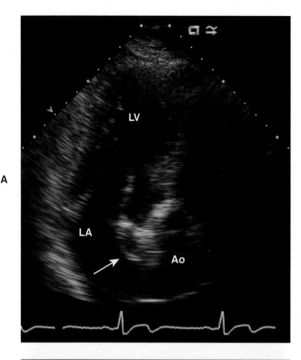

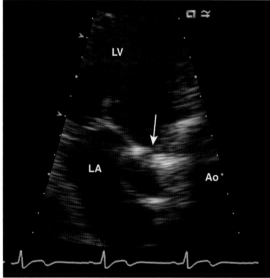

Figure 14–14 *A,* In the apical long axis view, a curved pulsatile echo-free space (*arrow*) is seen between the posterior aortic root and left atrium (*LA*). *B,* Using zoom mode, the narrow neck where this aneurysm of the aortic mitral intervalvular fibrosa communicates with the left ventricle (*LV*) is seen (*arrow*).

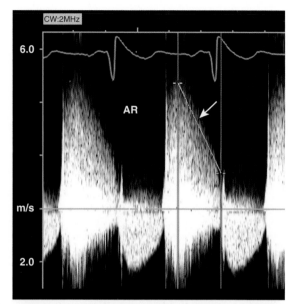

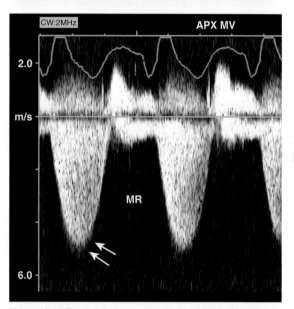

Figure 14–15 Regurgitation caused by endocarditis often has an acute onset. Acute aortic regurgitation (*AR, A*) shows a dense signal with a steep deceleration slope caused by rapid equalization of aortic and left ventricular pressures in diastole. *B,* With acute mitral regurgitation (*MR*), an early fall off from peak velocity is due to an increased left atrial systolic pressure and V wave.

❐ Pulmonary systolic pressure is estimated as described in Chapter 6.

❐ Early (mid-diastolic) closure of the mitral valve may be seen on M-mode when acute severe aortic regurgitation is present because of the rapid rise in diastolic LV pressure.

❐ The time course of the CW Doppler recording of valve regurgitation may show evidence of hemodynamic decompensation:

❐ A rapid decline in velocity in late systole with mitral (or tricuspid) regurgitation suggests a left (or right) atrial V wave.

❐ A steep diastolic deceleration slope with aortic regurgitation suggests acute regurgitation with an elevated LV end-diastolic pressure (Fig. 14–15).

❐ LV systolic function may be impaired, without LV dilation, with acute severe aortic regurgitation caused by endocarditis, possibly due to the effects of systemic infection; this may be combined with a shift to the steep segment of the LV pressure volume curve.

Step 7: Look for Other Complications of Endocarditis

■ More than one cardiac valve may be affected, either because of primary infection at more than one site or direct extension of infection to adjacent structures.

■ Septic coronary artery emboli, resulting in myocardial infarction, occur in 10% of patients.

■ Endocarditis may occur at intracardiac sites other than valve leaflets, including a mitral or tricuspid valve chord, a right atrial Chiari network or Eustachian valve, or the right atrial wall in a region abraded by the tip of a central catheter.

■ A pericardial effusion may be present, either as a nonspecific sign of systemic infection or because of direct extension of infection from the mitral annulus.

Key points:

❏ Once a vegetation has been detected on one valve, careful evaluation for infection of other valves is needed.

❏ The presence of a regional wall motion abnormality in a patient with endocarditis suggests a coronary embolus from a valve vegetation.

❏ Intracardiac sites subject to injury, such as the right atrial wall in patients with a central catheter or the tricuspid valve in patients with an indwelling right heart catheter, should be carefully examined for evidence of infection (Fig. 14–16).

SPECIAL SITUATIONS

Right-Sided Endocarditis

■ Only 6% to 13% of febrile intravenous drug users have endocarditis.

■ In intravenous drug users, infection affects the right heart (predominantly the tricuspid valve) in 75% of cases (Fig. 14–17).

■ Most cases of right-sided endocarditis in drug users are due to *Staphylococcus aureus*, and persistent infection or abscess formation requiring surgery occurs in less than 25% of cases.

■ Pulmonary emboli caused by right heart vegetations may result in elevated pulmonary pressures.

■ Left-sided involvement occurs in 25% to 35% of endocarditis cases in patients with a history of intravenous drug use.

■ TTE is adequate for evaluation of tricuspid valve endocarditis, but TEE may be needed to exclude left heart involvement.

Prosthetic Valves

■ Blood cultures should be drawn before any antibiotic therapy in febrile patients with a prosthetic heart valve.

■ TEE is indicated in all patients with a prosthetic heart valve and positive blood cultures.

■ TEE should be considered in patients with a prosthetic heart valve and suspected endocarditis, because transthoracic imaging is inadequate to exclude prosthetic valve infection.

■ More than 50% of patients with prosthetic valve endocarditis require surgical intervention.

Pacer or Defibrillator Leads

■ Late infection of permanent pacer or defibrillator leads is rare.

■ Vegetations on the pacer wire are detected in less than 25% of cases on transthoracic imaging but are seen in more than 90% on TEE when infection is present (Fig. 14–18).

■ The differential diagnosis of a mobile mass on a pacer lead includes thrombus. Thrombus and vegetation cannot be distinguished by echocardiography.

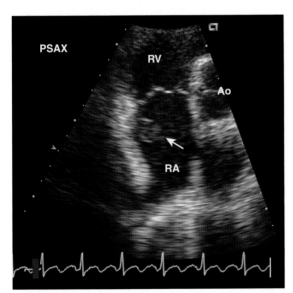

Figure 14–16 A rounded mass is seen in the right atrium (*RA*) attached to the free wall, near the distal tip of a central venous line, in this zoomed apical four-chamber view. This might be a thrombus or an infected vegetation, depending on blood culture results and clinical evidence of infection. *PSAX,* Parasternal short axis view.

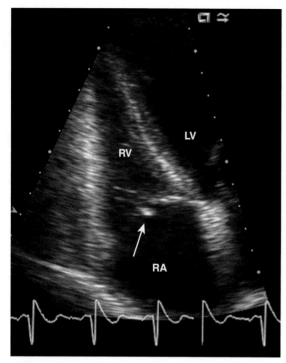
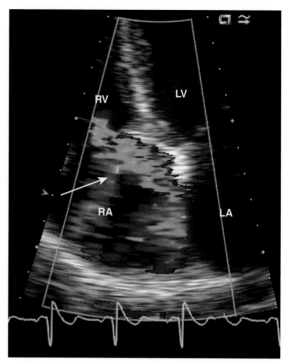

Figure 14–17 In this apical four-chamber view with angulation toward the right heart of an intravenous drug user with positive blood cultures for *Staph. aureus*, a small mobile echodensity is seen on the atrial side of the tricuspid valve (*A*). Color flow (*B*) shows an eccentric jet of moderate tricuspid regurgitation.

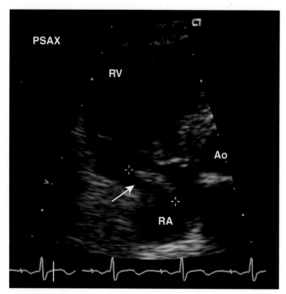

Figure 14–18 A linear mobile echo-density is seen attached to the transvenous pacer lead in a parasternal short axis (*PSAX*) view. The appearance is consistent with vegetation or a thrombus.

Staphylococcus aureus Bacteremia

- TEE is reasonable in patients with persistently positive blood cultures for *Staph. aureus*, even if the transthoracic study is negative.
- Chronic indwelling central venous catheters may be a source of thrombus or infection. TEE allows imaging of the catheter tip in the right atrium in the 90-degree longitudinal view.
- A mobile mass attached to the catheter tip is consistent with thrombus or vegetation.
- Thrombus or infection also may involve the adjacent right atrial wall.

NOTES

SELF-ASSESSMENT QUESTIONS

QUESTION 1

Echocardiography is requested in a 32-year-old man with a 2-week history of fevers and fatigue. He has known mitral valve prolapse and is followed with annual echocardiography. Physical examination is remarkable only for a temperature of 38.5° C, small conjunctival hemorrhages, and a murmur of mitral regurgitation. Laboratory data includes two blood cultures positive for *Streptococcus viridans* and microscopic hematuria.

Which additional finding on echocardiography is needed to meet the Duke criteria for definite endocarditis?

   A. A typical valvular vegetation
   B. Mitral regurgitation
   C. Evidence for a paravalvular abscess
   D. A ruptured chord
   E. None of the above

QUESTION 2

Echocardiography is requested in a 28-year-old woman with a murmur heard during the third month of pregnancy. The patient has no prior cardiac history, feels well, and denies fevers or malaise. Physical examination is normal, other than a systolic murmur at the cardiac base and her gravid state. Echocardiography is normal except for a small mobile linear echo at the aortic valve closure line in diastole.

The most appropriate next step is:

   A. TEE
   B. Blood cultures
   C. Reassurance
   D. Intravenous antibiotics
   E. Repeat echo in 2 weeks

QUESTION 3

A 67-year-old man in the intensive care unit with pneumonia and respiratory failure is referred for echocardiography for possible endocarditis, in the setting of fevers and positive blood cultures. A still-frame long axis view of the aortic valve is shown (Fig. 14–19). What feature of this aortic valve abnormality would help distinguish a vegetation from aortic valve sclerosis?

   A. Diffuse leaflet thickening
   B. Independent mobility
   C. Increased echodensity
   D. Number of cusps involved
   E. Antegrade aortic velocity

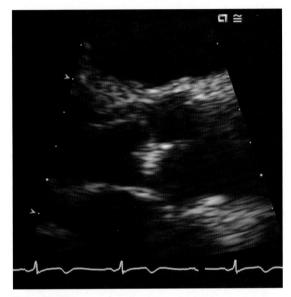

Figure 14–19

QUESTION 4

A 78-year-old man presented to the emergency department 5 days after shoulder surgery with fever, chills, and a cough. His shoulder surgery was performed for a chronic left shoulder fungal arthritis with *Candida parapsilosis,* with a left shoulder fusion 1 year previously and a persistent draining wound. His past medical history was remarkable for aortic homograft valve replacement 3 years earlier. The TEE images shown (Figs. 14–20*A* and *B*) were obtained.

Based on this data, the most likely diagnosis is:

A. Normal postoperative changes
B. Aortic pseudoaneurysm
C. Left atrial thrombus
D. Paravalvular abscess
E. Dehiscence of right coronary artery implantation site

QUESTION 5

Annual echocardiography was requested in this 39-year-old man with mitral valve prolapse and chronic mitral regurgitation. The image shown in Figure 14–21 was obtained. The patient feels well and denies any current symptoms. The most likely diagnosis is:

A. Vegetation
B. Anterior leaflet prolapse
C. Flail segment
D. Fibroelastoma
E. Nonbacterial thrombotic endocarditis

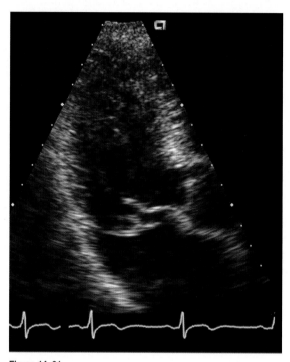

Figure 14–21

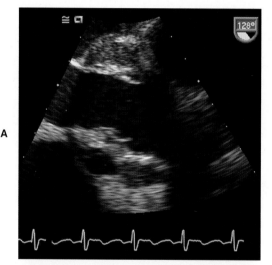

A

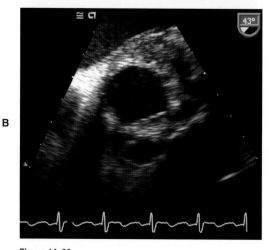

B

Figure 14–20

QUESTION 6

Echocardiography was requested in a 36-year-old man for a 1 week history of fever and a new murmur. He also complained of nausea and vomiting and was told he probably had viral gastroenteritis. He has no previous cardiac history, denies intravenous drug use, and is taking no medications. Physical exam shows an ill-appearing man with a temperature of 38.5° C, a blood pressure of 95/61 mm Hg, and a pulse of 110 beats per minute (bpm). Laboratory data and blood cultures are pending.

List five abnormal findings evident on his image (Fig. 14–22).

1. _____
2. _____
3. _____
4. _____
5. _____

QUESTION 7

Which of the following are seen in this image taken from a 26-year-old intravenous drug user referred for echocardiography for fevers and a new murmur (Fig. 14–23)?

  A. Tricuspid valve vegetation
  B. Atrial septal aneurysm
  C. Central line catheter tip
  D. Chiari network
  E. Cor triatriatum

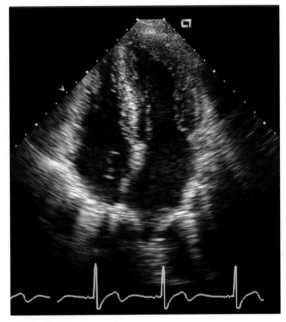

Figure 14–23

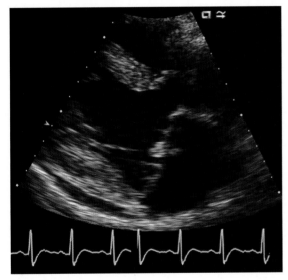

Figure 14–22

QUESTION 8

The TEE study shown in Figure 14–24 was requested in a 78-year-old woman for new onset atrial fibrillation to evaluate for left atrial thrombus prior to cardioversion. Her past medical history is remarkable for hypertension and hyperlipidemia. She has no history of neurologic events, and she is afebrile.

The most likely diagnosis is:

A. Bacterial endocarditis
B. Lambl's excrescence
C. Papillary fibroelastoma
D. Nonbacterial thrombotic endocarditis
E. Ultrasound artifact

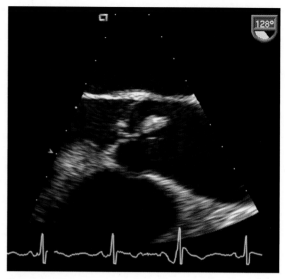

Figure 14–24

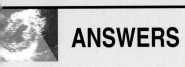

ANSWERS

ANSWER 1: E

This patient has one major criteria (typical blood cultures for endocarditis) and three minor criteria (predisposing condition, fever, and conjunctival hemorrhages) and thus meets the Duke criteria for endocarditis even before the echocardiogram is requested. In this setting, some clinicians would perform TEE first because the diagnosis is already certain, so the goal of echocardiography is to assess disease severity and detect complications. If the patient did not have three minor criteria for the diagnosis of endocarditis, the finding on echocardiography of typical vegetation or an abscess would constitute a second major criteria. A ruptured chord or atypical leaflet thickening would not add to the diagnostic criteria. The finding of mitral regurgitation is considered a major criterion only if this is new regurgitation, not just worsening of a preexisting condition.

ANSWER 2: C

A systolic ejection murmur, or "flow" murmur, can be appreciated in 80% of pregnant women. This benign finding is thought to be due to increased forward flow in the pulmonary artery caused by the increased cardiac output during pregnancy. Based on a normal physical examination and clinical history, it is very unlikely that she has endocarditis at the start of the echocardiographic study (low pretest likelihood). The finding described is consistent with a Lambl's excrescence, which is a normal variant. Thus the post-test likelihood of endocarditis also is very low, so reassurance is the most appropriate course. If the clinical features or echocardiographic findings were more typical for endocarditis, blood cultures and TEE would be reasonable. Empiric antibiotic therapy is reserved for cases in which the likelihood of endocarditis is very high and withholding therapy might negatively impact outcome. Repeat echocardiography in 2 weeks is most helpful in following treatment of endocarditis to ensure vegetation size is stable or decreasing with effective therapy.

ANSWER 3: B

Focal thickening of the leaflet occurs in both aortic valve sclerosis and a valve vegetation, and both often appear as echodense areas on the valve leaflets. Diffuse leaflet thickening is a non-specific finding that does not indicate aortic valve sclerosis or infection. However, independent mobility of a mass is highly suggestive of a valvular vegetation and is the most useful echocardiographic feature in this situation. An M-mode line through the area often helps determine independent motion. Distinguishing a Lambl's excrescence from a vegetation is problematic because both show independent mobility, although a Lambl's excrescence usually is thinner and shorter than a vegetation. The number of cusps involved is variable with both endocarditis and aortic sclerosis. The antegrade velocity is increased in aortic sclerosis when disease is severe enough to cause valve obstruction. However, antegrade velocity also may be increased with endocarditis caused by fever and a high cardiac output or concurrent aortic regurgitation. Mild regurgitation is common with aortic sclerosis; moderate or severe regurgitation is more likely with endocarditis.

ANSWER 4: D

In these long (A) and short (B) axis views of the aortic homograft, there is extensive thickening both anteriorly and posteriorly to the homograft valve and ascending aorta, with areas that are echodense (posteriorly) and echolucent (anteriorly). These findings are most consistent with a paravalvular abscess, even though blood cultures were negative in this patient on chronic suppressive antifungal therapy for his shoulder infection. Although extensive thickening caused by edema and hematoma often is seen early after surgery, these are unlikely to be normal postoperative changes 3 years after the cardiac procedure. Comparison with a previous echocardiogram would be helpful but was not available in this case. An aortic pseudoaneurysm more likely would be echolucent without areas of echodensity. Color Doppler would be helpful for demonstrating flow in a pseudoaneurysm. The posterior aspect of the paravalvular abscess protrudes into the left atrium, but the location and appearance are atypical for an atrial thrombus, and the mass clearly is part of the para-aortic precess. Dehiscence of the coronary implantation sites is a reasonable concern after replacement of the ascending aorta with a homograft, tissue, or prosthetic tube graft, because all require coronary reimplantation. Dehiscence can occur in the setting of infection, and the echolucent area in the region where the right coronary should be seen in these images is worrisome. However, the patient had no chest pain or electrocardiographic signs of ischemia in the right coronary distribution, and the posterior echodense region would not be explained by this diagnosis.

ANSWER 5: C

This apical long axis view shows prolapse of the posterior mitral leaflet with a partial flail segment seen behind the anterior mitral leaflet. The flail segment is attached to and has the same echogenicity as the posterior leaflet, and, unlike the prolapsed segment, the tip of the flail segment points away from the LV apex. The anterior and posterior leaflets fail to coapt normally because of the partial flail posterior leaflet; the anterior leaflet itself is relatively normal. Although a vegetation or fibroelastoma cannot be distinguished from a flail segment based on this image alone, the patient has no signs or symptoms of endocarditis and a flail segment is more likely than a valve tumor, especially since he has myxomatous mitral valve disease. The vegetations of marantic or nonbacterial thrombotic endocarditis often are smaller and more plaquelike and may be on the ventricular or atrial side of the leaflet.

ANSWER 6

This parasternal long axis image shows mitral valve prolapse with a small mass on the atrial side of the valve consistent with a *vegetation* in this febrile, ill patient. There is *LV enlargement* and *left atrial enlargement* suggestive of chronic mitral regurgitation. In addition, a *pericardial effusion* is seen. Blood cultures were positive for coagulase negative Staphylococcus. Despite prompt intravenous antibiotic therapy, his clinical course was complicated by severe mitral regurgitation, mild heart failure, and two transient ischemic neurologic events. After 1 week of hospitalization he underwent mechanical mitral valve replacement before completing the full 6 week course of antibiotics. At surgery, both the anterior and posterior leaflets showed evidence of infection, precluding valve repair, and a posterior

annular abscess was debrided. One year later he is asymptomatic with normal LV size and systolic function on echocardiography.

ANSWER 7: D

A linear series of irregular echoes is seen in the right atrium in this apical four-chamber view. This finding is most consistent with a Chiari network, a normal variant with a fine mesh of tissue extending from the inferior vena cava toward the superior vena cava. In real time, this tissue mesh moves erratically, sometimes appearing similar to spontaneous echo contrast in the right atrium. A tricuspid valve vegetation would be more clearly attached to the valve leaflets. Although the atrial septum bows slightly toward the right atrium, it does not meet criteria (excursion from the septal plane of more than 1.5 cm) for an atrial septal aneurysm. A central line catheter usually is brighter and more uniform in appearance, often with a double line caused by the fluid-filled lumen. The membrane that divides the atrium in cor triatriatum goes from the lateral wall of the atrium across to the septum, perpendicular to the echoes seen on this image.

ANSWER 8: C

This aortic valve has a large mass attached to the aortic side of the valve. Bacterial endocarditis is unlikely given the absence of evidence of infection, but blood cultures should be obtained with prolonged incubation to exclude fastidious organisms. A Lambl's excrescence is a small filamentous structure, more often seen on the ventricular side of the valve. Nonbacterial thrombotic endocarditis usually is diagnosed after an embolic event and occurs in patients with systemic inflammatory disorders. These vegetations tend to be multiple, sessile masses on the leaflets. This in not an ultrasound artifact, as there is no structure between the mass and transducer to cause a reverberation artifact. Thus the most likely diagnosis is a papillary fibroelastoma.

NOTES

15 Cardiac Masses and a Potential Cardiac Source of Embolus

THE ECHO EXAM

BASIC PRINCIPLES

STEP-BY-STEP APPROACH
Left Atrial Thrombi
Left Ventricular Thrombi
Right Heart Thrombi

Nonprimary Cardiac Tumors
Primary Cardiac Tumors
Vegetations
Patent Foramen Ovale
Evaluation for a Cardiac Source of Embolus

SELF-ASSESSMENT QUESTIONS

THE ECHO EXAM: CARDIAC MASSES AND SOURCE OF EMBOLUS

	STRUCTURES THAT MAY BE MISTAKEN FOR AN ABNORMAL CARDIAC MASS
Left atrium	Dilated coronary sinus (persistent left superior vena cava)
	Raphe between left superior pulmonary vein and left atrial appendage
	Atrial suture line after cardiac transplant
	Beam-width artifact from calcified aortic valve, aortic valve prosthesis, or other echogenic target adjacent to the atrium
	Interatrial septal aneurysm
Right atrium	Crista terminalis
	Chiari network (Eustachian valve remnants)
	Lipomatous hypertrophy of the interatrial septum
	Trabeculation of right atrial appendage
	Atrial suture line after cardiac transplant
	Pacer wire, Swan-Ganz catheter, or central venous line
Left ventricle	Papillary muscles
	Left ventricular web (aberrant chordae)
	Prominent apical trabeculations
	Prominent mitral annular calcification
Right ventricle	Moderator band
	Papillary muscles
	Swan-Ganz catheter or pacer wire
Aortic valve	Nodules of Arantius
	Lambl's excrescences
	Base of valve leaflet seen en face in diastole
Mitral valve	Redundant chordae
	Myxomatous mitral valve tissue
Pulmonary artery	Left atrial appendage (just caudal to pulmonary artery)
Pericardium	Epicardial adipose tissue
	Fibrinous debris in a chronic organized pericardial effusion

DISTINGUISHING CHARACTERISTICS OF INTRACARDIAC MASSES

CHARACTERISTIC	THROMBUS	TUMOR	VEGETATION
Location	LA (especially when enlarged or associated with MV disease)	LA (myxoma) Myocardium Pericardium	Usually valvular Occasionally on ventricular wall, pacer lead, or catheter tip
	LV (in setting of reduced systolic function or segmental wall abnormalities)	Valves	
Appearance	Usually discrete and somewhat spherical in shape *or* laminated against LV apex or LA wall	Various: may be circumscribed or may be irregular	Irregular shape, attached to the proximal (upstream) side of the valve with motion independent from the valve
Associated findings	Underlying etiology usually evident	Intracardiac obstruction depending on site of tumor	Valvular regurgitation usually present
	LV systolic dysfunction or segmental wall motion abnormalities (exception: eosinophilic heart disease)		Clinically: fevers, systemic signs of endocarditis, positive blood cultures
	MV disease with LA enlargement		

LA, *Left atrium;* LV, *left ventricle;* MV, *mitral valve.*

BASIC PRINCIPLES

- The first step in evaluation of a cardiac mass on echocardiography is to determine whether the findings are due to an ultrasound artifact or an actual anatomic finding (Fig. 15–1).
- A prominent normal cardiac structure or a normal anatomic variant may be mistaken for an abnormal mass.
- Ultrasound has limited utility for determination of tissue type; diagnosis of a cardiac mass is based on location, attachment, appearance, and any associated abnormalities.

Key points:

- ❏ Image quality for evaluation of a cardiac mass is optimized by using:
  - ❏ Highest transducer frequency with adequate tissue penetration
  - ❏ Acoustic access adjacent to the structure of interest (e.g., transthoracic apical for ventricular thrombi, transesophageal for atrial thrombi)
  - ❏ Visualization of the motion of the mass with the cardiac cycle
  - ❏ Use of a narrow sector and zoom mode once a mass is identified
  - ❏ Careful gain and processing adjustments (excessive or inadequate gain can obscure a mass)
  - ❏ Off-axis views from standard image planes
- ❏ A detailed knowledge of cardiac anatomy and normal variants allows recognition of structures that may mimic a cardiac mass.
- ❏ Echocardiography cannot identify the etiology of a cardiac mass based on appearance. A differential diagnosis for the echocardiographic finding is based on the location, appearance, size, mobility, physiologic effects, and other findings associated with the mass.
- ❏ Clinical data and other echocardiographic findings often provide clues about the identity of a cardiac mass (e.g., a left atrial mass in a patient with severe rheumatic mitral stenosis likely is an atrial thrombus).

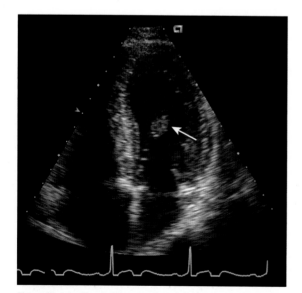

Figure 15–1 In this apical four-chamber view, an apparent mass is seen in the left ventricular chamber. Given the relationship of this mass to the anterior mitral leaflet, this most likely is a normal papillary muscle tip, seen in an oblique view. This diagnosis can be confirmed by scanning posteriorly to show its connection to the lateral left ventricular wall.

STEP-BY-STEP APPROACH

Left Atrial Thrombi

- Left atrial thrombi most often form in the atrial appendage, particularly in patients with atrial fibrillation (Fig. 15–2).
- Thrombi may be seen in the body of the left atrium with severe stasis of blood flow—for example, with mitral stenosis.
- Transesophageal echocardiography (TEE) is required to exclude left atrial thrombi when clinically indicated.

Key points:

- ❏ Transthoracic echocardiography is not sensitive for the diagnosis of left atrial thrombi because of the distance between the transducer and left atrium (limiting image quality at that depth) and the small size and atrial appendage location of most thrombi.
- ❏ The left atrial appendage may be visualized on transthoracic imaging in a parasternal short axis view or in an apical two-chamber view, but image quality often is limited.
- ❏ TEE images of the left atrial appendage are obtained from a high esophageal position. TEE evaluation includes:
  - ❏ Use of a high transducer frequency (typically 7 MHz)
  - ❏ A narrow image sector and zoom mode
  - ❏ Visualization in at least two orthogonal views, typically in views rotated to 0 degrees and 60 degrees
  - ❏ Pulsed Doppler recording of atrial appendage flow with the sample volume about 1 cm from the junction of the atrial appendage with the left atrial chamber
- ❏ The normal Doppler velocity with atrial contraction is more than 0.4 m/s; lower velocities in sinus rhythm suggest contractile dysfunction.
- ❏ The left atrial appendage has normal trabeculations that are distinguished from thrombi by their continuity with and echogenicity similar to the appendage wall and their lack of independent mobility (Fig. 15–3).

Left Ventricular Thrombi

- Left ventricular (LV) thrombus formation occurs in regions of blood flow stasis or low velocity flow.
- LV thrombi most often form in an akinetic or dyskinetic apex after myocardial infarction (Fig. 15–4).
- LV thrombi also are seen in patients with severely reduced LV systolic dysfunction.

Key points:

- ❏ Transthoracic echocardiography from the apical window is the optimal approach to

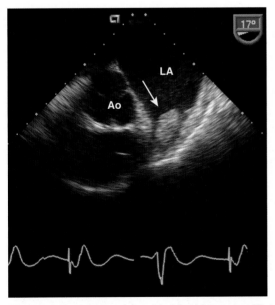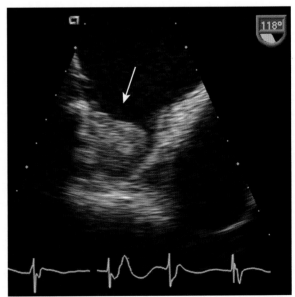

Figure 15–2 Transesophageal view of the left atrial appendage (A) shows an ovoid echodensity consistent with an atrial thrombus. B, This finding is confirmed in an orthogonal view at 118-degrees rotation using a magnified image.

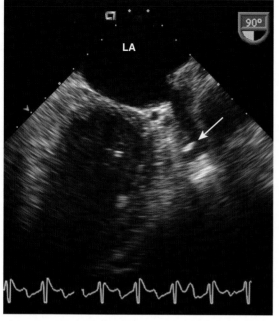

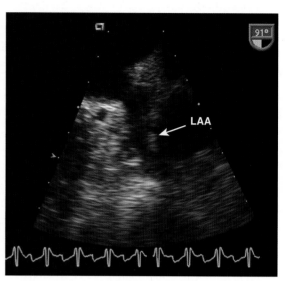

A

B

Figure 15–3 Transesophageal imaging of the left atrial appendage (*LAA*) at 90 degrees using a 7-MHz transducer frequency. *A,* There is a bright echo near the tip of the appendage that might be an atrial thrombus. *B,* In a close-up view, this echo appears to be a ridge attached to the wall of the appendage; thus it most likely is a prominent trabeculation.

detection of LV thrombi, with a sensitivity of 92% to 95% and a specificity of 86% to 88%.
- ❏ Detection of LV apical thrombi is enhanced by:
  - ❏ A steep left lateral decubitus patient position on a stretcher with an apical cutout
  - ❏ Use of a high transducer frequency (typically 5 to 7 MHz)
  - ❏ Standard and oblique image planes of the apex, especially medial angulation from a lateral transducer position
  - ❏ A shallow depth setting
- ❏ Myocardial trabeculations are differentiated from thrombi by their linear shape with an echodensity similar to and attachment to the myocardium (Fig. 15–5).
- ❏ Left-sided echo contrast is helpful in identifying thrombus when image quality is suboptimal.
- ❏ Transesophageal imaging is not sensitive for diagnosis of LV apical thrombi, because the apex is in the far field of the image and the true apex may not be included in the image plane.

Right Heart Thrombi

- ▪ Right atrial thrombi may be seen in patients with central lines that abrade the right atrial wall.
- ▪ Thrombi also may form on permanent pacer leads in the right atrium or ventricle.
- ▪ Peripheral venous thrombi may embolize to the right heart and become entangled in the tricuspid valve chords or a right atrial Chiari network (Fig. 15–6).

Key points:

- ❏ Normal echogenic structures in the right atrium that may be mistaken for a thrombus include:
  - ❏ Eustachian valve or Chiari network (Fig. 15–7)
  - ❏ Crista terminalis (Fig. 15–8A and B)
- ❏ Eustachian valves and Chiari networks are thin filamentous structures that extend from the region of the inferior vena cava toward the superior vena cava. The bright mobile echoes of a Chiari network may look similar to echo contrast in the right atrium.
- ❏ The right atrium and right ventricle are examined in parasternal short axis and right ventricular inflow views, in the apical four-chamber view, and from the subcostal window.
- ❏ Transesophageal imaging provides improved visualization of the right heart when thrombi are suspected.

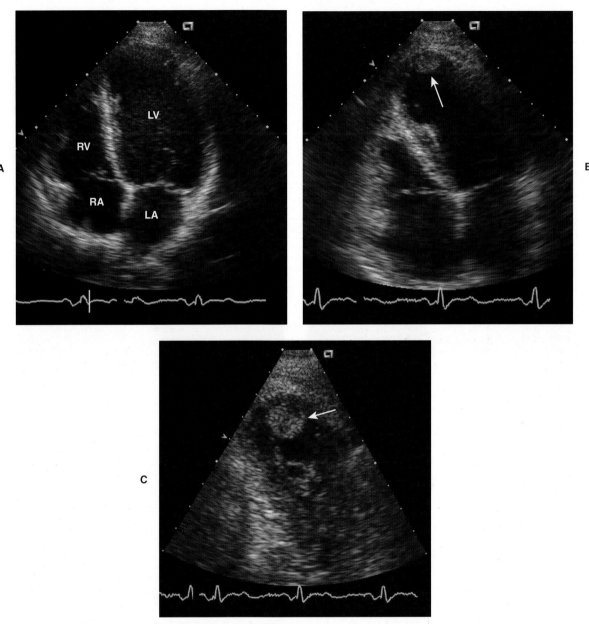

Figure 15–4 *A,* In the standard apical four-chamber view in the patient with a dilated cardiomyopathy, there is no evidence for thrombus formation in the akinetic apex, despite using harmonic imaging and a 4-MHz transducer frequency. *B,* However, with a slight decrease in depth, increase in gain, and posterior angulation of the image plane, a protruding apical thrombus now is evident. *C,* The apical thrombus is best seen at a shallower image depth with further posterior angulation of the image plane.

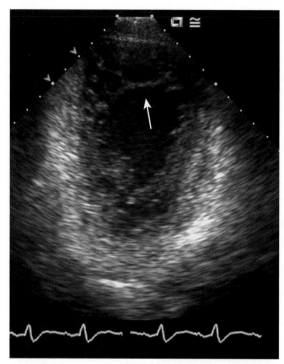

Figure 15–5 An echodensity was seen in the left ventricular apex. The transducer frequency was increased to 4 MHz, the focal depth decreased, and the transducer moved medially and angulated laterally from the apical position for further evaluation. The linear echo traversing the apex is consistent with prominent trabeculation, not thrombus, because it connected with myocardium at both ends.

Nonprimary Cardiac Tumors

- Nonprimary cardiac tumors are 20 times more common than primary cardiac tumors.
- Nonprimary tumors can involve the heart by:
  - Direct extension
  - Metastatic spread of disease
  - Production of biologically active substances
  - Side-effects related to treatment of the primary tumor
- Nonprimary cardiac tumors most often involve the pericardium but also may invade the myocardium. They rarely appear as intracardiac masses (Fig. 15–9).

Key points:

- The most common nonprimary cardiac tumors, in order of frequency, are:
  - Lung
  - Lymphoma
  - Breast
  - Leukemia
  - Stomach
  - Melanoma
  - Liver
  - Colon

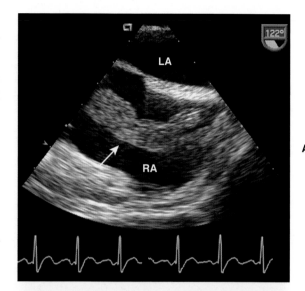
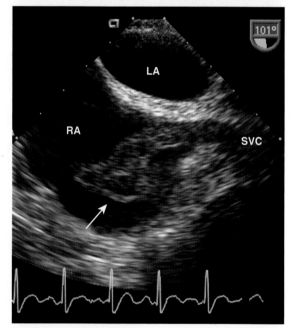

Figure 15–6 In this transesophageal echocardiography (TEE) long axis view of the right atrium, a large, echogenic, tubular, mobile mass is seen in the right atrium (*A*). Slight medial turning of the TEE probe (*B*) demonstrates that the mass originates from the region of the superior vena cava (*SVC*). By imaging in multiple planes, the attachment of this mass to a chronic indwelling catheter was demonstrated. The location, clinical setting, and appearance of the mass are most consistent with thrombus.

- All of these tumors may involve the pericardium by direct extension (breast, lung) or by metastatic spread, presenting with a pericardial effusion, sometimes with tamponade physiology. This is the most common cardiac presentation of tumor involvement (Fig. 15–10).

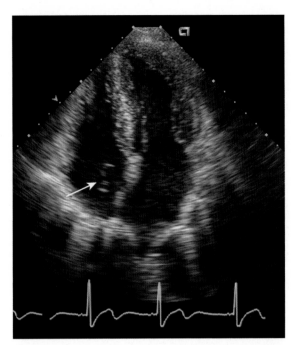

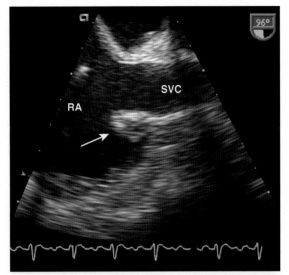

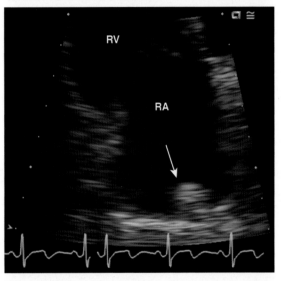

Figure 15–7 In an apical four-chamber view, several small echogenic targets are seen in the right atrium. In real time, these echoes showed chaotic motion, consistent with a Chiari network. A Chiari network consists of filamentous strands extending from the region of the inferior to the superior vena cava and represents a normal variant, most likely embryologic remnants. On transthoracic imaging, bright mobile echoes are seen in the right atrium, often best appreciated in parasternal right ventricular inflow and subcostal four-chamber views. On transesophageal echocardiography, the linear structure and attachments of the network are better appreciated.

□ Renal cell carcinoma may extend up the inferior vena cava into the right atrium and may be removed surgically "en bloc" with the primary tumor.

□ Carcinoid heart disease is characterized by thickening and shortening of the right-sided valve leaflets, resulting in pulmonic and tricuspid regurgitation.

□ Some chemotherapy affects the myocardium, so monitoring of ejection fraction by echocardiography often is needed in patients undergoing therapy.

□ Radiation therapy that includes cardiac structures in the treatment field may have very late (20 years or greater) adverse cardiac effects, including valve disease, accelerated coronary atherosclerosis, and myocardial fibrosis.

□ Transthoracic echocardiography (TTE) in standard views usually is adequate for evaluation of nonprimary cardiac tumors, but TEE provides improved image quality when needed.

Figure 15–8 This transesophageal long axis image (A) of the superior vena cava (SVC) and right atrium (RA) demonstrates the crista terminalis (arrow), the ridge at the junction of the trabeculated and smooth segments of the right atrial wall. The crista terminalis often is seen in the transthoracic apical four-chamber view (B) as a slight bump on the superior aspect of the right atrial wall.

Primary Cardiac Tumors

■ Primary cardiac tumors in adults usually are histologically benign.

■ Benign cardiac tumors result in adverse clinical outcomes as a result of:
□ Obstruction of blood flow
□ Embolization

■ Primary cardiac tumors most often present on echocardiography as an intracardiac mass.

A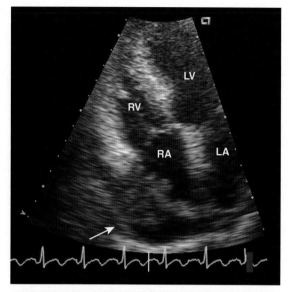

B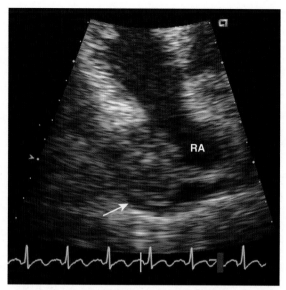

Figure 15–9 *A,* An apical four-chamber view shows an inhomogeneous mass either attached to or invading the right atrial free wall. *B,* A magnified view shows the anatomy in more detail but does not provide a tissue diagnosis. This mass clearly is not an artifact, thrombus, vegetation, or normal variant. A benign primary cardiac tumor is unlikely because the appearance is atypical for a myxoma or fibroma, given the apparent involvement of the atrial wall. Thus this most likely is a metastatic tumor to the heart or, less likely, a primary cardiac malignancy.

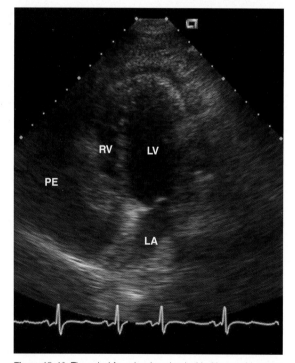

Figure 15–10 The apical four-chamber view in this 29-year-old woman with non-Hodgkin's lymphoma shows a large pericardial effusion (*PE*) that compresses the right ventricle (*RV*). The right atrium is nearly obliterated and could only be identified with color flow imaging. Cardiac tumors may present with an effusion, without a mass.

Key points:

❑ The most common primary cardiac tumors in adults, in order of frequency, are:
  ❑ Myxoma (Fig. 15–11)
  ❑ Pericardial cyst
  ❑ Lipoma
  ❑ Papillary fibroelastoma (Fig. 15–12)
  ❑ Angiosarcoma (malignant)
  ❑ Rhabdomyosarcoma (malignant)
❑ Myxomas most often are seen in the left atrium (75% of cases), attached by a narrow stalk to the center of the interatrial septum. Myxomas less often are seen in the right atrium and left and right ventricle.
❑ A pericardial cyst is a single-lobed or multi-lobed sac lined by mesothelium that communicates with the pericardial space. Pericardial cysts are rare but, when present, most often are seen adjacent to the right atrium.
❑ Papillary fibroelastomas typically are small masses attached to the downstream side of a cardiac valve. The appearance is similar to a vegetation (except that vegetations usually are on the upstream side of the valve), but blood cultures are negative and clinical signs of endocarditis are absent.
❑ Lipomatous hypertrophy of the interatrial septum is common with a typical appearance of sparing of the fossa ovalis. If in doubt, computed tomographic imaging confirms adipose tissue.

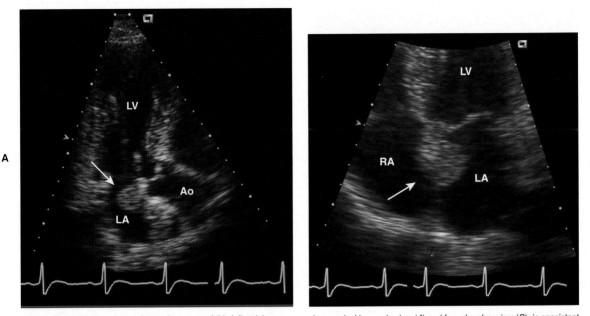

Figure 15–11 The location and smooth contour of this left atrial mass, seen in an apical long axis view (*A*) and four-chamber view (*B*), is consistent with an atrial myxoma.

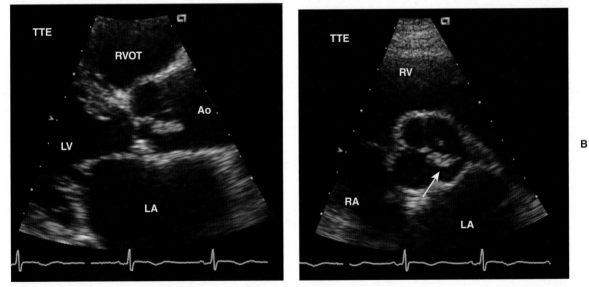

Figure 15–12 On transthoracic echocardiography (*TTE*), a mobile mass of echoes attached to the aortic valve leaflets is seen in long axis (*A*) and short axis (*B*) views. This patient had no clinical evidence of infective endocarditis and no evidence for a systemic inflammatory disease, so the most likely diagnosis is a papillary fibroelastoma. *RVOT,* Right ventricular outflow tract.

❑ Malignant primary cardiac tumors are rare, usually seen as an intracardiac mass.
❑ The goals of echocardiography in patients with a cardiac tumor are:
 ❑ Define the location and extent of tumor involvement
 ❑ Evaluate obstruction or regurgitation caused by the tumor

❑ Evaluate any associated pericardial effusion and signs of tamponade
❑ Often both transthoracic and transesophageal imaging are needed to fully evaluate a cardiac tumor. Masses located in the left atrium may be missed on transthoracic imaging (Fig. 15–13).

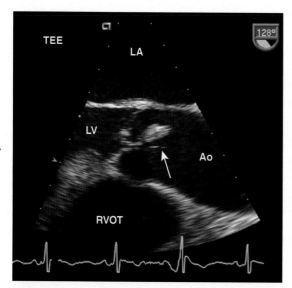
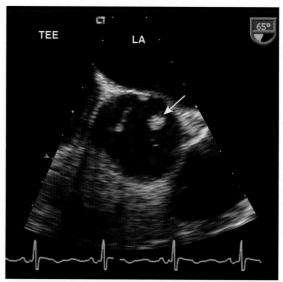

Figure 15–13 In the same patient as Figure 15–12, transesophageal echocardiography (*TEE*) in long (*A*) and short (*B*) axis views of the aortic valve appear similar to the transthoracic views, although image quality is improved because of use of a 7-MHz TEE transducer. *RVOT,* Right ventricular outflow tract.

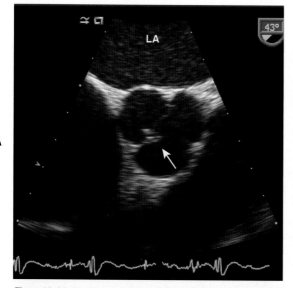
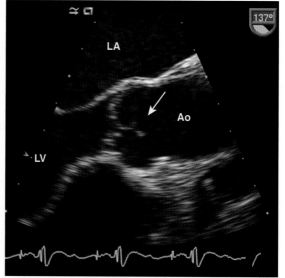

Figure 15–14 A small mass is seen on the aortic side of the valve on this transesophageal short axis image (*A*), with the long axis view (*B*) showing small masses at the leaflet base and at the leaflet tip. These masses showed independent motion in real time suggestive of vegetations. The patient had no clinical signs of endocarditis, and blood cultures were negative, so these findings may be due to nonbacterial thrombotic endocarditis.

Vegetations

- Vegetations are infected or noninfected masses of platelets and fibrin debris, typically attached to a valve leaflet.
- The vegetations of nonbacterial thrombotic endocarditis (NBTE) are small and attached to the downstream (compared with upstream with infective vegetations) side of the valve (Fig. 15–14).
- Infective vegetations are discussed in Chapter 14.

Key points:

- The most critical step in evaluation of a patient with an intracardiac mass, especially a valve vegetation, is to obtain blood cultures for possible infective endocarditis.
- Like infective endocarditis, nonbacterial thrombotic endocarditis is diagnosed based on a combination of clinical and echocardiographic findings.

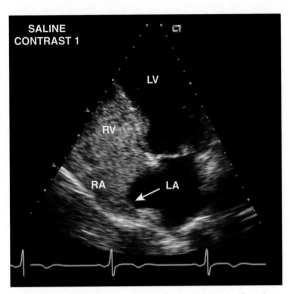

Figure 15–15 An atrial septal aneurysm is seen in this apical four-chamber view with saline contrast used to opacify the right heart. The atrial septum deviates from left to right in the region of the fossa ovalis with a radius of more than 2 cm at the maximum curvature point.

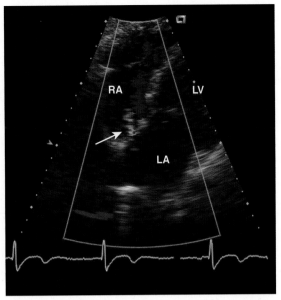

Figure 15–16 Color Doppler in an apical four-chamber view demonstrates a small jet of flow from left to right across the interatrial septum consistent with a patent foramen ovale. The direction of shunting depends on the relative right and left atrial pressures.

❏ TEE is more accurate for diagnosis of nonbacterial valve vegetations compared with transthoracic imaging.

❏ Valve involvement by noninfected vegetations is seen in patients with systemic inflammatory diseases (e.g., systemic lupus erythematosus) and some malignancies.

Patent Foramen Ovale

■ A small communication (patent foramen ovale) between the right and left atrium is present in 20% to 30% of adults.

■ A patent foramen ovale is associated with a contour abnormality of the septum with bulging from the midline larger than 15 mm (atrial septal aneurysm) in some patients (Fig. 15–15).

■ There is a higher prevalence of patent foramen ovale in patients with a cryptogenic stroke.

Key points:

❏ Shunting at the atrial level is sometimes seen with color Doppler but often requires a saline contrast injection for detection (Figs. 15–16 and 15–17).

❏ A patent foramen ovale allows blood flow from the right to left atrium when right atrial pressure exceeds left atrial pressure. In some patients, shunting occurs at rest; in others, a right to left shunt is seen only after a Valsalva

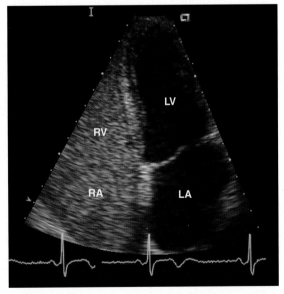

Figure 15–17 Saline contrast study in an apical four-chamber view in a patient with a systemic embolic event shows no evidence for contrast in the left heart, indicating the absence of a patent foramen ovale.

maneuver to transiently increase right atrial pressure.

❏ Appearance of echocontrast in the left atrium within 1 to 3 beats of right heart opacification is consistent with a patent foramen ovale. Later appearance of contrast may be due to transpulmonary passage.

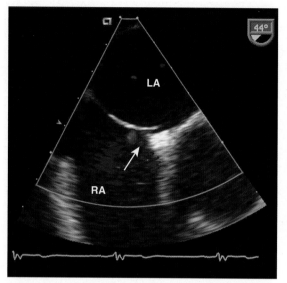 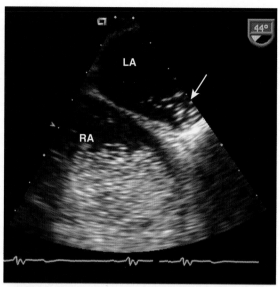

A

B

Figure 15–18 *A,* Transesophageal echocardiography in a patient with a cryptogenic stroke shows the typical "flap valve" appearance of a patent foramen ovale, with color Doppler demonstrating a narrow red flow signal in the slit-like orifice. *B,* With peripheral injection of saline contrast, there is prompt appearance of microbubbles in the left atrium (*arrow*) on the first cardiac cycle, consistent with passage across a patent foramen ovale.

❑ TEE is more sensitive than transthoracic imaging for detection of a patent foramen ovale (Fig. 15–18).

❑ In patients with chronically elevated right atrial pressures (such as severe pulmonary hypertension with right heart failure), persistent right to left shunting may result in arterial oxygen desaturation.

❑ Echocardiography (transesophageal or intracardiac) can be used to guide percutaneous closure of a patent foramen ovale (Fig. 15–19).

Evaluation for a Cardiac Source of Embolus

■ Echocardiography requested to evaluate for a cardiac source of embolus should include a saline contrast study for detection of patent foramen ovale.

■ A careful examination for cardiac thrombi, tumors, valvular vegetations, and aortic atheroma, often with TEE, is needed when a cardiac source of embolus is suspected.

Key points:

❑ If atrial fibrillation is present, a left atrial thrombus is a likely cause of clinical events, even if not detected on TEE.

❑ Embolic events in patients with mechanical prosthetic valves must be presumed to be related to the prosthetic valve, regardless of echocardiographic findings.

❑ Aortic atheroma, detected on TEE, are associated with an increased prevalence of embolic events.

❑ Transesophageal echocardiography is used to evaluate for a cardiac source of embolus in patients with:
  ❑ Abrupt occlusion of a major peripheral or visceral artery
  ❑ Cerebrovascular embolic events in patients younger than 45 years
  ❑ Cerebrovascular events without other evident causes in patients of any age
  ❑ Whenever clinical management would be altered based on the echocardiographic findings

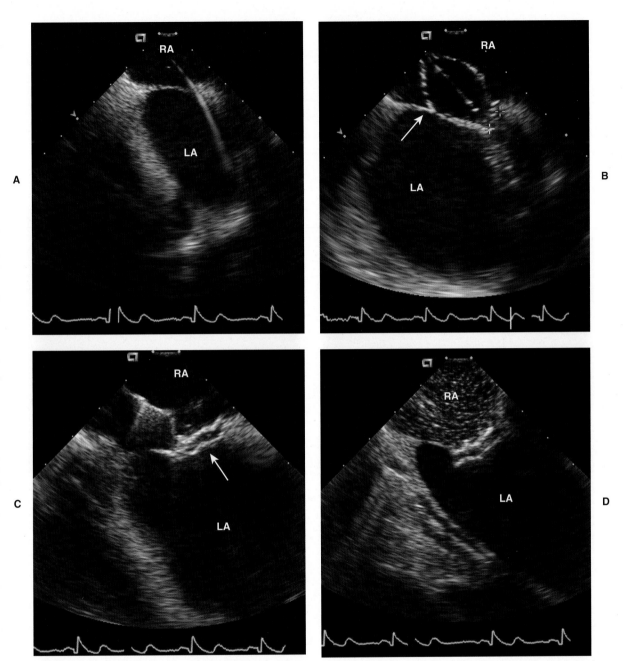

Figure 15–19 Intracardiac echocardiographic (ICE) guidance of percutaneous closure of a patent foramen ovale. The transducer tip (top of the sector) is in the right atrium (*RA*), with the septum in the mid-field and the left atrium (*LA*) in the far field of the images. *A,* The guiding catheter has been passed through the patent foramen ovale. *B,* A sizing balloon is inflated to measure the defect size. *C,* The closure device is in position but still attached to the catheter seen in the right atrium (*RA*). *D,* The guiding catheter has been removed and contrast injected into the right heart. The parallel linear echoes of the closure device are seen positioned on the atrial septum with no evidence for residual shunting.

QUESTION 1

The apical four-chamber view of a patient with an embolic stroke shown in Figure 15–20 demonstrates:

- A. No abnormalities
- B. Patent foramen ovale
- C. Atrial septal aneurysm
- D. Atrial septal defect
- E. Chiari network

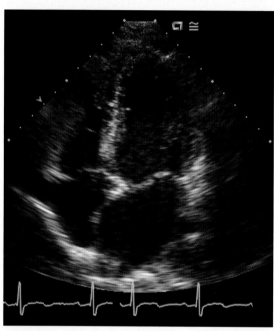

Figure 15–20

QUESTION 2

The transesophageal image shown in Figure 15–21 was obtained for a 54-year-old man with a cryptogenic stroke. These images are consistent with:

- A. Aortic atheroma
- B. Left atrial appendage thrombus
- C. Papillary fibroelastoma
- D. Patent foramen ovale
- E. Mitral valve prolapse

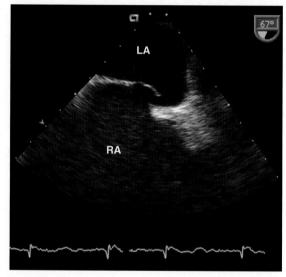

Figure 15–21

QUESTION 3

Figure 15–22 shows:

A. Atrial myxoma
B. Lipomatous hypertrophy of the interatrial septum
C. Eustachian valve
D. Atrial thrombus
E. Atrial septal occluder device

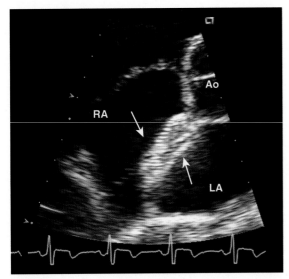

Figure 15–22

QUESTION 4

The echocardiographic image in Figure 15–23 was recorded from a 63-year-old obese woman who presented with acute shortness of breath. The rest of her echocardiographic images were unremarkable. The most likely cause of her shortness of breath is:

A. Pulmonary embolus
B. Cardiac tamponade
C. Left ventricular systolic dysfunction
D. Primary pulmonary disease
E. Aortic dissection

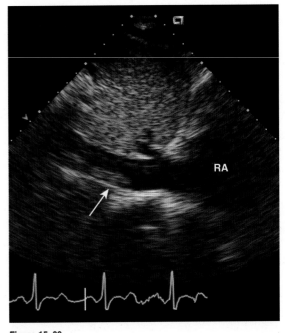

Figure 15–23

QUESTION 5

Transesophageal echocardiography was requested before an atrial flutter ablation procedure in this 62-year-old woman with a restrictive cardiomyopathy. The transesophageal view (Fig. 15–24) of the left atrial appendage is shown. The most appropriate next step in management of this patient is:

A. Proceed with atrial flutter ablation
B. Repeat TEE after 24 hours of intravenous heparin
C. Repeat TEE after 4 weeks of warfarin
D. Obtain other views of the atrial appendage
E. Record images using a higher transducer frequency

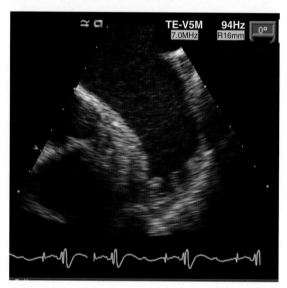

Figure 15–24

QUESTION 6

What is the structure indicated by the arrow in the transesophageal long axis view shown in Figure 15–25?

A. Right pulmonary artery
B. Pericardial effusion
C. Paravalvular abscess
D. Right atrial appendage
E. Superior vena cava

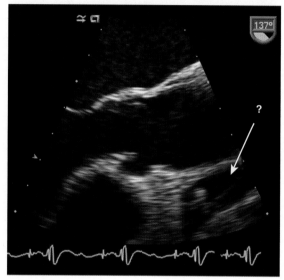

Figure 15–25

QUESTION 7

The transesophageal image in Figure 15–26 shows:

   A. Atrial myxoma
   B. Atrial septal defect
   C. Chiari network
   D. Persistent left superior vena cava
   E. Cor triatriatum

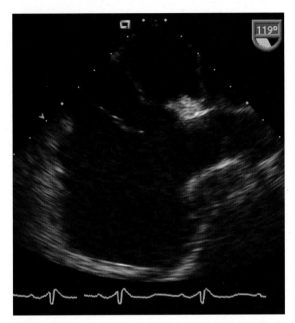

Figure 15–26

QUESTION 8

TEE was requested to evaluate for left atrial thrombus in a 61-year-old woman with a restrictive cardiomyopathy of unknown etiology. While examining the atrial appendage, a small echolucent structure was seen between the appendage (LAA) and left superior pulmonary vein (LSPV) with evidence of flow using color Doppler. Based on the pulsed Doppler signal in Figure 15–27, the echolucent structure most likely represents:

   A. Vascular tumor
   B. Pulmonary artery branch
   C. Coronary artery
   D. Pulmonary vein branch
   E. Persistent left superior vena cava

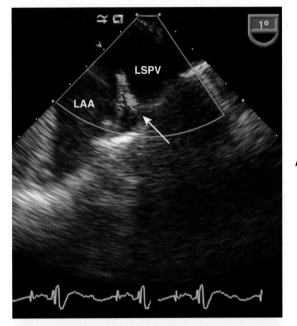

A

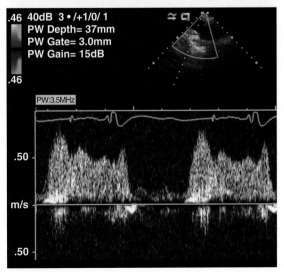

B

Figure 15–27

ANSWERS

ANSWER 1: A

In this apical four-chamber view, the atrial septum appears intact with slight bowing from left to right consistent with the normal hemodynamics of left atrial pressure slightly higher than right atrial pressure. The definition of an atrial septal aneurysm is deviation by 1.5 cm or more, which this image does not demonstrate. A patent foramen ovale may or may not be present, but diagnosis requires color Doppler and a saline contrast injection. If a secundum or primum atrial septal defect were present, the right heart chambers would be enlarged, and there would be discontinuity in the atrial septum. With a sinus venosus atrial septal defect, the septum might appear intact in this view, but the right heart would still be enlarged. There are no bright echoes in the right atrium to suggest a Chiari network.

ANSWER 2: D

These images show the interatrial septum with a slight discontinuity in the region of the foramen ovale. Color flow (Fig. 15–28) demonstrates right to left flow through this defect. A systematic and comprehensive TEE examination in this patient also would include imaging to exclude aortic atheroma, left atrial thrombus, papillary fibroelastoma, and mitral valve prolapse, because these cardiac findings also are associated with an increased risk of embolic events.

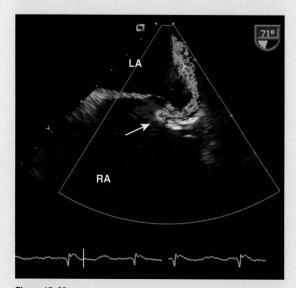

Figure 15–28

ANSWER 3: E

This transthoracic short axis view at the aortic valve level shows thickening and increased echogenicity in the interatrial septum. The bright parallel lines with regularly spaced echoes are consistent with artificial material, in this case, an atrial septal occluder device. The device is in the expected position. An atrial myxoma would be less echodense and protrude into the cardiac chamber. Lipomatous hypertrophy can be very echogenic but typically spares the fossa ovalis. An atrial thrombus could form along the atrial septum but would be less echogenic.

ANSWER 4: A

This subcostal view of the inferior vena cava (note the hepatic vein and entrance into the right atrium) shows a tubular echodensity in the lumen, suggestive of thrombus. Given this finding, it is likely that pulmonary embolism is the cause of acute shortness of breath. Cardiac tamponade occurs with a pericardial effusion, which should be visible in this view. Left ventricular systolic dysfunction would be evident on other 2D images. Primary pulmonary disease is not associated with deep venous thrombosis, as seen here. Aortic dissection typically presents with pain, rather than shortness of breath. On subcostal views, the aorta is posterior to the inferior vena cava and takes a more posterior course at the superior aspect of the image.

ANSWER 5: D

This view of the atrial appendage was correctly obtained with a 7-MHz transducer frequency and using a magnified view with the appendage centered in the image. The images show ridges in the tip of the triangular-shaped appendage that may be trabeculations, but it is difficult to exclude thrombus. Because 7 MHz already is the highest transducer frequency available with most TEE probes, the most useful maneuver is to obtain another view of the atrial appendage to see if the ridges connect to the wall or if there are areas more suggestive of thrombus. In Figure 15–29, a view at 58-degrees rotation in this patient shows a globular mass in the tip of the appendage, suggestive of thrombus. In addition, this patient had prominent spontaneous contrast in the atrial appendage and body of the left atrium, and the

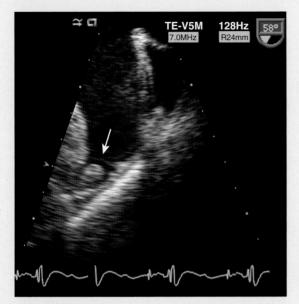

Figure 15–29

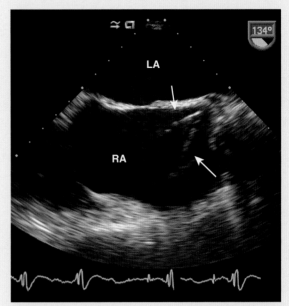

Figure 15–31

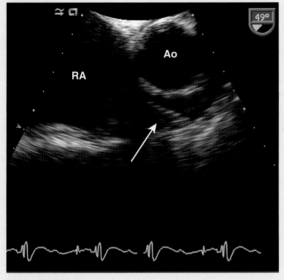

Figure 15–30

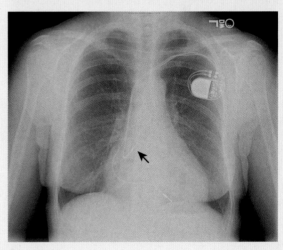

Figure 15–32

atrial flow velocity in the appendage was only 0.1 m/s (normal is more than 0.4 m/s).

ANSWER 6: D

This image shows (from posterior to anterior) the left atrium ascending aorta and right atrial appendage. Although it is unusual to recognize the atrial appendage in this view, the right atrial appendage is positioned just anterior to the aorta. Recognition was facilitated in this patient by the presence of right atrial pacer leads (the bright echo in the echolucent cavity). The pacer lead

could be followed by rotating the image plane (Fig. 15–30) to 49 degrees, showing the typical repetitive parallel echoes (*arrow*) of a pacer lead extending into the right atrial appendage, or by turning the probe rightward, while in the long axis view (Fig. 15–31) at 134 degrees, to show the lead entering the right atrium via the superior vena cava and then curving into the appendage. Her chest radiograph (Fig. 15–32) shows the position of the lead tip (*arrow*) in the right atrial appendage.

The right pulmonary artery would be seen posterior to the aorta and is cephalad to the superior edge of the image in this patient. A pericardial effusion rarely extends posteriorly around the base of the aortic root and pulmonary artery in the transverse sinus of the pericardium. A paravalvular abscess typically is located in the aortic annulus region. The superior vena cava runs parallel and lateral to the aorta, not anteriorly.

atrial membrane with cor triatriatum (which is more common in the left but can occur in the right atrium) typically traverses the atrium from the edge of the fossa ovalis on the septum to the lateral wall.

ANSWER 7: C

This is a TEE long axis view of the superior vena cava and right atrium showing a linear echo that arises from the junction of the inferior vena cava and right atrium. It is most consistent with a Chiari network. The term *Eustachian valve* is used for a small localized membrane at the inferior vena caval junction, and the term *Chiari network* is used when it extends (often with fenestrations) from the inferior vena cava to the superior vena cava. However, there is a range of sizes between these two extremes, as seen in this case. An atrial myxoma typically is a rounded mass, and an atrial septal defect would not be seen in this view. A persistent left superior vena cava usually is diagnosed based on a dilated coronary sinus. The

ANSWER 8: C

The Doppler signal shows low velocity (0.6 m/s) diastolic flow, which is most consistent with coronary artery flow, most likely the circumflex coronary artery, which lies in this area. A vascular tumor is unlikely and would have an arterial flow pattern, as would a pulmonary artery branch. A pulmonary vein branch would have the typical systolic and diastolic inflow patterns. A persistent left superior vena cava would have a venous flow pattern with systolic and diastolic inflow. This case exemplifies the additional value of the Doppler waveform in identification of unknown structures seen during an examination. The electrocardiogram shows an atrial paced rhythm.

NOTES

16 Echocardiographic Evaluation of the Great Vessels

THE ECHO EXAM: DISEASE OF THE GREAT VESSELS

EXAMINATION OF THE AORTA

AORTIC SEGMENT	MODALITY	VIEW	RECORDING	LIMITATIONS
Aortic root	TTE	Parasternal long axis	Images of sinuses of Valsalva, aortic annulus, and sinotubular junction	Shadowing of posterior aortic root
	TEE	High esophageal long axis	Standard long axis plane by rotating to about 120-130 degrees	
Ascending	TTE	Parasternal long axis	Move transducer superiorly to image sinotubular junction and ascending aorta.	Only limited segments visualized, variable between patients
	TTE Doppler	Apical	LVOT and ascending aorta flow recorded with pulsed or CW Doppler from an anteriorly angulated four-chamber view	Velocity underestimation if the angle between the Doppler beam and flow is not parallel
	TEE	High esophageal long axis	From long axis view, move transducer superiorly to image ascending aorta.	The distal ascending aorta may not be visualized.
Arch	TTE	Suprasternal	Long and short axis views of aortic arch	Descending aorta appears to taper as it leaves the image plane.
	TEE	High esophageal	From the short axis view of the initial segment of the descending thoracic aorta, turn the probe toward the patient's right side and angulate inferiorly.	View not obtained in all patients. The aortic segment at the junction of the ascending aorta and arch may not be visualized.
Descending thoracic	TTE	Parastenal and modified apical views	Rotate from long axis view to image thoracic aorta in long axis posterior to left ventricle or left atrium. From apical two-chamber view, use lateral angulation and clockwise rotation to image aorta.	Depth of thoracic aorta on TTE limits image quality. TEE usually needed for diagnosis.
	TTE Doppler	Suprasternal	Descending aorta flow recorded with pulsed Doppler from SSN view	Low wall filters needed to evaluate for holodiastolic flow reversal.
Proximal abdominal	TTE	Subcostal	Long axis of proximal abdominal aorta	Only the proximal segment is visualized.
	TTE Doppler	Transgastric	Proximal abdominal aorta flow recorded with pulsed Doppler	Low wall filters are needed to evaluate for holodiastolic flow reversal.
	TEE	Transgastric	From the transgastric position, portions of the abdominal aorta may be seen posteriorly.	Does not allow evaluation of entire abdominal aorta.

CW, *Continuous wave;* LVOT, *left ventricular outflow tract;* SSN, *suprasternal notch;* TEE, *transesophageal echocardiography;* TTE, *transthoracic echocardiography.*

AORTIC DISSECTION

Dissection Flap
  In aortic lumen
  Independent motion
  True and false lumen
  Entry sites
  Thrombosis of false lumen
Indirect Findings
  Aortic dilation
  Aortic regurgitation
  Coronary ostial involvement
  Pericardial effusion

COMPLICATIONS OF THORACIC AORTIC DISSECTION

Aortic valve regurgitation
  Due to aortic root dilation
  Due to leaflet flail
Coronary artery occlusion due to dissection at the orifice
  Ventricular fibrillation
  Acute myocardial infarction
Distal vessel obstruction or occlusion
  Carotid (stroke)
  Subclavian (upper limb ischemia)

COMPLICATIONS OF THORACIC AORTIC DISSECTION—cont'd

Aortic rupture
  Into the pericardium
    Pericardial effusion
    Pericardial tamponade
  Into the mediastinum
  Into the pleural space
    Pleural effusion
    Exsanguination

SINUS OF VALSALVA ANEURYSM

Congenital
  Complex shape
  Protrusion into RVOT
  Fenestrations
Acquired
  Infection or inflammation
  Symmetric shape
  Communication with aorta
  Potential for rupture

AORTIC ATHEROMA

Complex ($\geq$4 mm or mobile)
Associated with
  Coronary artery disease
  Cerebroembolic events

RVOT, *Right ventricular outflow tract.*

BASIC PRINCIPLES

- A systematic approach is needed for echocardiographic evaluation of the great vessels.
- Transesophageal imaging is more sensitive than transthoracic imaging for detection of aortic aneurysm and dissection.
- Wider field of view tomographic imaging techniques, including chest computed tomography (CT) or cardiac magnetic resonance (CMR) imaging, provide optimal evaluation of the great vessels.

Key points:

- ❏ Many segments of the aorta and pulmonary artery can be visualized on transthoracic imaging, but:
  - ❏ Evaluation of branch pulmonary arteries and the branching of systemic arteries from the aorta often is not possible.
  - ❏ Ultrasound imaging artifacts must be distinguished from an intraluminal dissection flap.
- ❏ The term "aortic root" includes the aortic annulus, sinuses of Valsalva, sinotubular junction, and ascending aorta.
- ❏ When the echocardiogram is nondiagnostic or equivocal, additional imaging techniques should be recommended, based on the clinical signs and symptoms.

STEP-BY-STEP APPROACH

Transthoracic Echocardiography

- Examination of the aorta is based on visualization of several segments from different acoustic windows.
- The sequence suggested here follows the sequence of the standard transthoracic study; other exam sequences may be appropriate with an acute clinical presentation.

Step 1: Record Blood Pressure and Ensure the Patient Is Medically Stable

- Aortic disease often presents as a medical/surgical emergency, so appropriately trained health care providers should be available during the study.
- Blood pressure is recorded at the beginning of the study, because findings may change with altered loading conditions.

Key points:

- ❏ When time is of the essence, limited imaging and Doppler data should be focused on the specific clinical question.

- ❏ It may be appropriate to proceed directly to transesophageal imaging when aortic dissection is suspected; the echocardiographer should consult with the referring provider to ensure the most appropriate test is performed in a timely manner.

Step 2: Assess the Aortic Root from the Parasternal Window

- The aortic root is seen in the standard and high parasternal long axis view (Figs. 16–1 and 16–2).
- Diameter measurements typically are reported at end-diastole for the aortic annulus, sinuses of Valsalva, sinotubular junction, and in the mid-ascending aorta (Fig. 16–3).
- Color Doppler allows detection of aortic regurgitation and evaluation of the flow pattern in the ascending aorta.

Key points:

- ❏ After recording the standard parasternal long axis view of the aortic root, the transducer is moved up one or more interspaces to visualize as much of the ascending aorta as possible.
- ❏ The sinotubular junction is defined as the top of the sinuses of Valsalva and is recognized by the acute angle at the transition from the curved sinuses to the tubular ascending aorta.

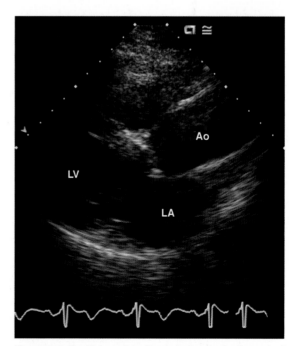

Figure 16–1 Standard parasternal long axis view showing the proximal ascending aorta.

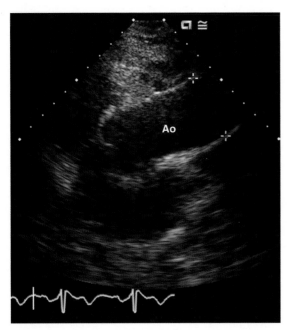

Figure 16–2 In the same patient as Figure 16–1, additional segments of the ascending aorta are seen when the transducer is moved cephalad one or two interspaces.

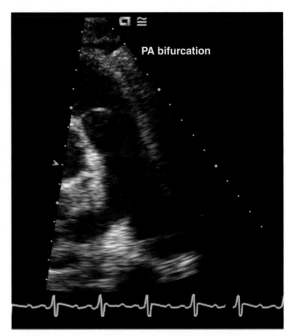

Figure 16–4 In the parasternal short axis view of the aortic valve, the pulmonary artery (*PA*) is seen. Often the lateral wall is difficult to delineate in adults.

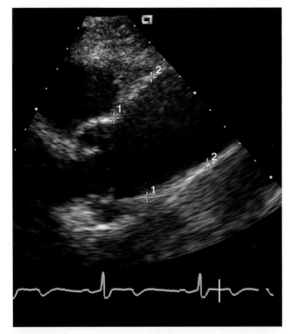

Figure 16–3 In addition to standard measurement at the annulus and sinuses of Valsalva, the sinotubular junction (1) and midascending aorta (2) are measured when the aorta is dilated.

- ◻ Aortic dimensions also may be measured in systole or at the largest diameter during the cardiac cycle.
- ◻ Comparison of measurements on serial studies or by different modalities should be at the same time point in the cardiac cycle.

Step 3: Assess the Pulmonary Artery from the Parasternal Window

- ▪ The pulmonary artery is visualized in the short axis view by angulation superiorly to demonstrate the bifurcation of the main pulmonary artery (Fig. 16–4).
- ▪ Images also can be obtained in the right ventricular outflow view.
- ▪ Color, pulsed, and continuous wave Doppler allow detection of pulmonic regurgitation and abnormal pulmonary artery flow patterns.

Key points:

- ◻ In adults, visualization of the lateral wall of the pulmonary artery is difficult because the acoustic window is limited by the adjacent lung.
- ◻ Pulmonary artery diameter measurements are mainly helpful in adults with congenital heart disease and may be better made by other imaging techniques (such as CT or CMR imaging).
- ◻ A small amount of pulmonic regurgitation is normal and is characterized by a narrow jet on color Doppler and a low intensity, low velocity spectral Doppler signal.
- ◻ With pulmonary hypertension, the pulmonic regurgitant velocity is increased, reflecting the elevation of pulmonary diastolic pressure. The antegrade systolic flow shows a

shortened time to peak velocity and mid-systolic deceleration.

❑ With branch pulmonary artery stenosis, a high velocity signal may be detected with spectral Doppler, even when image quality is suboptimal (Fig. 16–5).

❑ With a patent ductus arteriosus, the continuous systolic and diastolic flow from the descending aorta into the pulmonary artery is seen with color and spectral Doppler.

❑ Full evaluation of the main pulmonary artery and branches in patients with congenital heart disease usually requires CMR or CT imaging.

Step 4: Assess the Descending Thoracic Aorta from the Parasternal and Apical Window

■ The mid-portion of the descending thoracic aorta can be visualized from the parasternal long axis view, posterior to the left atrium, by rotating the image plane to obtain a longitudinal view of the aorta (Fig. 16–6).

■ The descending thoracic aorta also can be imaged from the apical two-chamber view by lateral angulation of the image plane (Fig. 16–7).

■ Color Doppler is helpful in distinguishing image artifacts from an intraluminal flap in these views.

Key points:

❑ Dilation of the descending aorta and dissection flaps can be identified in these views when image quality is adequate.

❑ Only some segments of the descending thoracic aorta are visualized, so significant pathology may be missed.

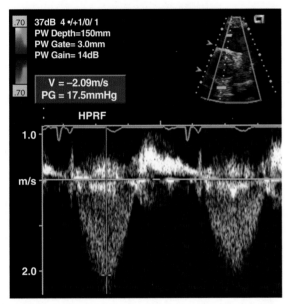

Figure 16–5 Stenosis of the distal right pulmonary artery in this patient with a repaired tetralogy of Fallot is demonstrated using high pulse repetition frequency Doppler to localize the origin of the high velocity jet.

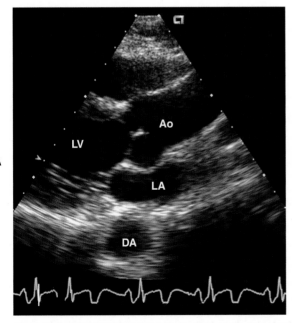

A

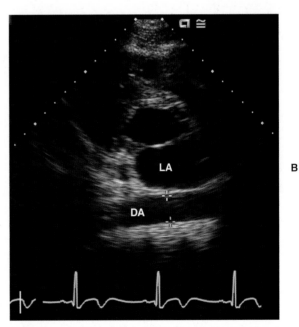

B

Figure 16–6 A, Parasternal long axis view in a Marfan patient showing the descending aorta (DA) posterior to the left atrium. B, A long axis view of the descending thoracic aorta can be obtained by rotating the transducer clockwise into a parasternal short axis plane.

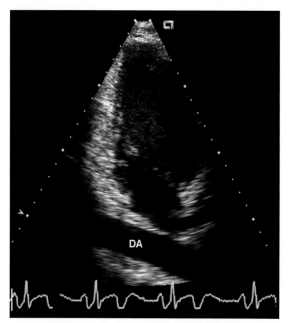

Figure 16–7 Another segment of the descending thoracic aorta (*DA*) is imaged in the same patient as Figure 16–6 from the apical two-chamber view with lateral angulation of the image plane.

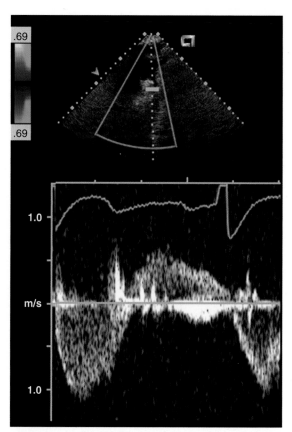

Figure 16–9 In a patient with severe aortic regurgitation, holodiastolic flow is seen in the descending thoracic aorta. The diastolic flow signal is above the baseline from the end of ejection up to the start of the next ejection period.

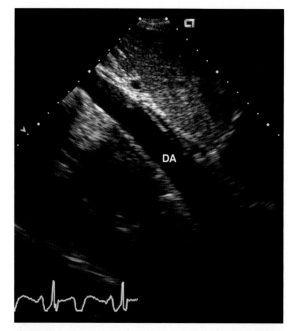

Figure 16–8 The proximal abdominal aorta seen from the subcostal window. *DA,* Descending aorta.

❐ The aorta is in the far field of the image in these views, limiting evaluation for aortic atheroma.

❐ In patients with a large left pleural effusion, the descending aorta can be imaged from the posterior chest wall, using the pleural effusion as an acoustic window.

Step 5: Assess the Proximal Abdominal Aorta from the Subcostal Window

■ The proximal abdominal aorta is seen in the subcostal view by slight lateral angulation from the inferior vena cava image plane (Fig. 16–8).

■ Holodiastolic flow reversal is seen in the proximal abdominal aorta in patients with severe aortic valve regurgitation (Fig. 16–9).

Key points:

❐ Diameter of the proximal abdominal aorta is routinely measured in patients with aortic disease, such as Marfan syndrome.

❐ With a normal pattern of flow, antegrade systolic flow is followed by early diastolic flow reversal, mid-diastolic low velocity antegrade flow, and a very brief late diastolic flow signal resulting from elastic recoil of the aorta (Fig. 16–10).

❐ To detect the holodiastolic flow reversal seen with severe aortic regurgitation, the filters are adjusted to show low velocity flow.

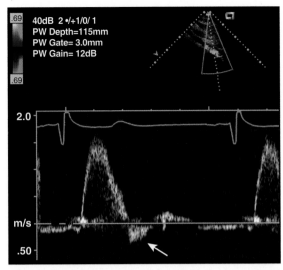

Figure 16–10 Normal flow in the proximal abdominal aorta is characterized by antegrade flow in systole, brief early diastolic reversal (*arrow*), low velocity forward flow in mid–diastole, and then a slight flow reversal at end-diastole.

❑ Holodiastolic flow reversal also is seen with other aortic diastolic flow abnormalities, such as a patent ductus arteriosus, surgical systemic–to–pulmonary shunt (e.g., Blalock Taussing shunt), or aorto-pulmonary window.

Step 6: Assess the Aortic Arch and Proximal Descending Thoracic Aorta from the Suprasternal Notch Window

■ The aortic arch is visualized in long and short axis views from the suprasternal notch window (Fig. 16–11).
■ Pulsed Doppler recordings of flow in the proximal descending thoracic aorta show holodiastolic flow reversal when moderate to severe aortic regurgitation is present (Fig. 16–12).

Key points:

❑ The aortic arch is measured in its midsection, where the ultrasound beam is perpendicular to the aortic walls.
❑ The descending aorta appears to "taper," even when normal, because of the oblique plane of the ultrasound image compared with the curvature of the aorta.
❑ The distance from the aortic valve that holodiastolic flow reversal persists correlates with regurgitant severity. Thus reversal in the proximal descending aorta is seen with moderate regurgitation, but reversal in the abdominal aorta indicates severe regurgitation.
❑ The right pulmonary artery is seen in cross section, under the arch, in the long axis view of the aortic arch.

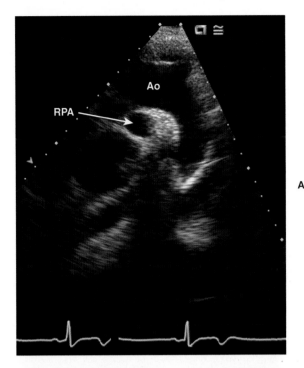

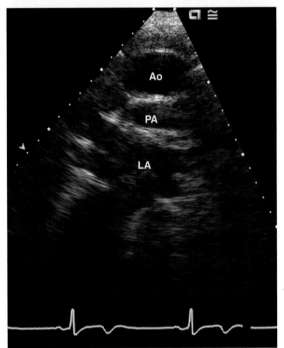

Figure 16–11 The long axis view of the aortic arch (*A*) shows segments of the ascending and descending thoracic aorta, the arch, and the origins of the head and neck vessels. The right pulmonary artery (*RPA*) is seen under the curve of the arch. In the short axis view of the arch (*B*), the left atrium (*LA*) and pulmonary veins are seen inferior to the right pulmonary artery (*PA*).

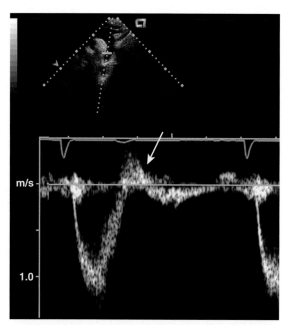

Figure 16–12 Normal flow in the descending thoracic aorta shows early diastolic flow reversal (corresponding to diastolic coronary blood flow, *arrow*), low velocity forward flow in mid-diastole, and slight reversal at end-diastole. This patient had no aortic regurgitation.

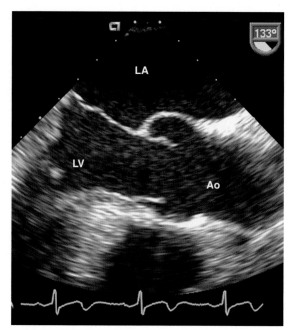

Figure 16–13 A long axis view of the ascending aorta is obtained by transesophageal echocardiography at about 120 to 140 degrees rotation, with the probe withdrawn in the esophagus to see the ascending aorta.

❐ A longitudinal view of the left pulmonary artery can be obtained by leftward rotation and angulation of the image plane.

Step 7: Decide Whether Transesophageal Echocardiography or Other Imaging Procedures Are Needed

■ Echocardiographic interpretation should first describe the imaging and Doppler findings, along with a differential diagnosis for these findings. The level of confidence in any diagnosis should be indicated.

■ Second, the interpretation should indicate any areas of uncertainly and, in conjunction with the referring physician, suggest additional diagnostic procedures.

Key points:

❐ Complete evaluation of the aorta and pulmonary artery may require additional imaging procedures, including:
  ❐ Transesophageal echocardiography
  ❐ Chest computed tomography
  ❐ CMR imaging
  ❐ Cardiac catheterization with aortography.
❐ Selection of the most appropriate diagnostic modality depends on several clinical factors, including the differential diagnosis, acuity of symptoms, concurrent diseases, and local expertise in imaging.

Transesophageal Echocardiography

Step 1: Image the Aortic Root from a High Esophageal Position

■ Long axis views of the ascending aorta provide excellent image quality for detection of aortic dilation or dissection.

■ Short axis images provide confirmation of findings and are helpful in distinguishing artifact from intraluminal abnormalities.

■ Color Doppler evaluation of the flow pattern in the aortic root helps identify dissection flaps.

Key points:

❐ The long axis view typically is obtained at 120 degrees rotation, but there is individual variability, so the image plane should be adjusted to show the aortic root in a long axis orientation (Fig. 16–13).

❐ From the long axis view, the transducer is moved up in the esophagus to image as much of the ascending aorta as possible.

❐ Slow medial and lateral turning of the image plane from the long axis view may identify abnormalities not seen in the centered long axis view.

❐ The short axis view is used to provide an orthogonal image plane. The short axis view should be recorded from the aortic valve level to as high as possible in the ascending aorta (Fig. 16–14).

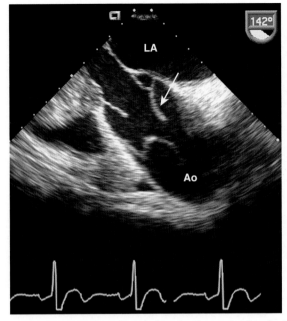
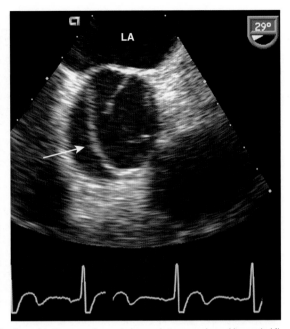

Figure 16–14 In a patient with aortic dissection, the complex dissection flap (*arrow*) in the ascending aorta is seen in transesophageal long axis (*A*) and short axis (*B*) views of the ascending aorta.

❒ Color Doppler in long and short axis views may show flow in two lumens when a dissection is present.

❒ Imaging artifacts often seen in the ascending aorta include linear reverberations from the aorta itself or adjacent structures.

❒ Artifacts are distinguished from anatomic abnormalities by examination in at least two imaging planes; their location, appearance, and pattern of motion relative to the aortic wall; and correlation with color Doppler flow patterns.

Step 2: Evaluate Aortic Valve Anatomy and Function

■ The presence of aortic valve disease prompts careful evaluation for associated disease of the aortic root.

■ Conversely, aortic root disease may result in aortic valve regurgitation.

Key points:

❒ The risk of aortic dilation and dissection is higher in patients with a congenital bicuspid or unicuspid valve, compared with those with a trileaflet valve (Fig. 16–15).

❒ Aortic disease may result in aortic regurgitation either from dilation of the aortic root and central noncoaptation of the leaflets or from extension of a dissection flap into the valve, resulting in a flail leaflet.

❒ Aortic valve anatomy and function is evaluated with two-dimensional (2D) and color Doppler in a long axis view at about 120 degrees rotation and in the short axis view at about 30 degrees rotation.

❒ Additional scanning medially and laterally from the long axis view, and superiorly and inferiorly from the short axis view, also is helpful.

Step 3: Examine the Descending Thoracic Aorta

■ The descending thoracic aorta is well visualized on transesophageal echocardiography (TEE) by turning the image plane toward the patient's back.

■ The short axis view is recorded with the transducer slowly withdrawn from the transgastric level to the high esophagus (Fig. 16–16).

■ The aortic arch is visualized from the high TEE position by turning the image plane medially with caudal angulation.

Key points:

❒ Long axis views of the descending aorta supplement short axis views and are helpful for evaluation of any abnormal findings. However, the long axis view alone may miss abnormalities that are located medial and lateral to the image plane.

❒ Color flow provides visualization of flow in the true and false lumens when dissection is present.

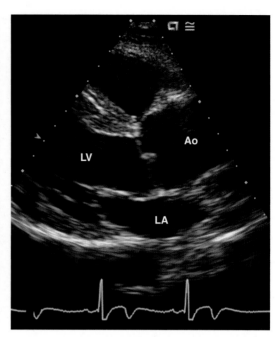

A   **B**

Figure 16–15 Transthoracic imaging of a bicuspid aortic valve in short axis view (*A*) often is associated with dilation of the aortic root, as seen in the corresponding long axis view (*B*).

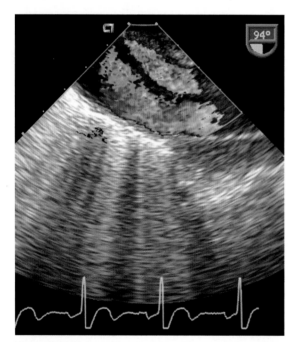

Figure 16–16 Transesophageal imaging of the descending thoracic aorta in a longitudinal view in a patient with aortic dissection, obtained by turning the transducer toward the patient's back and then rotating the image plane by about 90 degrees.

❑ Color flow also is helpful in distinguishing image artifacts from dissection flaps and atheroma.
❑ When the aorta is tortuous, care is needed to distinguish intraluminal abnormalities from an oblique image plane.

SPECIAL CONSIDERATIONS

Chronic Aortic Dilation

■ There are many causes of aortic dilation, including:
  ❑ Hypertension
  ❑ Annuloaortic ectasia
  ❑ Marfan syndrome and other connective tissue disorders
  ❑ Aortic dilation associated with congenital unicuspid and bicuspid aortic valves
  ❑ Inflammatory diseases of the aorta, including tertiary syphilis and Takayasu's aortitis
  ❑ Systemic inflammatory disease, including ankylosing spondylitis
■ Echocardiography provides accurate measurement of the aortic root and often provides anatomic clues about the cause of disease.

Key points:
  ❑ Hypertensive aortic dilation usually is mild and accompanied by left ventricular (LV) hypertrophy, aortic valve sclerosis, and mitral annular calcification.

❏ Marfan syndrome is characterized by loss of the normal acute angle at the sinotubular junction. Early in the disease, this finding may be subtle; late in the disease, the aortic root appears globular with no discernible sinotubular junction (Fig. 16–17).

❏ Aortic dilation associated with congenital valve abnormalities is independent of valve hemodynamics.

❏ Aortic dilation resulting from an inflammatory process usually is characterized by increased thickness of the aortic walls.

❏ In ankylosing spondylitis, the increase in aortic wall thickness extends into the base of the anterior mitral valve leaflet, with the appearance of a subaortic "bump" in a long axis view.

❏ Takayasu's aortitis typically involves the aortic arch and branches, resulting in areas of stenosis and dilation, but the descending aorta also may be involved.

Aortic Dissection

Step 1: Use the Basic Approach for Evaluation of the Aorta to Identify the Dissection Flap

■ The characteristics of a dissection flap (Fig. 16–18) are:
   ❏ A thin, linear, mobile intraluminal echo
   ❏ Motion independent of the aortic walls
   ❏ Separation of the lumen into two channels
■ The entry site of the dissection from the true into the false lumen may be identified with color Doppler.
■ An ascending aortic dissection usually requires surgical intervention, so it is especially important to determine whether a dissection flap is present in the ascending aorta.
■ TEE is more sensitive than transthoracic imaging for detection of aortic dissection and should be the initial echo procedure when this diagnosis is suspected.

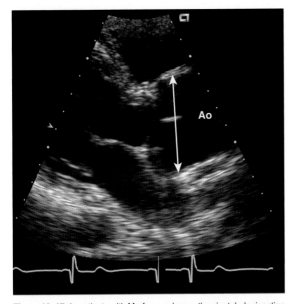

Figure 16–17 In patients with Marfan syndrome, the sinotubular junction is lost with a "water balloon" appearance of the aortic root.

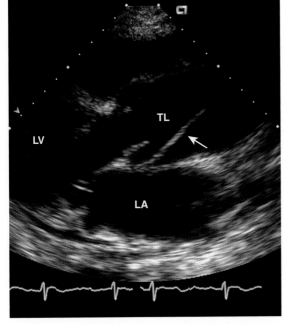
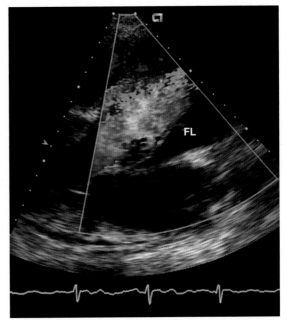

Figure 16–18 Transthoracic parasternal long axis view showing a linear echo in the lumen of a dilated ascending aorta (A), with a dissection flap (arrow) separating the true lumen (TL) from the false lumen (FL). In real time, this linear echo showed motion separate from the motion of the aortic wall and was seen in multiple image planes. Color Doppler (B) shows flow only in the true lumen.

Key points:

❏ Imaging artifacts may be mistaken for a dissection flap. Approaches to avoiding a false positive diagnosis include imaging the flap in more than one imaging plane, documenting flow in two separate lumens, and demonstrating the three key characteristics of a dissection flap.

❏ There may be more than one entry site from the true into the false lumen, and multiple exit sites may be detected distally.

❏ The false lumen may be thrombosed. In this situation, the flap does not move and the false lumen is filled with an irregular echodensity, consistent with thrombus.

❏ Localized dissection into the aortic wall may result in a crescent-shaped intramural hematoma, without a dissection flap (Fig. 16–19).

❏ Outcomes with intramural hematoma and dissection are similar.

Step 2: Look for Complications of Aortic Dissection

■ Complications of aortic dissection include:
  ❏ Pericardial effusion
  ❏ Aortic regurgitation
  ❏ Extension of the dissection flap into a coronary artery
  ❏ Involvement of arteries that arise from the aorta
■ Echocardiography may detect the central complications of aortic dissection, but evaluation of branch vessels typically require other imaging techniques.

Key points:

❏ Pericardial effusion may be due to rupture of the dissection into the pericardial space. Because the effusion is acute, tamponade physiology may be present with only a small effusion.

❏ Aortic regurgitation may be due to aortic dilation with central noncoaptation of the leaflets or due to a flail leaflet from extension of the dissection flap into the valve (Fig. 16–20).

❏ Extension of a dissection flap into the coronary artery may be visualized on transthoracic or TEE imaging in some cases. More often, the key finding is a regional wall motion caused by ischemia in the myocardium supplied by the dissected vessel.

❏ The proximal segments of the left carotid and subclavian and right brachiocephalic arteries may be seen by echocardiography in some cases. However, accurate evaluation of these vessels and more distal arteries (renal, mesenteric, etc.) requires other imaging approaches.

Sinus of Valsalva Aneurysm

■ A congenital sinus of Valsalva aneurysm is an irregularly shaped, thin-walled, outpouching of the sinus.
■ Rupture into adjacent chambers results in a fistula from the aorta into the right ventricle, right atrium, or left atrium, depending on which sinus is affected.
■ Acquired sinus of Valsalva aneurysms usually are due to endocarditis and typically have a rounded, symmetric shape (Fig. 16–21).

Key points:

❏ Rupture of a right coronary sinus aneurysm is into the right ventricle, left coronary sinus

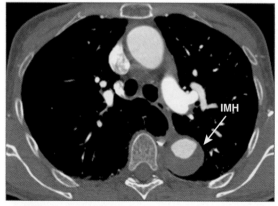

Figure 16–19 Intramural hematoma (*IMH*) seen on a chest computed tomography scan in the descending thoracic aorta. This finding can be seen on transesophageal echocardiography but may be difficult to distinguish from atheromatous or extra-aortic disease.

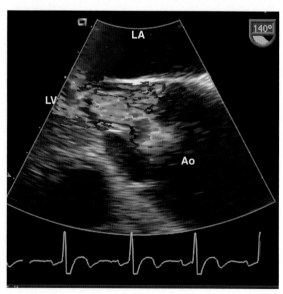

Figure 16–20 An aortic dissection can result in severe aortic regurgitation, as seen in this diastolic frame in a TEE long axis view, because of extension of the dissection flap into the aortic valve leaflet.

into the left atrium, and noncoronary sinus into the right atrium.

◻ Flow in the fistula from the aorta is continuous with high velocity flow in both systole and diastole, reflecting the systolic and diastolic pressure differences between the aorta and receiving chamber.

◻ Acquired aneurysms caused by infection may extend below the aortic valve, into the base of the septum. Imaging in long axis views helps determine the level and extent of involvement.

Aortic Pseudoaneurysms

■ An aortic pseudoaneurysm is a contained aortic rupture (Fig. 16–22).

■ Pseudoaneurysms may occur after aortic surgery because of dehiscence at the proximal or distal anastomosis or at a coronary reimplantation site.

Key points:

◻ A pseudoaneurysm is detected as an echolucent space adjacent to the aorta. The pseudoaneurysm may be echodense if hematoma is present.

◻ A pseudoaneurysm should be suspected when a para-aortic mass is found in a patient with recent or remote surgery on the ascending aorta.

◻ Although often initially diagnosed by echocardiography, evaluation of the size and origin of the pseudoaneurysm often requires a wide field of view imaging approach, such as CMR imaging or CT.

Atherosclerotic Aortic Disease

■ Aortic atheroma may be detected on TEE imaging of the ascending and descending thoracic

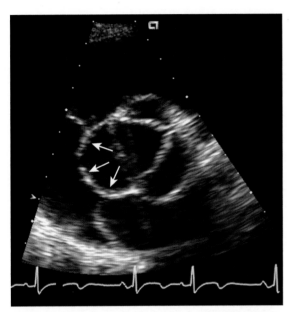

Figure 16–21 This short axis view of the aortic valve shows the valve leaflets open to a triangular shape in systole. There is asymmetric dilation of the sinuses of Valsalva, most prominently involving the noncoronary sinus (*arrows*), consistent with a sinus of Valsalva aneurysm.

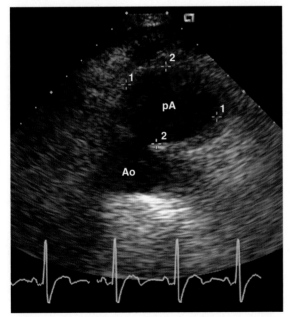

A

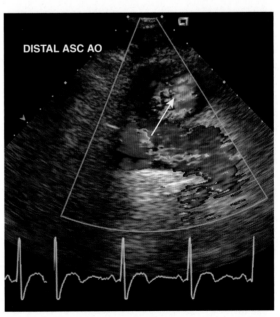

B

Figure 16–22 In a patient with a Dacron tube graft replacement of the ascending aorta (*ASC AO*), an abnormal echo-lucent space is seen adjacent to the ascending aorta, near the distal anastomosis site. The 3.5-by-4.5–cm diameter (1 and 2) space appears lined by thrombus (*A*). Color Doppler demonstrates flow from the aorta into this space (*B*), consistent with a contained aortic rupture or pseudoaneurysm (*pA*).

aorta and are a marker of coronary disease (Fig. 16–23).

- Atheromas that protrude into the aortic lumen and atheroma associated with mobile thrombus are associated with an increased risk of embolic events.

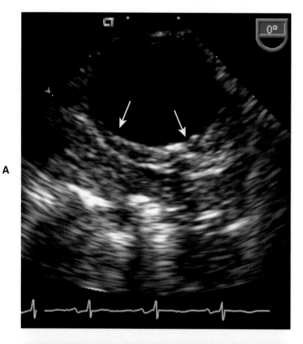

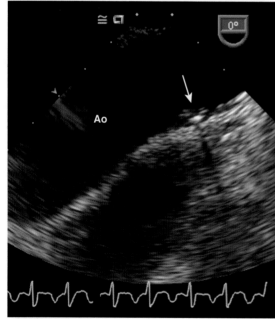

Figure 16–23 The descending thoracic aorta was evaluated in sequential short axis images (*A*) as the transducer was withdrawn in the esophagus. From a high esophageal position, the image plane was turned medially and angulated caudally to show the aortic arch and ascending aorta (*B*). The irregular thickening of the aortic wall with an area of calcification (with shadowing) is consistent with an aortic atheroma.

Key points:
- ❑ Atheroma are identified as irregular focal areas of thickening of the aortic wall, with or without associated calcification.
- ❑ Images of the aortic arch are limited, even with TEE imaging, but atheroma may be detected from a high TEE position in some cases.

Pulmonary Artery Abnormalities

- Isolated abnormalities of the pulmonary artery are rare; most pulmonary artery disease is associated with congenital heart disease (Fig. 16–24).
- Idiopathic dilation of the pulmonary artery is an uncommon abnormality in which a dilated pulmonary artery is seen in the absence of other congenital lesions.
- Thrombus in the pulmonary artery may be seen on transesophageal or transthoracic imaging in some cases, but echocardiography is not an accurate approach for diagnosis of pulmonary embolism.

Key points:
- ❑ Abnormalities of the pulmonary artery associated with other congenital heart disease include pulmonary artery dilation and branch pulmonary artery stenosis.
- ❑ Pulmonary artery dissection is rare.

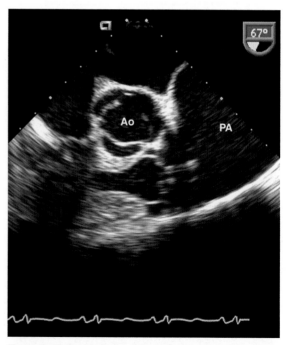

Figure 16–24 Severe dilation of the pulmonary artery (*PA*) seen on transesophageal echocardiography in a patient with congenital heart disease.

SELF-ASSESSMENT QUESTIONS

QUESTION 1

Identify the structures numbered 1-5 in Figure 16–25 by matching with the following list:

  A. Descending aorta
  B. Ascending aorta
  C. Left ventricle
  D. Left atrium
  E. Right pulmonary artery
  F. Left pulmonary artery
  G. Brachiocephalic vein
  H. Azygous vein

1. _____
2. _____
3. _____
4. _____
5. _____

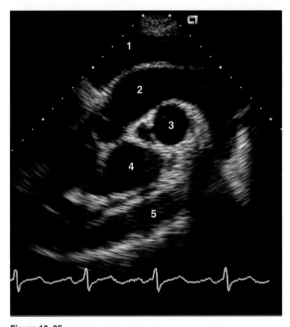

Figure 16–25

QUESTION 2

Identify the structures numbered 1-3 in Figure 16–26 by matching with the following list:

  A. Descending aorta
  B. Ascending aorta
  C. Aortic arch
  D. Pulmonary artery
  E. Left atrium
  F. Pulmonary vein

1. _____
2. _____
3. _____

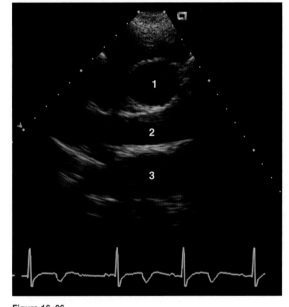

Figure 16–26

QUESTION 3

What is the structure indicated by the arrow in Figure 16–27?

_____

How would you confirm this diagnosis? _____
_____

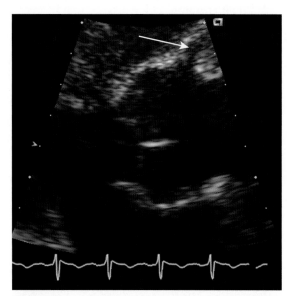

Figure 16–27

QUESTION 4

Which of the following diagnoses is most likely in the patient with the image shown in Figure 16–28?

   A. Dilated pulmonary artery
   B. Paravalvular abscess
   C. Aortic intramural hematoma
   D. Pulmonary embolism
   E. Aortic dissection

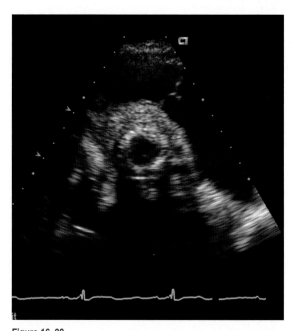

Figure 16–28

QUESTION 5

The image in Figure 16–29 was obtained from a 48-year-old man with the acute onset of chest pain. The most likely diagnosis is:

- A. Pulmonary embolism
- B. Acute myocardial infarction
- C. Mediastinal hematoma
- D. Aortic dissection
- E. Costochondritis

QUESTION 6:

The echocardiographic image in Figure 16–30 was recorded from a 22-year-old man. The most likely diagnosis is:

- A. Normal aorta
- B. Sinus of Valsalva aneurysm
- C. Aortic dissection
- D. Marfan syndrome
- E. Takayasu's aortitis

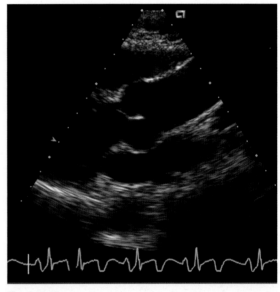

Figure 16–30

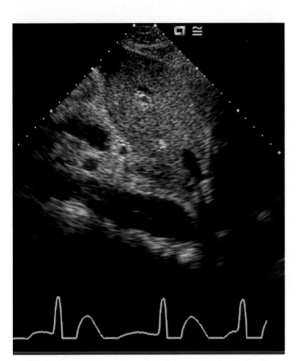

Figure 16–29

QUESTION 7

A 74-year-old man was referred for echocardiography for new onset chest pain and a chest CT suggesting an ascending aortic dissection. The most likely mechanism of the finding shown in Figure 16–31 is:

A. Dilation of the aortic root
B. Right coronary artery dissection
C. Rupture into the pericardium
D. Thromboembolism
E. Valvular vegetation

QUESTION 8

The flow signal in Figure 16–32 is most consistent with the diagnosis of:

A. Aortic coarctation
B. Aortic regurgitation
C. Patent ductus arteriosus
D. Branch pulmonary stenosis
E. Persistent left superior vena cava

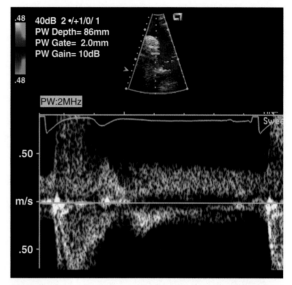

Figure 16–32

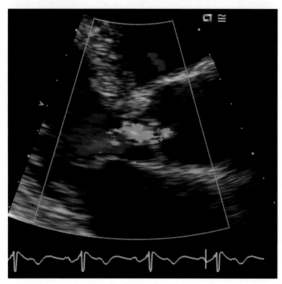

Figure 16–31

ANSWERS

ANSWER 1

This suprasternal notch long axis view of the aortic arch shows the:

1: G. Brachiocephalic vein
2: B. Ascending aorta
3: E. Right pulmonary artery
4: D. Left atrium
5: A. Descending aorta

The left ventricle is not well seen in this view. The right pulmonary artery is seen in cross section under the aortic arch, but the image plane does not include the left pulmonary artery. The azygous vein arises from the inferior vena cava, courses superiorly adjacent to the spine receiving the drainage of the intercostal veins, and then enters the superior vena cava above the right mainstem bronchus. When normal in size, it is rarely seen by echocardiography and lies medial to the descending thoracic aorta.

ANSWER 2

This suprasternal notch short axis view of the aortic arch shows:

1: C. Aortic arch
2: D. Pulmonary artery
3: E. Left atrium

The arch appears circular in cross section. The section of pulmonary artery imaged is predominantly the right pulmonary artery but includes the origin of the left pulmonary artery. Sometimes the entrances of the four pulmonary veins into the left atrium can be seen, but they are not well visualized in this case.

ANSWER 3: RIGHT CORONARY ARTERY

This is a zoomed image of the aortic valve and sinuses of Valsalva in a long axis transthoracic view. The closed aortic leaflets are seen with a prominent closure line. The anterior sinus typically is the right coronary sinus, with the posterior sinus being either the left or noncoronary sinus, depending on the exact medial-lateral angulation of the image plane. The tubular structure arising from the top of the right coronary sinuses has the typical location and appearance of a right coronary artery. Confirmation of this diagnosis would include pulsed Doppler interrogation showing typical diastolic coronary flow.

ANSWER 4: B

This is a transthoracic parasternal short axis view of the aortic valve, just above the leaflet level, in a young man with a tissue aortic valve and root replacement for endocarditis with recurrent infection. The bright circular aortic graft is seen in the center of an irregular echodensity consistent with a hematoma or abscess. The pulmonary artery and valve are seen well, and this image shows no evidence for dilation or thrombus formation in the pulmonary artery. An aortic intramural hematoma is in the wall of the aorta, not around the aorta, as in this image, but it can be problematic to distinguish between these two diagnoses. There is no evidence of an intimal flap to suggest dissection on this image.

ANSWER 5: D

This subcostal view of the proximal abdominal aorta shows a dissection flap in the aorta. This patient also has a dissection flap identified in the ascending aorta (shown in Fig. 16–18), and he underwent emergency root replacement. The pulmonary artery is not seen in this view. Thrombi are rarely seen in the pulmonary artery by echocardiography. Although specific, they are not a sensitive finding for diagnosis of pulmonary embolism. A diagnosis of acute myocardial infarction would require imaging of the left ventricular wall motion. An aortic dissection might present with a mediastinal hematoma, which would be seen from the parasternal window. Costochondritis does not have any associated echocardiographic findings.

ANSWER 6: D

This image shows a mildly dilated aorta (4.0 cm at the sinuses), with mild early effacement of the sinotubular junction consistent with Marfan syndrome. The patient's mother and brother both have a definite diagnosis of Marfan syndrome, and he has musculoskeletal findings consistent with this diagnosis. This aorta is not normal for a 22-year-old man. A sinus of Valsalva aneurysm is characterized by asymmetric dilation of one of the sinuses, not symmetric as in this case. There is no intimal flap to suggest aortic dissection. Takayasu's (and other forms of aortitis such as syphilis) are associated with increased thickness of the aortic wall resulting from the inflammatory process.

ANSWER 7: A

This image shows aortic regurgitation. Although this may be an incidental finding related to aortic valve sclerosis in a 74-year-old man, in a patient with aortic dissection, this finding is of concern because the aortic valve may become incompetent because of dilation of the root or extension of the dissection flap into the valve leaflets. The dissection flap also can extend into the right or left coronary artery, resulting in myocardial infarction. Rupture into the pericardium occurs when the dissection extends into the pericardial reflection at the base of the aorta. Thromboembolism is not associated with dissection—distal ischemia is due to occlusion of flow by the dissection flap—and would not explain aortic regurgitation. There is no evidence for a valvular vegetation on this image.

ANSWER 8: C

This pulsed Doppler recording in the descending thoracic aorta from a suprasternal notch window shows antegrade flow in systole and then a continuous flow signal in diastole. The sample volume is at the inner edge of the aorta, in the region of the ductus arteriosus, and this flow signal indicates continuous flow from the aorta into the pulmonary artery via a patent ductus. With aortic coarctation, antegrade velocity is increased and there is continuous forward flow in diastole. With aortic regurgitation, the diastolic reversal is more laminar, with a smooth velocity curve (see Fig. 16–9). Branch pulmonary stenosis might be detected from this window but would be associated with high velocity systolic flow. A persistent left superior vena cava would have a typical venous flow pattern with low velocity antegrade systolic and diastolic flow.

NOTES

17 The Adult with Congenital Heart Disease

CATEGORIES OF CONGENITAL HEART DISEASE

CONGENITAL STENOTIC LESIONS
Subvalvular
Valvular
Supravavular
Peripheral great vessels (aortic coarctation)

CONGENITAL REGURGITANT LESIONS
Myxomatous valve disease
Ebstein's anomaly

ABNORMAL INTRACARDIAC COMMUNICATIONS
Atrial septal defect
Ventricular septal defect
Patent ductus arteriosus

ABNORMAL CHAMBER AND GREAT VESSEL CONNECTIONS
Transposition of the great arteries
Ventricular inversion (congenitally corrected transposition)
Tetralogy of Fallot
Tricuspid atresia
Truncus arteriosus

CLUES TO THE IDENTIFICATION OF CARDIAC STRUCTURES IN ADULTS WITH CONGENITAL HEART DISEASE

STRUCTURE	ANATOMIC FEATURE	ECHO APPROACH
Right atrium	Inferior vena cava enters right atrium	Start with subcostal approach to identify RA
Right ventricle	Prominent trabeculation Moderator band Infundibulum Tricuspid valve Apical location of annulus	Apical four-chamber view to compare annular insertions of two valves, parasternal for valve anatomy and infundibulum
Pulmonary artery	Bifurcates	Parasternal long-axis view or apical four-chamber view angulated very anteriorly
Left atrium	Pulmonary veins usually enter left atrium	Transesophageal imaging for pulmonary vein anatomy
Left ventricle	Mitral valve Basal location of annulus Fibrous continuity between anterior mitral leaflet and semilunar valve	Apical four-chamber view and parasternal long- and short-axis views
Aorta	Gives rise to aortic arch and arterial branches	Start with parasternal long-axis view and move transducer superiorly to follow vessel to its branches

RA, *Right atrium.*

APPROACH TO THE ECHOCARDIOGRAPHIC EXAMINATION IN ADULTS WITH CONGENITAL HEART DISEASE

BEFORE THE EXAMINATION
Review the clinical history
Obtain details of any surgical procedures
Review results or prior diagnostic tests
Formulate specific questions

SEQUENCE OF EXAMINATION
Identify cardiac chambers, great vessels, and their connections
Identify associated defects, and evaluate the physiology of each lesion
    Regurgitation and/or stenosis (quantitate as per Chapters 11 and 12)
    Shunts (calculate $Q_p{:}Q_s$)
    Pulmonary hypertension (calculate pulmonary pressure)
    Ventricular dysfunction (measure ejection fraction if anatomy allows)

AFTER THE EXAMINATION
Integrate echo and Doppler findings with clinical data
Summarize findings
Identify which clinical questions remain unanswered, and suggest appropriate subsequent diagnostic tests

EXAMPLES
1. A 24 year old with a history of a cardiac murmur has an echocardiogram, which shows:

Right ventricular outflow velocity	1.6 m/s
Pulmonary artery velocity	3.1 m/s
Tricuspid regurgitant jet	3.4 m/s
Estimated right atrial pressure	5 mm Hg (small IVC with normal respiratory variation)

Because the right ventricular outflow velocity is elevated, the maximum pulmonic valve gradient should be calculated using the proximal velocity in the Bernoulli equation:

$$P = 4(V^2_{jet} - V^2_{prox})$$

$$P = 4[(3.1)^2 - (1.6)^2] = 4[9.6 - 2.6] = 28 \text{ mm Hg}$$

If the proximal velocity is not included, the gradient would be overestimated at 38 mm Hg.

Estimated pulmonary systolic pressure is calculated by subtracting the pulmonic valve gradient from the tricuspid valve gradient because pulmonic stenosis is present:

$$PAP = (P_{RV\text{-}RA} + P_{RA}) - (P_{RV\text{-}PA})$$

$$PAP = (4V^2_{TR} + P_{RA}) - (P_{RV\text{-}PA} = [4(3.4)^2 + 5)] - 28 = 23 \text{ mm Hg}$$

Thus pulmonary artery systolic pressure is normal even though the tricuspid regurgitant jet indicates a right ventricular systolic pressure of 51 mm Hg.

2. A 26-year-old woman undergoes echocardiography for symptoms of decreased exercise tolerance. She is found to have an enlarged right atrium and ventricle with paradoxic septal motion and the following Doppler data:

Right ventricular outflow	
Velocity	1.8 m/s
Velocity time integral (VTI_{RVOT})	32 cm
Diameter	2.6 cm
Left ventricular outflow	
Velocity	1.1 m/s
Velocity time integral (VTI_{LVOT})	16 cm
Diameter	2.4 cm

The right heart enlargement suggests an atrial septal defect may be present. The shunt ratio is calculated from the ratio of pulmonary flow (Q_p), measured in the right ventricular outflow tract and systemic flow (Q_s), measured in the left ventricular outflow tract. At each site, cross-sectional area is calculated as the area of a circle:

$$CSA_{RVOT} = \pi(D/2)^2 = 3.14(2.6/2)^2 = 5.3 \text{ cm}^2$$

$$CSA_{LVOT} = \pi(D/2)^2 = 3.14(2.4/2)^2 = 4.5 \text{ cm}^2$$

Flow at each site then is calculated:

$$Q_p = CSA_{RVOT} \times VTI_{RVOT} = 5.3 \text{ cm}^2 \times 32 \text{ cm} = 170 \text{ cm}^3 \text{ or ml}$$

$$Q_s = CSA_{LVOT} \times VTI_{LVOT} = 4.5 \text{ cm}^2 \times 16 \text{ cm} = 72 \text{ cm}^3 \text{ or ml}$$

so that $Q_p{:}Q_s = 170/72 = 2.4$

These calculations are consistent with a significant shunt that most likely will require closure to prevent progressive right heart dysfunction.

BASIC PRINCIPLES

Identification of Cardiac Chambers and Great Vessels

■ Identification of the chambers, the great vessels, and their connections is the first step in echocardiographic evaluation of the patient with congenital heart disease (see the Echo Exam tables at the beginning of the chapter).

Key points:

□ The right and left ventricle are distinguished based on the atrioventricular valve anatomy and position, the presence or absence of a moderator band, and the presence or absence of a muscular infundibular region (Fig. 17–1).

□ The size and location of the ventricular chamber is not reliable for distinguishing the anatomic left from right ventricle.

□ The right ventricle tends to have a more triangular shape, whereas the left ventricle is more ellipsoid, but shape can be unreliable when severe dilation is present.

□ The aorta and pulmonary artery are identified by their distal anatomy, with bifurcation into two pulmonary arteries or continuation into an aortic arch (Fig. 17–2).

□ In addition to anatomic definitions, the ventricle that pumps oxygenated blood into the aorta is termed the "systemic ventricle," and the ventricle that pumps systemic venous re-

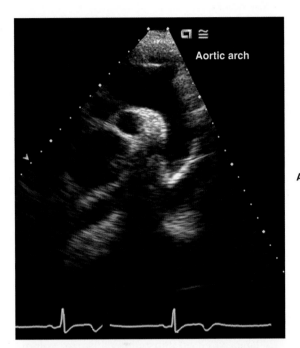

A

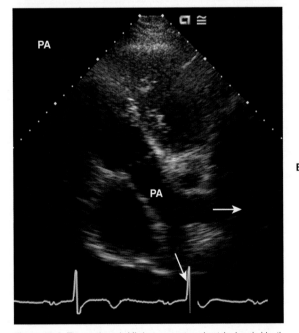

B

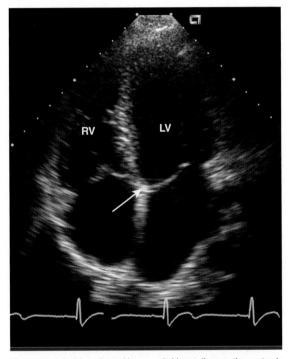

Figure 17–1 In this patient with congenital heart disease, the anatomic right and left ventricle are identified in the apical four-chamber view based on morphologic features that include a more apical position of the tricuspid versus mitral annulus (*arrow*) and the moderator band and trabeculations in the right ventricle. The atrioventricular valves are associated with the correct anatomic ventricle, even when atrial or great vessel connections are discordant. Mitral and tricuspid valve anatomy were confirmed in other views. This patient with a patent ductus arteriosus has mild left ventricular and left atrial enlargement but an otherwise unremarkable four-chamber view.

Figure 17–2 The aortic arch (*A*), in a suprasternal notch view, is identified by the arch and head and neck vessels. The pulmonary artery (*B*), from a low parasternal apical view, is identified based on its bifurcation.

turn into the pulmonary artery is termed the "pulmonic ventricle."

Valve Involvement

■ Valve stenosis and regurgitation are evaluated using the same methods as are used for acquired valve disease.

Key points:

❑ Congenital valve stenosis may be valvular, subvalvular, or supravalvular.
❑ Delineation of the level of obstruction using pulsed and color Doppler is necessary in addition to continuous wave (CW) Doppler measurements.

Intracardiac Shunts

■ Intracardiac shunts are detected and quantitated using multiple Doppler modalities.

Key points:

❑ Intracardiac shunts are detected based on the presence of a flow disturbance on the downstream side of the shunt with color or pulsed Doppler.
❑ The velocity and shape of the CW Doppler signal across an intracardiac shunt reflects the pressure difference across the shunt and is a key factor in determining shunt location.
❑ The pulmonic-to-systemic flow ratio is calculated based on transpulmonic stroke volume and transaortic stroke volume.

Complex Disease

■ Complex congenital heart disease should be evaluated at centers with established adult congenital heart disease programs.
❑ This chapter includes a basic approach for simple conditions or patients with a well-established diagnosis.
❑ More complex cases require additional data acquisition by sonographers and physicians with expertise in congenital heart disease.

STEP-BY-STEP APPROACH

Basic Transthoracic Echocardiographic Examination for Congenital Heart Disease

■ A structured study sequence is needed to ensure that all the images and Doppler flows needed for diagnosis are recorded.
■ Most adult echocardiography laboratories acquire images and Doppler data in a similar sequence as for a standard adult study.

■ With complex disease, the sonographer and physician work together during image acquisition to ensure the needed data are obtained.

Step 1: Review the Clinical History

■ Review the details of any previous surgical or percutaneous procedures.
■ Obtain reports (and images when possible) of any previous diagnostic tests.
■ Determine the specific objectives of the current examination.

Key points:

❑ Knowledge of previous procedures and diagnostic studies ensures the current exam provides additional information and focuses on the key clinical issues.
❑ Complete evaluation of the adult with congenital heart disease often requires multiple diagnostic modalities; the echocardiographic examination provides only part of the needed information.

Step 2: Acquire Images and Doppler Data from the Parasternal Window

Parasternal long axis view

■ The position and angle of the transducer needed to obtain a long axis view help identify an abnormal cardiac position in the chest (dextroversion or dextrocardia).
■ The great vessel identities and location are evaluated in the long axis view.
■ The connections of the great vessels to the ventricles are determined.
■ Doppler is used to evaluate for valve regurgitation, areas of stenosis, and intracardiac shunts.

Key points:

❑ Medial and lateral angulation of the transducer shows the relationship of the great vessels to each other and to the ventricular chambers.
❑ The pulmonary artery normally is anterior to the aorta; an anteriorly located aorta suggests transposition of the great vessels (Fig. 17–3).
❑ The transducer is moved up one or more interspaces to follow the great vessel(s) seen in the long axis view, allowing differentiation of the aorta from the pulmonary artery.
❑ Ventricular and atrial septal defects can be identified with color Doppler during slow scanning from lateral to medial in the long axis image plane and from apex to base in the short axis plane.
❑ Standard measurements of great vessels and cardiac chambers are recorded in the long axis view.

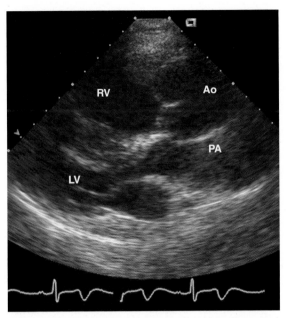

Figure 17–3 In a parasternal long axis image of a patient with transposition of the great arteries, the anterior-posterior locations of the aorta (*Ao, larger and anterior*) and pulmonary artery (*PA, smaller and posterior*) are opposite the normal position, and the vessels lie parallel to each other, rather than in the normal criss-cross relationship.

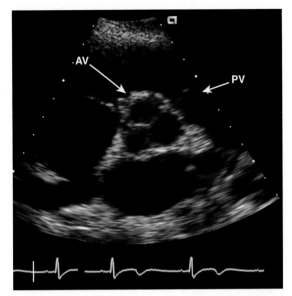

Figure 17–4 The normal aortic valve and pulmonic valve planes are perpendicular to each other, so the aortic valve (*AV*) is seen in short axis when the pulmonic valve (*PV*) is seen in long axis. The most anterior great vessel at the base of the heart is the pulmonary artery.

☐ The transducer location for image acquisition is recorded, because this information cannot be determined from the images themselves.

☐ An enlarged coronary sinus suggests a persistent left superior vena cava.

Parasternal short axis view

■ The short axis view shows the relationship of the semilunar (aortic and pulmonic) valves (Fig. 17–4).

■ Basal ventricular size, systolic function, and septal motion are evaluated.

■ Ventricular and atrial septal defects are demonstrated using color Doppler.

Key points:

☐ The normal relationship of the aortic and pulmonic valve planes is perpendicular to each other. When both are seen in short axis in the same image plane, transposition of the great vessels is present (Fig. 17–5).

☐ The anterior-posterior and medial-lateral locations of the aorta and pulmonary artery at the base are evaluated; the aortic root is anterior to the pulmonary artery when transposition is present.

☐ Atrial and ventricular septal defects typically are clearly visible in the short axis view.

☐ The location of the ventricular septal defect relative to the aortic valve helps distinguish a

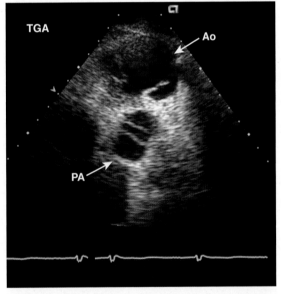

Figure 17–5 With transposition of the great arteries (TGA), the aorta (*Ao*) is anterior to the pulmonary artery (*PA*) with a side-by-side (instead of criss-cross) relationship of the great arteries. The semilunar valves are both in the same image plane, so the aortic and pulmonic valves are both seen in cross section in a short axis view.

membranous from subpulmonic (or supracristal) ventricular septal defect.

☐ Pulsed and CW Doppler interrogation of any abnormal color flow signals is helpful for diagnosis based on the time course and velocity of flow.

☐ Standard measurements of great vessels and cardiac chambers are recorded in the long axis view.

Parasternal right ventricular inflow and outflow views

■ The right ventricular (RV) inflow view is helpful for evaluation of the right atrium, pulmonary atrioventricular valve, and annulus (Fig. 17–6).

■ CW Doppler measurement of atrioventricular valve regurgitant velocity allows measurement of right ventricular (or pulmonary) systolic pressure.

■ The RV outflow view allows visualization of RV outflow obstruction, at the subvalvular, pulmonic valve, or supravalvular level.

■ Doppler evaluation allows localization of the level of RV outflow obstruction and calculation of the gradient between the ventricle and pulmonary artery.

Key points:

❐ Standard RV inflow and outflow views may be difficult to obtain when transposition is present.

❐ Slow angulation from the long axis view toward the RV inflow view and RV outflow view, using color Doppler, may be helpful for diagnosis of atrial and ventricular septal defect.

❐ When right (or pulmonic) ventricular outflow tract obstruction is present, ventricular systolic pressure does *not* equal pulmonary systolic pressure; instead, the transpulmonic gradient is subtracted from ventricular systolic pressure to determine pulmonary systolic pressure (Fig. 17–7).

❐ Evaluation of RV outflow obstruction requires color and pulsed Doppler (to determine the anatomic location of the increase in velocity) and CW Doppler (to measure the peak velocity).

Step 3: Acquire Images and Doppler Data from the Apical Window

■ The size and function of both ventricles are evaluated in the four-chamber, two-chamber, and long axis views.

■ The atrioventricular valves are evaluated using two-dimensional (2D) imaging and color and CW Doppler.

■ Anterior angulation from the four-chamber view often allows imaging of the connection from each ventricle to the great vessels (Fig. 17–8).

■ Ventricular inflow and outflow signals are recorded using pulsed and CW Doppler.

Key points:

❐ The normal transducer orientation is used to ensure correct identification of the location and anatomy of each ventricle.

❐ The apical view often allows recognition of the anatomic left and right ventricles, based on the distance from the annulus to the apex, as well as the presence of the moderator band.

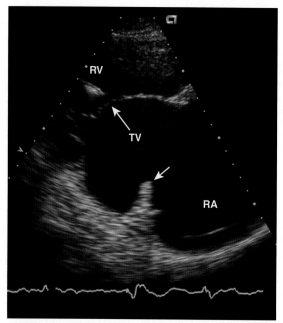

Figure 17–6 The right ventricular inflow view in a patient with Ebstein's anomaly of the tricuspid valve (*TV; short arrow*) shows the apical displacement of the septal leaflet from the annulus (*short arrow*), with the atrialized portion of the right ventricle (*RV*) between the annulus and leaflet attachment level.

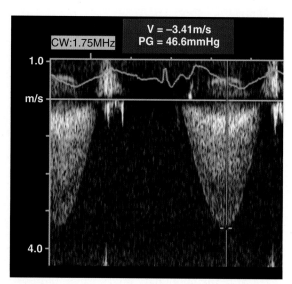

Figure 17–7 From a parasternal window, continuous wave Doppler was used to record this high velocity systolic ejection signal from the region of the pulmonic valve in a patient with pulmonic stenosis. This signal might be due to subpulmonic or valvular stenosis; two-dimensional imaging and color Doppler are helpful in localizing the level of obstruction.

❏ The atrioventricular valves are evaluated using standard Doppler approaches.

❏ With anterior angulation to image the great vessels, the bifurcation of the pulmonary artery and the curve of the aortic arch may be visualized, helping with identification of the ventricular to great vessel connections.

❏ With posterior angulation, the size and location of the coronary sinus are evaluated.

❏ Atrial anatomy and size may be evaluated, although the distance of these chambers from the transducer may limit detailed evaluation, particularly in patients with an interatrial baffle repair.

❏ Evaluation of the interatrial septum may be limited by ultrasound drop out, because the atrial septum is parallel to the ultrasound beam.

Step 4: Acquire Images and Doppler Data from the Subcostal Window

■ The subcostal four-chamber view allows evaluation of the interatrial septum (Fig. 17–9).

■ The right ventricular size and systolic function often are best evaluated from the subcostal view.

■ The entrance of the inferior vena cava identifies the right atrial chamber.

Key points:

❏ The ultrasound beam is perpendicular to the interatrial septum from the subcostal view, so ultrasound dropout, simulating an atrial defect, is less likely. This view is optimal for 2D and color Doppler detection of an atrial septal defect or patent foramen ovale.

❏ In adults, the free wall of the right ventricle may not be easily visible in apical views, limiting evaluation of RV size and function.

❏ The subcostal view provides a more standard image plane of the right ventricle, with the ultrasound beam perpendicular to the RV free wall, and thus is more reliable for evaluation of RV size and function.

❏ The junction of the inferior vena cava and right atrium provides anatomic information on atrial situs, in addition to allowing estimation of right atrial pressure.

Step 5: Acquire Images and Doppler Data from the Suprasternal Notch Window

■ A standard transducer orientation allows identification of aortic arch position and anatomy.

■ Aortic coarctation is evaluated (or excluded) based on CW Doppler of descending aortic flow (Figs. 17–10 and 17–11).

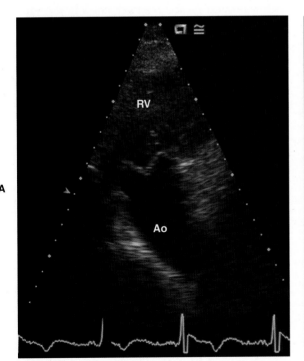
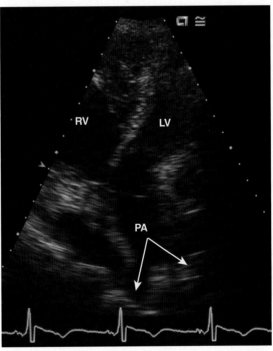

Figure 17–8 From the apical four-chamber view, the transducer is angulated anteriorly to show (*A*) the ascending aorta (*Ao*), which has coronary ostia and an arch, and then (*B*) the pulmonary artery (*PA*) with its bifurcation (*arrows*). This view is helpful for documenting which ventricle ejects into each great vessel. In this patient with transposition of the great vessels and an interatrial baffle repair, the right ventricle ejects into the anteriorly located aorta and the left ventricle ejects into the more posteriorly located pulmonary artery.

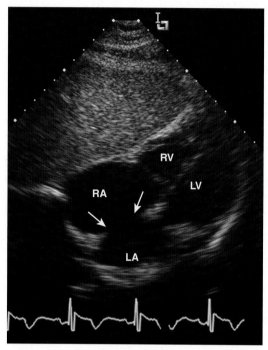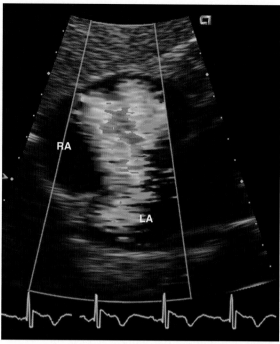

Figure 17–9 The subcostal view is ideal to evaluate for a secundum atrial septal defect. In this patient, the right atrium (*RA*) and right ventricle (*RV*) are enlarged, and there is an apparent defect in the center of the atrial septum (*arrows; A*). Because the ultrasound beam is perpendicular to the atrial septum from this window, this likely is a true defect and not echo drop-out. Color flow imaging (*B*) confirms the large defect with left to right flow.

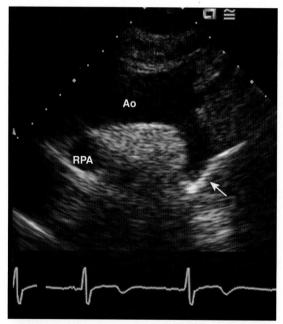

Figure 17–10 The suprasternal notch view is used to evaluate aortic coarctation. However, on two-dimensional imaging, even a normal descending aorta (*Ao*) appears to taper (*arrow*), because the curvature of the vessel results in an oblique plane through the vessel. Thus evaluation by two-dimensional imaging is limited. *RPA*, Right pulmonary artery.

■ Images and pulsed Doppler flows in the superior vena cava are useful in many types of congenital heart disease.

Key points:
❏ A right-sided aortic arch may be missed if the transducer or image orientation is reversed.
❏ Normal systolic and diastolic flow in the descending aorta excludes a diagnosis of aortic coarctation.
❏ The superior vena cava typically is to the right of the ascending aorta. Flow patterns are particularly important when obstruction is present or when the superior vena caval flow has been redirected into the pulmonary artery.
❏ The right pulmonary artery is seen inferior to the arch. When ultrasound penetration is optimal, the left atrium and pulmonary veins also may be identified.
❏ The branch pulmonary arteries may be seen in the short axis view in some patients.
❏ An aortic-to-pulmonary artery shunt may be evaluated from the suprasternal notch view in some cases (e.g., patent ductus arteriosis, aortic-to-pulmonary window).

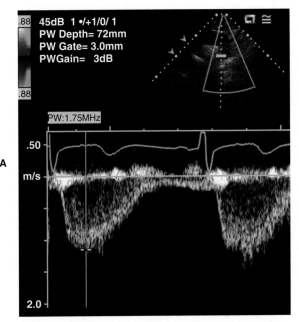

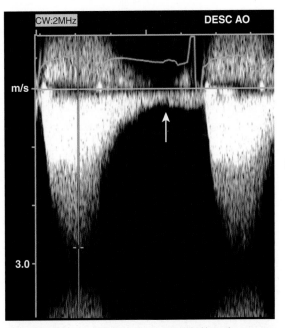

A

B

Figure 17–11 Flow is recorded using pulsed Doppler in the descending aorta (*DESC AO*) proximal to (*A*) the coarctation and with continuous wave Doppler as blood passes through the narrowed segment (*B*). When a severe coarctation is present, there is persistent antegrade flow in diastole (*arrow*) caused by a higher diastolic pressure proximal, compared with distal, to the coarctation.

Step 6: Pulmonary Pressure Estimation

■ In the absence of pulmonic stenosis, RV (and pulmonary) systolic pressure is calculated by the standard approach based on tricuspid regurgitant jet velocity and estimated right atrial pressure (Fig. 17–12).

■ With complex congenital heart disease, estimation of pulmonary pressures depends on the exact cardiac anatomy.

Key points:

❑ When pulmonic stenosis is present, the transpulmonic systolic gradient is subtracted from the estimated RV systolic pressure.

❑ With a large unrestricted ventricular septal defect and Eisenmenger's physiology, pulmonary artery and aortic pressures are equalized, even if there is no tricuspid regurgitation.

❑ With tricuspid atresia and Fontan physiology (direct connection of systemic venous return to the pulmonary artery), pulmonary pressures are low, with a venous-type blood flow pattern.

❑ Pulmonary diastolic pressure can be estimated from the end-diastolic pulmonic regurgitant velocity, plus an estimate of RV diastolic pressure (Fig. 17–13).

❑ The velocity through a ventricular septal defect reflects the left ventricular (LV) to RV systolic pressure difference.

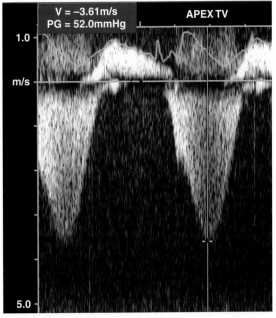

Figure 17–12 This tricuspid regurgitant jet shows a maximum velocity of 3.6 m/s consistent with a right ventricular (RV) to right atrial (RA) systolic pressure difference of 52 mm Hg, or an estimated RV systolic pressure of 62 mm Hg, assuming an RA pressure of 10 mm Hg. However, this patient has pulmonic stenosis, so the RV to pulmonary artery (PA) systolic gradient must be subtracted from the estimated RV pressure to estimate PA systolic pressure. This is the same patient as Figure 17–7, so estimated PA systolic pressure is 62 mm Hg − 47 mm Hg, or 15 mm Hg.

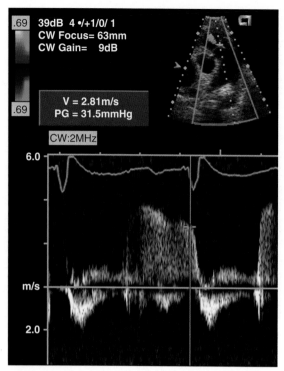

Figure 17–13 The end-diastolic pulmonic regurgitant velocity reflects the diastolic pulmonary artery (PA) to right ventricular (RV) pressure gradient, 32 mm Hg in this case. Assuming an RV diastolic pressure of 10 mm Hg, estimated PA diastolic pressure is 32 mm Hg + 10 mm Hg = 42 mm Hg, consistent with severe pulmonary hypertension.

Step 7: Study Review and Reporting

- Most adult studies are reported in the standard format, with additional sections for the congenital findings.
- The report describes the anatomy and physiology, with an indication of the level of certainty of each finding, depending on data quality.
- The echocardiographic findings are interpreted in view of the clinical history, previous surgical procedures, and current clinical indication.

Key points:

- The findings in most patients with congenital disease can be described using a standard report format; however, with complex congenital heart disease, a more detailed narrative description is needed.
- The echocardiographic study is not used to deduce the surgical history; instead, the surgical history is reviewed to ensure the echocardiographic study provides a complete evaluation.
- The echocardiographic study seeks to answer the specific clinical question articulated by the referring physician.

- The current study is compared with previous examinations (with side-by-side review of images when possible).

Step 8: Determine Remaining Anatomic/ Physiologic Questions

- Initial evaluation of simple congenital heart disease and follow-up studies of more complex disease may require only transthoracic echocardiography.
- Additional diagnostic procedures often are needed for evaluation of complex congenital heart disease.

Key points:

- Transthoracic echocardiography often cannot fully evaluate atrial level anatomy and flow in patients with Fontan physiology or an interatrial baffle repair because of the distance of the transducer from the structures of interest (Fig. 17–14).
- Extracardiac connections, such as arterial-to-pulmonary shunts, are difficult to assess by transthoracic echocardiography.
- Previous surgical procedures may result in shadowing or reverberations resulting from prosthetic valves, conduits, or patch material.
- Evaluation of branch pulmonary artery stenosis usually requires other diagnostic approaches.
- Quantitation of RV volumes and systolic function is problematic with standard echocardiographic approaches.
- These areas of uncertainty or issues that cannot be addressed by echocardiography are identified at the end of the study with suggestions for appropriate additional diagnostic approaches.

Basic Transesophageal Approach

Step 1: Assess the Risk of Transesophageal Echocardiography and Institute Appropriate Modification in the Study Protocol

- The risk of conscious sedation is higher in some patients with congenital heart disease.
- Additional monitoring and sedation by an anesthesiologist may be needed in some cases.

Key points:

- Risk of sedation is highest in patients with cyanosis, severe pulmonary hypertension, or Eisenmenger's physiology.
- Concurrent pulmonary or other medical conditions also may be present that increase procedural risk.
- Baseline oxygen saturation is assessed before beginning the procedure, because patients

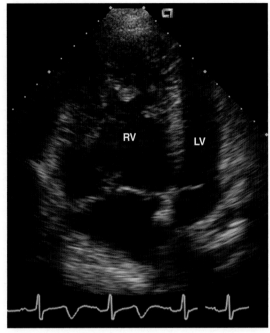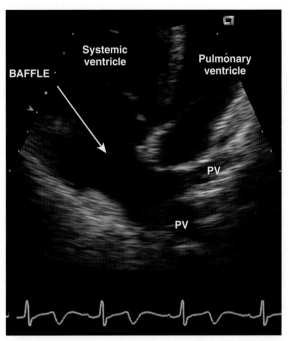

A   B

Figure 17–14 Apical four-chamber view of a patient with transposition of the great arteries and an interatrial baffle repair. The systemic (anatomic right, *RV*) ventricle is dilated and hypertrophied as expected, and the pulmonic (anatomic left, *LV*) ventricle is relatively normal size (*A*). The interatrial baffle is not easily seen in the four-chamber view, but the pulmonary venous channel is better seen by posterior angulation of the transducer with pulmonary veins (*PV*) draining into the baffle and then the systemic ventricle (*B*).

may have significant chronic desaturation resulting from an intracardiac shunt.
- When risk is high or uncertain, a cardiac anesthesiologist should be asked to assist with the procedure.
- All the health care providers involved in the study (e.g., physician, nurse, and sonographer) should understand and review any potential risks.

Step 2: Determine the Objectives of the Transesophageal Echocardiography Study

- In consultation with the referring physician, the clinical data and transthoracic echocardiogram are reviewed to determine the specific areas of interest on the transesophageal echocardiography (TEE) study.
- A complete TEE study is performed whenever possible, putting priority on key elements if study length is constrained.

Key points:
- TEE provides better visualization of posterior structures, such as the atrial septum, pulmonary veins, and interatrial baffle repairs (Fig. 17–15).
- TEE provides improved images when prosthetic material shadows posterior structures from the transthoracic approach.

- Anterior and extracardiac structures, such as systemic venous return conduits, branch pulmonary stenosis, and arterial-to-pulmonic shunts may be difficult to visualize on TEE (Fig. 17–16).
- Be sure all individuals involved in the TEE study understand the study objectives.

Step 3: Transesophageal Echocardiography Imaging Sequence

- The standard imaging sequence, described in Chapter 3, is appropriate for adults with congenital heart disease.
- The examiner should ensure that all cardiac structures are evaluated by imaging and Doppler, preferably in at least two orthogonal views.

Key points:
- Start with the standard TEE four-chamber, two-chamber, long axis rotational series of images to provide an overview of cardiac anatomy.
- Follow a checklist to ensure all structures are evaluated:
  - Systemic and pulmonary ventricles (including anatomic identity, location, great vessel connections, and systolic function)
  - Aorta and pulmonary artery (including size, location, and connections to the ventricles)

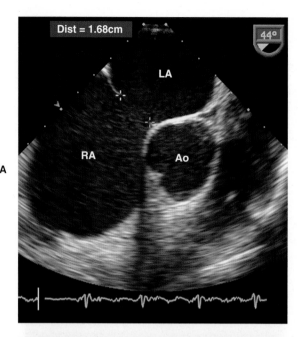

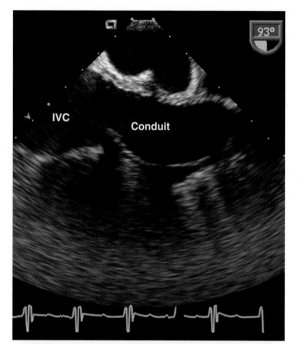

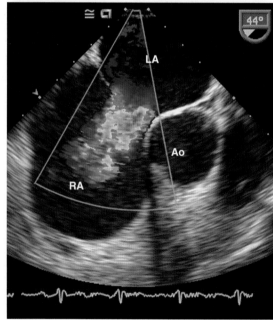

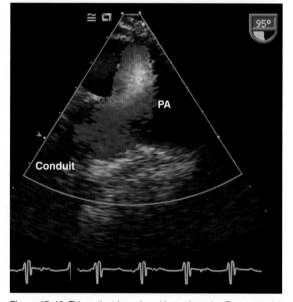

Figure 17–15 Transesophageal echocardiography provides superior images of the atrial septum. In this patient with a secundum atrial septal defect, the exact location and size of the defect can be measured (A) and the flow across the defect visualized with color Doppler (B).

Figure 17–16 This patient has tricuspid atresia and a Fontan conduit from the inferior vena cava (IVC) to the pulmonary artery. The conduit is seen on transesophageal echocardiography in a vertical image plane by turning the probe toward the patient's right side. The junction of the IVC and the conduit (A) is seen, and then the probe is slowly withdrawn in the esophagus, keeping the conduit centered in the image plane (B) to show the flow from the conduit into the pulmonary artery (PA).

❏ Aortic and pulmonic valves (including anatomy and Doppler flows)
❏ Systemic and pulmonary atrioventricular valves (anatomy and function)
❏ Left and right atrium (or interatrial baffle, Fontan conduit, etc.)
❏ Atrial and ventricular septums
❏ Location and flow patterns in all four pulmonary veins

❏ Superior and inferior vena cava
❏ Coronary sinus
❏ Descending aorta
❏ Transgastric views may provide alternate views of the ventricles, atrioventricular valves, and aortic and pulmonic valves.

- ❑ Before completing the study, ask the nurse and sonographer if any imaging views or Doppler flows have been missed and if they have any other suggestions.

SPECIAL CONSIDERATIONS IN COMMONLY SEEN CONDITIONS

Atrial Septal Defects

- ■ RV volume overload resulting from an atrial septal defect (ASD) results in the characteristic findings of RV enlargement and paradoxical septal motion (Fig. 17–17).
- ■ ASDs are classified as:
  - ❑ Secundum (center of atrial septum)
  - ❑ Primum (adjacent to the atrioventricular valves)
  - ❑ Sinus venosus (near junction of superior or inferior vena cava)
- ■ Anomalous pulmonary venous draining into the right atrium or cavae also results in right-sided volume overload.
- ■ Both the anatomic size of an ASD (measured directly) and the physiology effects (based on the amount of flow across the defect) are useful measures of disease severity.

Key points:

- ❑ A secundum or primum ASD may be visualized on transthoracic imaging in parasternal short axis, apical four-chamber, and subcostal four-chamber views (see Figs. 17–9 and 17–15).
- ❑ Color Doppler evidence of transatrial flow prevents mistaking echo dropout from an ASD, but care is needed to distinguish normal inflow from the superior and inferior vena cava from flow across the atrial septum.
- ❑ A primum ASD may be accompanied by a cleft anterior mitral leaflet (Fig. 17–18).
- ❑ An endocardial cushion defect is the association of a primum ASD with an adjacent ventricular septal defect.
- ❑ A sinus venosus ASD may be difficult to visualize on transthoracic imaging and often is suspected based on unexplained right-sided enlargement.
- ❑ The presence of RV dilation mandates a careful search for an ASD or anomalous pulmonary venous return using 2D imaging, color Doppler, and an intravenous saline contrast study.
- ❑ When visualized, the diameter of the ASD can be directly measured from two images.

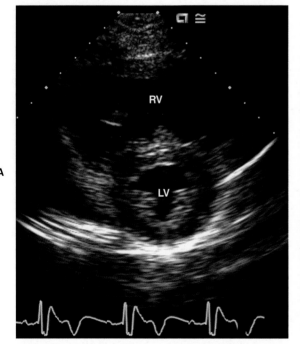

A

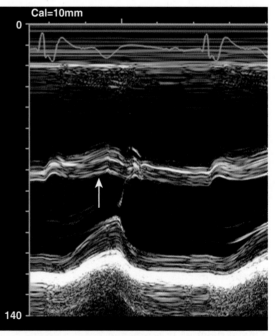

B

Figure 17–17 With right-sided volume overload (but normal pulmonary pressures) caused by an atrial septal defect, there is significant right heart enlargement on two-dimensional imaging with a normal septal curvature at end-systole (*A*), and there is paradoxical septal motion seen on M-mode with anterior motion of the septum during systole and rapid posterior motion during diastole because of the increased right-sided diastolic filling volume (*B*).

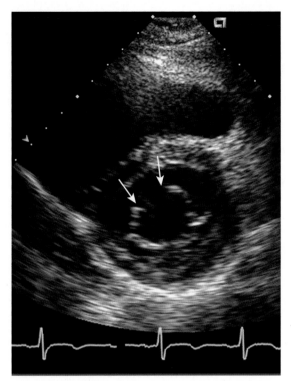

Figure 17–18 A cleft anterior mitral valve seen in a parasternal short axis image with differing maximal excursion of the medial and lateral aspects of the cleft leaflet (*arrows*).

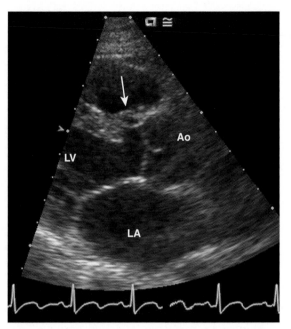

Figure 17–19 In a patient referred for a systolic murmur, the region of the membranous septum (*arrow*) appears abnormal in the standard parasternal long axis view.

❏ Shunt flow, defined as the ratio of pulmonary blood flow (Qp) to systemic blood flow (Qs), is determined by calculating stroke volume in the pulmonary artery and aorta, with a ratio of more than 1.5:1 considered significant.

❏ Transesophageal imaging is more sensitive than transthoracic imaging for detection of a sinus venosus ASD or anomalous pulmonary venous return.

Ventricular Septal Defects

■ Ventricular septal defects (VSDs) are classified as:

❏ Membranous (from just beneath the aortic valve to under the septal tricuspid leaflet)

❏ Supracristal (from just beneath the aortic valve to under the pulmonic valve)

❏ Inlet (between the mitral and tricuspid valves)

❏ Muscular (anywhere in the muscular part of the ventricular septum)

■ Large uncorrected VSDs result in severe pulmonary hypertension early in life with equalization of pulmonary and systolic pressures and bidirectional shunting (Eisenmenger's physiology).

■ Small VSDs are associated with a high pressure difference (and high velocity) between the left and right ventricle in systole.

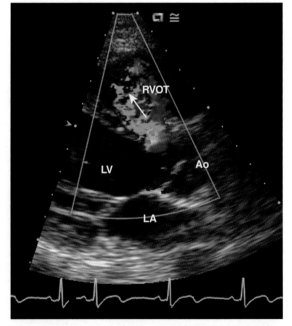

Figure 17–20 In the same patient as Figure 17–19, color Doppler confirms right-to-left flow consistent with a membranous ventricular septal defect. *RVOT,* Right ventricular outflow tract.

Key points:

❏ The anatomic site of a VSD is detected using a combination of 2D imaging and color Doppler to demonstrate systolic turbulence on the right side of the ventricular septum (Figs. 17–19 and 17–20).

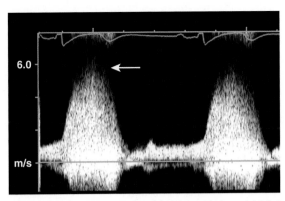

Figure 17–21 Continuous wave Doppler of the ventricular septal defect flow from the parasternal window in the same patient as Figure 17–20 shows a very high velocity signal consistent with a small defect and a large pressure gradient between the left and right ventricles in systole.

❐ The VSD is confirmed using CW Doppler to demonstrate the high velocity systolic ejection–type Doppler curve (Fig. 17–21).

❐ The peak velocity of the VSD jet is related to the LV to RV systolic pressure difference as stated in the Bernoulli equation: $\Delta P = 4v^2$.

❐ A low velocity diastolic signal also may be seen corresponding to the diastolic pressure difference between the left and right ventricle.

❐ With Eisenmenger's physiology, a large VSD is seen on 2D imaging with bidirectional flow on color and spectral Doppler. RV and LV size and wall thickness are similar, and the velocities in the mitral and tricuspid regurgitant jets are equal (Fig. 17–22).

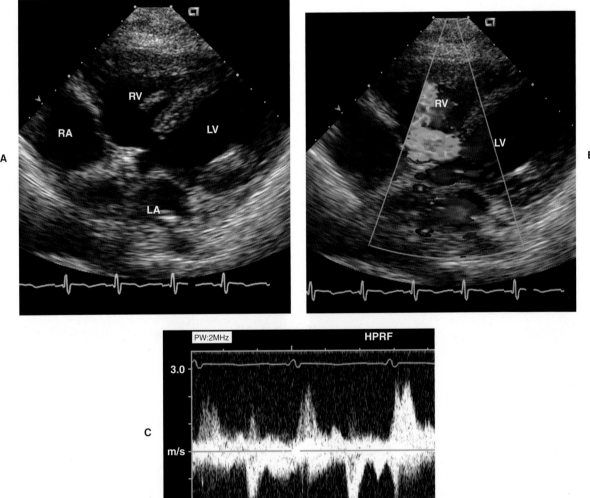

Figure 17–22 A, With a large ventricular septal defect, as seen in this low parasternal four-chamber view in a patient with trisomy 21, Eisenmenger's physiology is present with equalization of right and left ventricular pressures, significant systemic oxygen desaturation, and cyanosis. Color flow shows both right-to-left (B) and left-to-right flow, and spectral Doppler shows relatively low velocity bidirectional flow (C).

Patent Ductus Arteriosus

■ Most cases of patent ductus arteriosus (PDA) are diagnosed and treated early in life, with only rare cases diagnosed in adults.

■ Continuous systolic and diastolic flow into the main pulmonary artery is the key finding in adults with a PDA.

Key points:

❏ Color Doppler of the main pulmonary artery shows the diastolic flow from the PDA originating near the pulmonary artery bifurcation (Fig. 17–23).

❏ Pulsed Doppler evidence of continuous flow in the pulmonary artery is diagnostic; this flow differs from pulmonic regurgitation because it is distal to the pulmonic valve and the diastolic components extend into systole (Fig. 17–24).

❏ Diastolic flow reversal also may be seen in the descending thoracic aorta and should not be mistaken for aortic regurgitation.

Aortic Coarctation

■ An aortic coarctation results in an increased systolic velocity and persistent diastolic ante-

grade flow in the descending thoracic aorta (Fig. 17–25).

■ Descending aortic flow is recorded with CW Doppler from the suprasternal notch view.

Key points:

❏ Doppler may underestimate the severity of coarctation because of the nonparallel intercept angle between the eccentric jet and ultrasound beam.

❏ When the proximal velocity is also increased, the proximal velocity should be included in the pressure gradient calculation: $\Delta P = 4(V_{max}^2 - V_{prox}^2)$ (see Fig. 17–11).

❏ Imaging of the coarctation is rarely possible by transthoracic imaging in adults; TEE may be helpful in select cases.

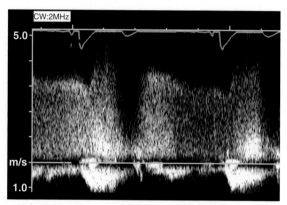

Figure 17–24 Continuous wave Doppler shows continuous flow from the aorta into the pulmonary artery with the shape and velocity reflecting the pressure difference between the two vessels. For example, the increase systolic velocity corresponds to the increase in systemic blood pressure during systole.

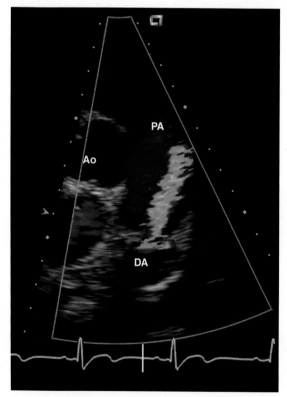

Figure 17–23 Patent ductus arteriosus seen in a parasternal short axis image of the pulmonary artery. A color jet of diastolic flow is seen entering the pulmonary artery near its bifurcation with the flow originating from the descending aorta (*DA*) just posterior to pulmonary artery (*PA*).

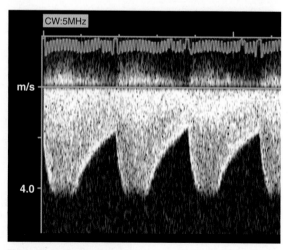

Figure 17–25 Continuous wave Doppler flow in the descending aorta in a patient with a severe aortic coarctation. The antegrade velocity of more than 4 m/s is consistent with a pressure gradient of at least 64 mm Hg (possibly higher if the intercept angle is not parallel to blood flow), and persistent antegrade flow in diastole confirms severe obstruction.

❑ Further evaluation of aortic coarctation with computed tomographic (CT) imaging or cardiac catheterization typically is needed.

Ebstein's Anomaly

■ Ebstein's anomaly is characterized by apical displacement of one or more tricuspid valve leaflets (Fig. 17–26; see also Fig. 17–6).
■ Imaging the tricuspid annulus and leaflets in parasternal RV inflow and apical four-chamber views usually is diagnostic.
■ The segment of the right ventricle between the annulus and displaced leaflet is "atrialized"; for example, ventricular myocardium is physiologically part of the atrial chamber.

Key points:

❑ Ebstein's anomaly may be isolated or associated with an ASD and is common (about 15% to 40%) in patients with congenitally corrected transposition of the great vessels.
❑ Ebstein's anomaly is associated with ventricular pre-excitation resulting from an accessory atrioventricular pathway (e.g., Wolf-Parkinson-White [WPW] syndrome).
❑ In the apical four-chamber view, a distance of >10 mm between the mitral and tricuspid leaflet insertions is diagnostic of Ebstein's anomaly.
❑ Ebstein's anomaly typically results in moderate or severe tricuspid regurgitation.

Complex Congenital Heart Disease

Tetralogy of Fallot

■ Tetralogy of Fallot (TOF) is characterized by:
  ❑ A membranous (anteriorly misaligned) VSD
  ❑ An aorta that straddles the ventricular septum
  ❑ RV outflow obstruction resulting in right ventricular hypertrophy
■ Most adults with TOF have undergone previous surgical repair with VSD closure and relief of RV outflow obstruction (Fig. 17–27).
■ The most common long-term issue after TOF repair is severe pulmonic regurgitation with progressive RV enlargement and eventual dysfunction.

Key points:

❑ RV outflow obstruction may be subvalvular, valvular, or supravalvular or may occur at more than one site, including branch pulmonary artery stenoses.
❑ Occasionally an adult patient with an untreated TOF will be diagnosed by echocardiography because the RV outflow obstruction prevents pulmonary hypertension.
❑ Severe pulmonic regurgitation typically is low velocity with a to-and-fro flow pattern by

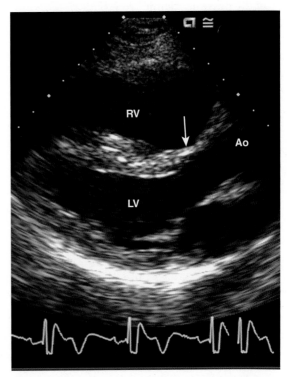

Figure 17–27 Parasternal long axis view in a typical patient with repaired tetralogy of Fallot. The right ventricular outflow tract is enlarged, the basal septum is intact but has increased echogenicity (*arrow*) suggestive of ventricular septal defect patch repair, and the aorta (*Ao*) is mildly enlarged and slightly overrides the septum.

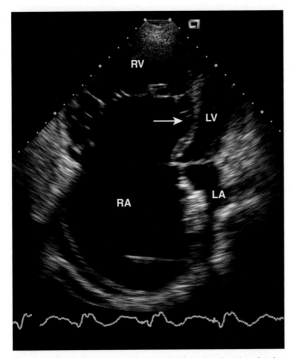

Figure 17–26 Ebstein's anomaly in an apical four-chamber view showing severe apical displacement of the septal tricuspid valve leaflet (*arrow*).

pulsed, CW, and color Doppler that may be overlooked because of the absence of turbulence (Fig. 17–28).

❑ Additional evaluation with cardiac magnetic resonance (CMR) imaging often is needed for quantitation of RV size and function.

Transposition of the Great Arteries

■ Transposition of the great arteries (TGA) is treated in childhood with one of the following:
  ❑ An interatrial baffle repair that redirects systemic and pulmonary venous inflow to restore a normal pattern of circulation, but with the anatomic right ventricle serving as the systemic ventricle (Mustard or Senning repair)
  ❑ More recently, an arterial switch procedure with the aorta and pulmonary artery transected and reconnected to the correct ventricles (Jatene procedure)
■ The aorta is anterior and the great vessels are parallel to each other when TGA is present (see Figs. 17–3 and 17–4).
■ With an interatrial baffle repair, a major long-term issue is systolic dysfunction of the systemic (anatomic right) ventricle.
■ With an arterial switch repair, a few patients develop systemic semilunar valve regurgitation, particularly of the neoaortic valve with dilation of the proximal "aortic" root (Fig. 17–29).

Key points:

❑ With an interatrial baffle repair, the circulatory pattern of oxygenated and unoxygenated blood is normal, but the systemic ventricle is the anatomic right ventricle and the pulmonary ventricle is the anatomic left ventricle (Fig. 17–30).

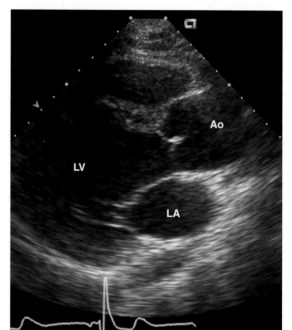

A

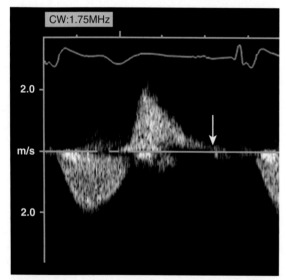

Figure 17–28 Continuous wave Doppler signal of severe pulmonic regurgitation in a patient with repaired tetralogy of Fallot and persistent pulmonic regurgitation after surgical pulmonic valvotomy. The retrograde flow in diastole has a signal density similar to antegrade flow consistent with similar volume flow rates. The diastolic deceleration slope is steep and reaches the baseline before the end of diastole (*arrow*), consistent with equalization of diastolic pulmonary artery and right ventricular pressures.

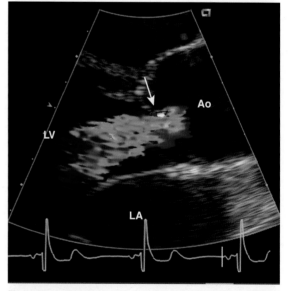

B

Figure 17–29 This 19-year-old man with transposition of the great arteries underwent a great vessel switch repair as an infant. The ventricular great vessel relationships now are relatively normal, as seen in this long axis view. However, the sinuses of the transposed pulmonic valve (neoaorta) are dilated to 4.6 cm (*A*), and central "aortic" regurgitation is present (*B*) with a vena contracta width of 0.5 cm.

- ❐ The atrioventricular valves are associated with each ventricle, so the systemic atrioventricular valve is the tricuspid valve and the pulmonary atrioventricular valve is the mitral valve.
- ❐ Atrial baffle leaks and stenosis are difficult to evaluate by transthoracic imaging, typically requiring TEE or other imaging approaches.
- ❐ A lower Nyquist limit (i.e., signal aliasing at a lower velocity) and use of variance mode on the color display enhance detection of baffle leaks.
- ❐ With an arterial switch procedure, the neoaorta–the systemic semilunar valve and sinuses–was the anatomic pulmonic valve. The coronary arteries also were transposed to the neoaorta.
- ❐ Branch pulmonic stenosis can occur after an arterial switch repair related to moving the pulmonary artery anteriorly during the repair procedure.

Fontan Physiology with Tricuspid Atresia

- ■ Fontan physiology refers to a direct, valveless surgical connection from the systemic venous return to the pulmonary artery, without an intervening right ventricle.
- ■ A Fontan repair is used for patients with only a single functional ventricle, including those with tricuspid atresia (Fig. 17–31).
- ■ Flow in a Fontan conduit is driven by the pressure gradient from the systemic venous return to the pulmonary artery, with a flow pattern similar to a normal systemic venous inflow (Fig. 17–32).

Key points:

- ❐ There are many variations of the Fontan procedure:
  - ❐ Early Fontan repairs connected the right atrium to the pulmonary artery. These patients often have a severely enlarged right atrium with significant arrhythmias and may have obstruction of the pulmonary veins posterior to the dilated atrium.
  - ❐ More recent repairs include a direct connection of the superior vena cava to the right pulmonary artery, with the inferior vena cava connected to the pulmonary artery by a conduit. This repair leaves the small residual right atrium (with the coronary sinus) in communication with the left atrium via an ASD.

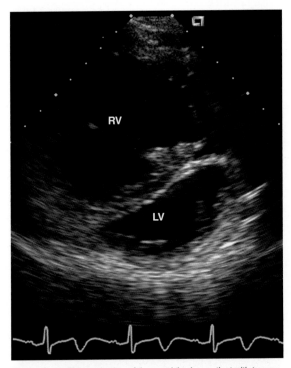

Figure 17–30 Short axis view of the ventricles in a patient with transposition of the great arteries and an interatrial baffle repair. The right ventricle (*RV*) is located anteriorly but serves as the systemic ventricle and is appropriately dilated and hypertrophied. The smaller posteriorly located left ventricle (*LV*) is the low pressure pulmonic ventricle, with systolic curvature of the septum reflecting the physiologic functions of each ventricle.

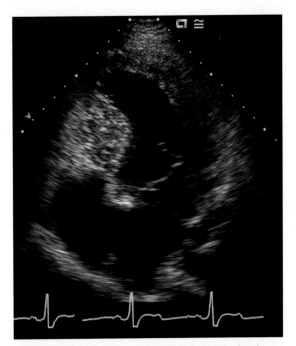

Figure 17–31 Apical view in a patient with tricuspid and pulmonic atresia shows only one ventricle and atrioventricular valve. The tricuspid valve is absent, with the small residual right ventricular chamber (not visible in this view) communicating with the left ventricle via a ventricular septal defect. The right and left atrium are connected by a large atrial septal defect. Pulmonary blood flow in this patient is provided by a right subclavian artery–to–pulmonary artery shunt.

❏ TTE and TEE of a Fontan conduit is challenging and depends on the exact surgical repair and location of the conduit (see Fig. 17–16).

❏ Valved conduits connecting the right ventricle to the pulmonary artery are used for other types of complex congenital heart disease.

These patients do not have Fontan physiology, because the right ventricle provides pulsatile systolic pulmonary blood flow.

Congenitally Corrected Transposition of the Great Arteries

■ The pathway of blood flow with congenitally corrected transposition of the great vessels (CCTGA) is:
  ❏ Systemic venous return to the right atrium, then into the left ventricle and out the pulmonary artery
  ❏ Pulmonary venous return to the left atrium, then into the right ventricle and out the aorta

■ Some patients with CCTGA remain undiagnosed until adulthood because the flow of oxygenated and unoxygenated blood is physiologic, even though the anatomic right ventricle serves as the systemic ventricle.

■ Defects commonly associated with CCTGA include a ventricular septal defect, pulmonic stenosis, Ebstein's anomaly of the systemic (tricuspid) atrioventricular valve, and complete heart block.

Key points:
  ❏ CCTGA also is called "ventricular inversion" or l-TGA, because the pattern of blood flow is normal other than the reversed positions of the ventricles (and the associated atrioventricular valves).

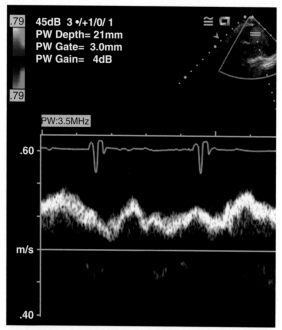

Figure 17–32 Flow in a Fontan conduit is similar to systemic venous flow, with low velocity forward flow in systole and diastole.

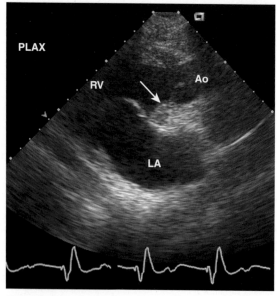

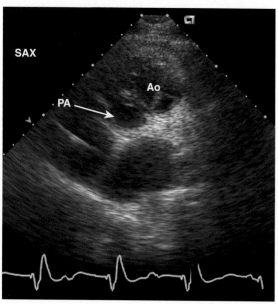

Figure 17–33 *A*, Parasternal long axis (*PLAX*) view in a patient with congenitally corrected transposition of the great arteries (ventricular inversion) shows the muscular ridge (*arrow*) between the systemic atrioventricular valve and aorta consistent with an anatomic right ventricle (*RV*) serving as the systemic ventricle. *B*, In the short axis (*SAX*) view, the position of the aorta (*Ao*) anterior to the pulmonary artery (*PA*) and the side-by-side relationship of the great arteries is evident.

❑ CCTGA is evident on echocardiography based on the systemic ventricle having the anatomic features of a right ventricle (moderate band, apical annulus, and tricuspid valve [Fig. 17–33]).

❑ As with TGA, in CCTGA the atrioventricular valves are associated with each ventricle, so the systemic atrioventricular valve is the tricuspid valve and the pulmonary atrioventricular valve is the mitral valve.

❑ Long-term, systolic dysfunction of the systemic ventricle may complicate CCTGA.

❑ Typically the aortic annulus is anterior and to the left of the pulmonic valve.

❑ Dextroversion (apex pointed toward the right) or mesocardia often is present with CCTGA, which limits acoustic access because of the retrosternal cardiac position.

NOTES

SELF-ASSESSMENT QUESTIONS

QUESTION 1

A 23-year-old asymptomatic man is referred for echocardiography to evaluate a murmur. In the parasternal short axis view just below the aortic valve, an area of systolic turbulence from the left ventricle into the right ventricle is seen in the 10 o'clock position around the LV outflow tract circumference.

The most likely diagnosis is:

A. Membranous ventricular septal defect
B. Muscular ventricular septal defect
C. Supracristal ventricular septal defect
D. Eccentric aortic regurgitant jet
E. Coronary artery flow

QUESTION 2

In evaluating a patient with complex congenital heart disease, two ventricles are visible in the apical four-chamber view.

Which of the following features is most helpful in identification of the anatomic right ventricle?

A. Triangular shape
B. Size relative to the other ventricle
C. Rightward and anterior location in chest
D. Wall thickness
E. Distance from apex to annulus

QUESTION 3

A 27-year-old woman undergoes echocardiography for a murmur during pregnancy and is found to have an atrial septal defect. The following measurements are made:

Pulmonary artery
    Velocity   1.6 m/s
    Velocity time integral (VTI_{RVOT})   28 cm
    Diameter   2.5 cm
Left ventricular outflow
    Velocity   1.2 m/s
    Velocity time integral (VTI_{LVOT})   24 cm
    Diameter   2.1 cm
Mitral valve
    Velocity time integral (VTI_{MV})   11 cm
    Annulus diameter   3.2 cm

Calculate the pulmonic-to-systemic shunt ratio:

QUESTION 4

In a 23-year-old woman with a history of surgery to close an atrial septal defect in childhood, parasternal views show a cleft in the anterior mitral valve leaflet with mild to moderate mitral regurgitation.

Which of the following is most likely to be found in this patient?

A. Aortic coarctation
B. Bicuspid aortic valve
C. Ventricular septal defect
D. Ebstein's anomaly
E. Pulmonic stenosis

QUESTION 5

A patient with an uncorrected tetralogy of Fallot presents for echocardiographic evaluation. His blood pressure is 120/80 mm Hg, pulse is 80 beats per minute (bpm), and estimated right atrial pressure is 10 mm Hg. The following maximum systolic velocities are recorded with CW Doppler:

Aortic valve	1.2 m/s
Mitral valve	5.1 m/s
Pulmonic valve	4.0 m/s
Tricuspid valve	4.7 m/s

Calculate:
LV systolic pressure ____mm Hg
RV systolic pressure ____mm Hg
Pulmonary artery (PA) systolic pressure ___mm Hg
Velocity in the ventricular septal defect ____m/s

QUESTION 6

A 23-year-old patient with trisomy 21 is referred for echocardiography. On exam, the blood pressure is 125/76 mm Hg, pulse is 88 bpm, and respiratory rate is 18 per min. His hands show clubbing and cyanosis, and the room air oxygen saturation is 79%. On echocardiography, an endocardial cushion defect is seen with an ostium primum ASD and a large nonrestrictive VSD. The mitral regurgitant jet velocity is 5.0 m/s, the antegrade aortic velocity is 1.3 m/s, and the pulmonary artery systolic flow velocity is 0.9 m/s. Estimated right atrial pressure is 5 mm Hg based on normal size and respiratory variation in the inferior vena cava. There is only trace tricuspid regurgitation, and a CW Doppler tricuspid velocity could not be recorded.

Based on this data, estimated pulmonary systolic pressure is:

A. Not possible to determine
B. 125 mm Hg
C. 100 mm Hg
D. 75 mm Hg
E. 50 mm Hg

QUESTION 7

On a transthoracic echocardiogram requested for evaluation of a murmur in a 27-year-old woman, the right atrium and right ventricle are enlarged. Careful evaluation shows no evidence of an ASD or pulmonic valve disease. Tricuspid regurgitant jet velocity is 2.1 m/s. Left heart anatomy and function are normal.

Which of the following may have been missed and would explain right heart enlargement?

A. Membranous ventricular septal defect
B. Patent ductus arteriosus
C. Aortic coarctation
D. Persistent left superior vena cava
E. Anomalous pulmonary venous return

QUESTION 8

While doing an echocardiogram on a 22-year-old man referred for evaluation of a murmur, a color Doppler signal is seen (Fig. 17–34A). You interrogate this region with pulsed Doppler and record the spectral display shown (Fig. 17–34B). The color Doppler signal most likely is due to:

A. Coronary blood flow
B. Supracristal ventricular septal defect
C. RV outflow obstruction
D. Pulmonic regurgitation
E. Artifact

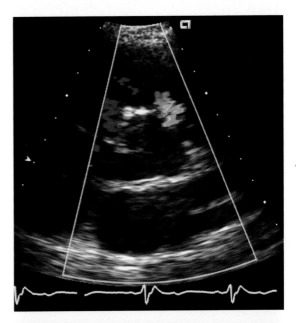

A

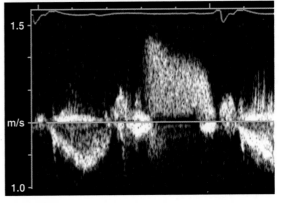

B

Figure 17–34

QUESTION 9

This Doppler signal (Fig. 17–35) was obtained for a 28-year-old woman with a history of repaired tetralogy of Fallot.

The most likely diagnosis is:

A. Residual ventricular septal defect
B. Severe tricuspid regurgitation
C. Large atrial septal defect
D. Moderate mitral stenosis
E. Severe pulmonic regurgitation

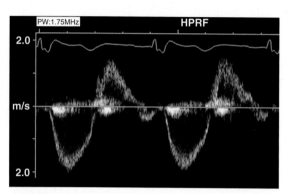

Figure 17–35

QUESTION 10

A 19-year-old pregnant woman is referred for evaluation of a murmur, and this flow signal is obtained (Fig. 17–36).

The most likely diagnosis is:

A. Normal flow murmur of pregnancy
B. Persistent left superior vena cava
C. Ventricular septal defect
D. Patent ductus arteriosus
E. Atrial septal defect

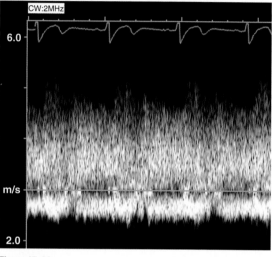

Figure 17–36

ANSWERS

ANSWER 1: A

In the short axis view just below the aortic valve, a membranous VSD is seen in about the 10 o'clock position, entering the right ventricle adjacent to the septal leaflet of the tricuspid valve. Many membranous VSDs spontaneously close in childhood related to adherence of the tricuspid valve leaflet to the septum. A supracristal VSD would be seen in the 1 or 2 o'clock position in the short axis view, entering the RV outflow tract adjacent to the pulmonic valve. Muscular VSDs would not be seen in this view, as they occur more apically, anywhere in the muscular part of the ventricular septum. Both an aortic regurgitant jet and coronary blood flow would occur in diastole, not systole, although both might be seen in this location and could be mistaken for a different flow signal if timing is not carefully assessed.

ANSWER 2: E

The atrioventricular valves go with the corresponding ventricles, so the anatomic right ventricle has a tricuspid valve. The tricuspid valve annulus usually is slightly more apical than the mitral valve annulus, so this is a reliable feature for identifying the right ventricle. Occasionally, the tricuspid and mitral valve annuli are at the same level and other features must be used for anatomic identification of the ventricular chambers. The normal triangular shape, smaller size, and thinner walls of the right ventricle are all altered when the anatomic right ventricle serves as the systemic ventricle. With systemic pressures, the right ventricle appropriately enlarges, hypertrophies, and changes shape, similar to an anatomic left ventricle. The location of the right and left ventricles in the chest is abnormal in some complex congenital heart disease and is not a reliable indicator of anatomy.

ANSWER 3: The Q_p:Q_s is 1.63

The shunt ratio is calculated from the ratio of pulmonary flow (Q_p), measured in the RV outflow tract (RVOT), and systemic flow (Q_s), measured in the LV outflow tract (LVOT). At each site, cross-sectional area (CSA) is calculated as the area of a circle:

$$CSA_{RVOT} = \pi(D/2)^2 = 3.14(2.5/2)^2 = 4.9 \ cm^2$$

$$CSA_{LVOT} = \pi(D/2)^2 = 3.14(2.1/2)^2 = 3.5 \ cm^2$$

Flow at each site then is calculated:

$$Q_p = CSA_{RVOT} \times VTI_{RVOT} = 4.9 \ cm^2 \times 28 \ cm = 137 \ cm^3 \ (or \ ml)$$

$$Q_s = CSA_{LVOT} \times VTI_{LVOT} = 3.5 \ cm^2 \times 24 \ cm = 84 \ cm^3 \ (or \ ml)$$

so that Q_p:Q_s = 137/84 = 1.63

These calculations are consistent with a moderate shunt that likely will require further evaluation and consideration of closure after pregnancy.

The transmitral volume flow rate should equal transaortic flow in the absence of aortic or mitral regurgitation and might provide an alternate site for calculation of systemic blood flow.

$$Q_{MV} = CSA_{MV} \times VTI_{MV} = 8.0 \ cm^2 \times 11 \ cm = 88 \ cm^3 \ (or \ ml)$$

In this case, there is only a slight (4 ml) difference between transaortic and transmitral flow rates, which is within measurement error. Transmitral flow is rarely used for shunt ratio calculations, because reproducible measurement of mitral annulus diameter is problematic.

ANSWER 4: C

A cleft mitral valve is most often associated with a primum atrial septal defect or an atrioventricular canal defect with a ventricular and atrial septal defect. The other conditions listed are not known to be associated with a cleft mitral valve. Thus the most likely other finding on this study would be a small residual (or missed) ventricular septal defect. In patients with an aortic coarctation, about 50% have a bicuspid aortic valve. Conversely, in patients with a bicuspid aortic valve, about 10% have an aortic coarctation, so the presence of either of these conditions mandates a search for the other. Ebstein's anomaly and pulmonic stenosis often accompany congenitally corrected transposition of the great vessels. Ebstein's anomaly of the tricuspid valve is associated with secundum atrial septal defects, arrhythmias caused by pre-excitation and bypass tract, and transposition of the great vessels.

ANSWER 5

LV systolic pressure is the same as systolic blood pressure (120 mm Hg) because there is no significant transaortic systolic gradient.

RV systolic pressure is calculated from the tricuspid regurgitant (TR) jet velocity to determine the RV to right atrial (RA) systolic pressure difference and then adding estimated right atrial pressure:

$$RV \text{ pressure} = \Delta P_{RV-RA} + P_{RA} =$$
$$4V^2_{TR} + P_{RA} = [4(4.7)^2 + 10)] = 98 \text{ mm Hg}$$

Pulmonary artery pressure (PAP) in systole is calculated by subtracting the pulmonic valve gradient from the estimated RV systolic pressure because pulmonic stenosis is present:

$$\Delta P_{RV-PA} = 4V^2_{PA} = 64 \text{ mm Hg}$$

$$PAP = RV \text{ pressure} - \Delta P_{RV-PA} =$$
$$RV \text{ pressure} - 4V^2_{PA} = 98 - 64 = 34 \text{ mm Hg}$$

The velocity in the ventricular septal defect (VSD) reflects the systolic LV to RV pressure gradient.

Since,

$$LV \text{ pressure} - RV \text{ pressure} =$$
$$120 - 98 = 22 \text{ mm Hg}$$

and

$$\Delta P_{VSD} = 4(V_{VSD})^2$$

Then,

$$V_{VSD} = \sqrt{(\Delta P_{VSD}/4)} = \sqrt{(22/4)} = 2.5 \text{ m/s}$$

ANSWER 6: B

This patient has a large nonrestrictive ventricular septal defect with clinical evidence of Eisenmenger's physiology, including cyanosis, clubbing, and resting arterial oxygen desaturation. Laboratory data likely include polycythemia. Given that pulmonary and systemic pressures are equalized with Eisenmenger's physiology, the best estimate of pulmonary pressure in this patient is the same as the systolic blood pressure. When an adequate tricuspid regurgitant jet is not available, the velocity in the pulmonic regurgitation jet and the time to peak velocity in antegrade pulmonary flow may provide clues that pulmonary hypertension is present.

ANSWER 7: E

Possible explanations for right heart enlargement include pressure overload, volume overload, and primary contractile dysfunction of the right ventricle. Contractile dysfunction might be due to a cardiomyopathy or to a RV infarction, neither of which are likely or listed as possible answers. RV pressure overload resulting from pulmonary hypertension or pulmonic valve disease was not present based on the tricuspid regurgitant jet velocity. Thus, this patient is likely to have volume overload as the cause of right heart enlargement. If the transthoracic study shows no evidence for significant pulmonic or tricuspid regurgitation or an ASD, it is likely that a sinus venosus ASD and/or anomalous pulmonary venous return is present. The next step should be TEE.

Left to right flow through a membranous VSD enters the RVOT in systole and thus flows directly into the pulmonary vascular bed without volume overload of the right ventricle. Indeed, the chambers that are enlarged with a VSD are the left atrium and left ventricle. Similarly, a patent ductus arteriosus is associated with left heart (not right heart) volume overload. Aortic coarctation results in pressure overload and hypertrophy of the left ventricle but does not affect the right heart. A persistent left superior vena cava is an incidental finding that results in dilation of the coronary sinus but does not cause right heart dilation, because the total volume of systemic venous return to the right atrium is normal.

ANSWER 8: D

These color and spectral Doppler images are typical for physiologic pulmonic regurgitation. In the short axis view of the aortic valve, any of these flow signals might be seen at the location identified by the color Doppler signal. However, although the right coronary ostium is found near this location (usually closer to the 12 o'clock position) and coronary blood flow would occur in diastole with a similar flow pattern and velocity, it would not be accompanied by a systolic ejection curve. This is a typical location for a supracristal VSD, but the velocity in a small VSD would be very high in systole (4 to 5 m/s) because of the large pressure gradient between the left ventricle and right ventricle in systole. RV outflow obstruction is excluded based on the normal systolic ejection signal and the spectral Doppler showing a diastolic flow signal. An artifact would be associated with only noise on the pulsed Doppler tracing, rather than a typical flow signal. This example illustrates the importance of using the spectral Doppler display to establish the correct reason for an abnormal color Doppler flow pattern.

ANSWER 9: E

This Doppler signal was recorded with high pulse repetition frequency (HPRF) Doppler in the

RVOT at the level of the pulmonic valve. Antegrade flow in systole is laminar (smooth velocity envelope) with a maximum velocity of about 2 m/s, consistent with either mild stenosis or a high antegrade volume flow rate. In diastole, low velocity retrograde flow is seen with a steep deceleration slope and cessation of flow before the end of diastole, consistent with severe pulmonic regurgitation and equalization of pulmonary and RV diastolic pressures by end-diastole. In fact, this flow signal is consistent with "to and fro" flow in the pulmonary artery and the absence of an effective pulmonic valve.

This signal cannot be mistaken for a residual VSD, which would have a high systolic velocity in a patient with previous surgery for tetralogy of Fallot. In a patient with tetralogy of Fallot without previous surgery, low velocity VSD flow may be seen in association with a high transpulmonary gradient. Severe tricuspid regurgitation can result in low velocity antegrade and retrograde flow across the tricuspid valve when pulmonary pressures are low. However, the diastolic flow signal would show an A velocity, because this patient is in sinus rhythm on the electrocardiogram. A large ASD is associated with lower velocity, less organized flow across the atrial septum. With mitral stenosis, the accompanying flow in systole would be high velocity (e.g., mitral regurgitation).

ANSWER 10: D

This Doppler tracing shows continuous high velocity (about 4 m/s) flow in both systole and diastole. The presence of a pressure gradient of at least 64 mm Hg and continuous flow are typical for a patent ductus arteriosus. With the normal increased flow volumes of pregnancy, higher flow rates may be seen in the inferior and superior vena cava, but the flow velocities are low (about 1 m/s), and patterns would be similar to normal venous flow. Flow in a persistent left superior vena cava would be similar to any other venous inflow pattern; more often this diagnosis is based on finding a dilated coronary sinus. A VSD is associated with a high velocity in systole and a long duration of systolic flow but not with continuous high velocity flow, because there is only a small diastolic pressure difference between the right and left ventricles. An ASD is associated with low velocity flow reflecting the low pressure difference between the atrial chambers.

NOTES

INDEX